ISSUES AND TRENDS IN NURSING

CONTRIBUTORS

Diane M. Billings, RN, EdD
Professor of Nursing
Indiana University
Bloomington, Indiana

Vicki L. Black, RN, MSn, CS
Doctoral student,
University of Arizona-Tucson
Case Manager
Carondelet St. Joseph's Hospital
Tucson, Arizona

Patricia A. Calico, RN, DNS
Assistant Professor
College of Nursing and Health
University of Cincinnati
Cincinnati, Ohio

Luther Christman, RN, PhD
Nurse Consultant
Chapel Hill, Tennessee

Cheryl Hall Harris, RN, BSN
Consultant Nursing Department
Children's Mercy Hospital
Kansas City, Missouri

Fred Hendrickson, PhD
Professor of Philosophy
Bellarmine College
Louisville, Kentucky

Philip Jacobs, PhD
Department of Health Service Administration
   and Community Medicine
University of Alberta
Edmonton, Alberta

Sandra L. Jamison, RN, DNS
Professor, Division of Nursing Education
Director, Graduate Nursing Program
Indiana Wesleyan University
Indianapolis, Indiana

Janet W. Kenney, RN, PhD
Associate Professor
Arizona State University
College of Nursing
Tempe, Arizona

Sharon Minton Kirkpatrick, RN, MN, PhD
Assistant Professor of Nursing
Graceland College
Independence, Missouri

Iris R. Shannon, RN, PhD
Associate Professor
College of Nursing
Rush University
Chicago, Illinois

Heidi R. Sulis, MPH
Director of Community Health Outreach
Porter Medical Center
Middlebury, Vermont

Barbara Talento, RN, PhD
Associate Professor
Department of Nursing
California State University-Fullerton
Fullerton, California

Carmen Germaine Warner,
RN, MSN, FAAN

Hospital and University Publishing
    Consultant
Consultant, Emergency Health Care
Spirituality and Health Care Integrator
San Diego, California

Sharon M. Weisenbeck,
RN, MS

Executive Director
Kentucky Board of Nursing
Louisville, Kentucky

Gloria Y. York, RN, MA(ed)

Vice President, Continuing Education
Professional update
San Diego, California

PREFACE

The educational preparation of today's nursing student is varied and complex. Students must grasp a wealth of physiologic and technologic information, and they must also understand the theoretical base on which competent clinical practice depends. It is critical that students understand the rich heritage of nursing and the many factors that interact to influence nursing care. From this understanding, students can become informed practitioners who can effect positive growth and change thoughout their careers.

ISSUES AND TRENDS IN NURSING is a text designed for nursing students in all types of programs. The book is the result of an extensive survey of over 100 instructors who were asked to rate over 200 distinct issues according to perceived importance, interest, and/or need. In the final compilation of issues and trends, some important threads emerged, which serve as the unifying framework for the entire text. These threads include historical, social, political, cultural, and economic factors.

Chapters 1 and 2 present an overview of the history and evolution of nursing science and practice. Included is an overview of past struggles, issues, controversies, and positive growth, which lay the foundation for discussion of issues in the chapters that follow. The next unit, Chapters 3 through 7, presents economic, social, political, cultural, legal, and ethical dynamics that interact to influence health care in general and nursing specifically. Discussions emphasize the important role nurses can play in effecting change.

Chapters 8, 9, and 10 focus on issues related to nursing education, including licensure and the ever-increasing emphasis on continuing education. Expanding environments of nursing practice are presented in three evolving realms of nursing care: rural (Chapter 11), urban (Chapter 12), and international (Chapter 13). Changing demographics and access to health care are addressed in each chapter, and exciting opportunities for nurses are presented. The final two chapters are devoted to the special challenges of nursing: changing images and future perspectives. Both chapters synthesize important threads presented throughout the text and suggest directions for future growth.

ACKNOWLEDGMENTS

Sincere appreciation is extended to the individuals who have contributed their study and insights to *Issues and Trends in Nursing*. The contributors to this book have vast experience and possess deep understanding of the specific areas about which they write. Appreciation is also given to Linda Duncan, Linda Stagg, and the entire Mosby–Year Book editorial staff who gave encouragement and support throughout the preparation of the manuscript. Gratitude remains in my heart for my late husband who was always enthusiastic and helpful with my writing endeavors. Appreciation is especially extended to my son Paul for our stimulating discussions, his valuable input, and his ongoing interest and encouragement during the development of this project.

Grace L. Deloughery

CONTENTS

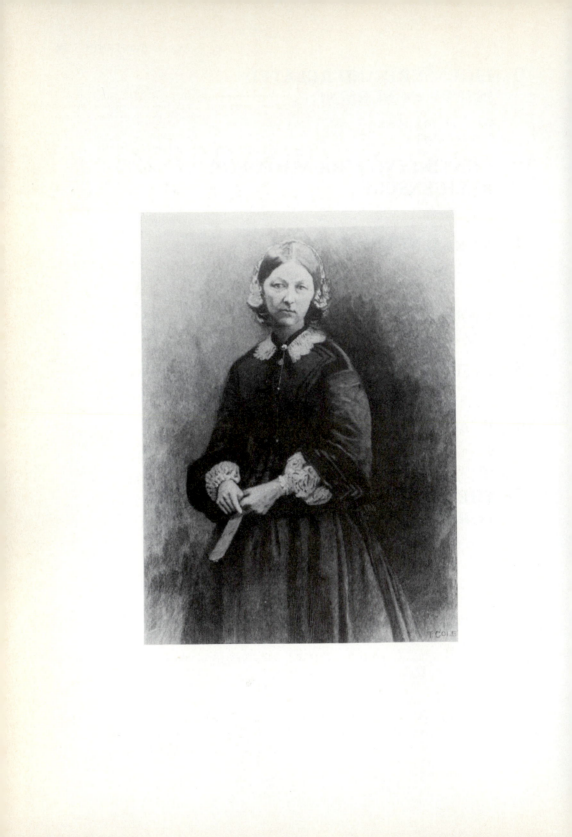

CHAPTER 1

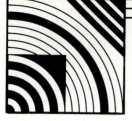

HISTORICAL OVERVIEW

Grace L. Deloughery

OBJECTIVES

After completing this chapter the reader should be able to:

- Describe nursing care in prehistoric times

- Summarize major events, developments, and struggles of each period in nursing history

- Describe how nursing today is related to the development of education for women, and when and how education for women evolved

- Discuss the contribution of Florence Nightingale and other leaders in nursing before the twentieth century

- Discuss the impact that social reform, Karl Marx, and other political philosophers of the nineteenth century had on nursing

- Describe nursing in pioneer America and how it evolved through the various wars that followed

- List six major factors influencing health care and provision of health/nursing services since World War II

Important historical developments profoundly conditioned and influenced the evolution of nursing. Primarily these are the Crusades, the Renaissance, the Reformation, the Industrial Revolution, the development of modern science and health facilities, two

1

World Wars, various types of research in social and basic science, social welfare, rapid technological advances, and the Equal Rights Movement. Perhaps more important than any of these, the liberation of women served as a catalyst and critical component of the evolution of the nursing profession. The new freedom enabled women to develop a profession and achieve recognition. Today, they continue to strive for additional freedom to develop individual and professional potentials.

ANCIENT BEGINNINGS

Nursing dates from prehistoric times, when those who proved themselves adept in caring for the sick naturally were asked to nurse friends or acquaintances; some established a practice of nursing through reputation.

Though separate and distinct from medicine, nursing is closely allied to medical progress and practice. Just as one cannot understand modern nursing without some understanding of medicine and surgery, one cannot understand the evolution of nursing without an awareness of the primitive beginnings of medicine. Medicine progressed from witchcraft to the birth of the rediscovery of Hippocratic principles by the English clinicians of the seventeenth century. Remember that modern medicine rests on the physiological principles that Harvey discovered and the correlation of symptoms with organic changes that Morgagni taught. When these great principles became integrated with clinical medicine, they gave it impetus under which present understanding, cure, and prevention of disease continues to progress.

Egyptian Medicine

Medicine originated in the practice of magic. In early Egypt certain empirical knowledge regarding sickness slowly accumulated from witchcraft. The practice of medicine never entirely outgrew the superstitions that surrounded its origins. Well-educated patients today look to physicians for something more than the logical application of a technical science. Medicine in Egypt reached a surprisingly advanced stage of knowledge. The custom of embalming enabled the Egyptians to become well acquainted with organs of the body. From clinical observation they learned to recognize some 250 different diseases, and to treat them they developed a number of drugs and procedures, including surgery. By about 480 BC neurosurgery was advanced beyond the imagination of the Greeks. However, Egyptian lack of knowledge regarding normal and pathological physiology and of experimental investigation limited their theories.

Greek Medicine and Hospitals

With the decline of Egyptian civilization, medicine came under Greek influence. Hippocrates (about 400 BC) changed the magic of medicine into a science of medicine. He taught physicians to use their eyes and ears and to reason from facts rather than from gratuitous assumptions. His writings on fractures and dislocations were unexcelled until the discovery of the x-ray. The Oath of Hippocrates is used today to admit many to the practice of medicine, and the Hippocratic school has, perhaps erroneously, been given credit for the first ethical guide on medical conduct.

In ancient Greece there were two refuges for the sick; secular and religious. Physicians directed the secular, which corresponded roughly to spas or health resorts of today. Some were endowed and had outpatient departments, and some were used for the instruction of medical students. The secular places of healing and the sanctuaries of the Gods, especially Aesculapius, were closely associated. Importance was placed on the role of emotions in bringing about cure, and also included the role of wholesome food, physiotherapy, and fresh air and sunshine, perhaps on porches overlooking the blue Mediterranean while the patient awaited the appearance of the god in dreams.

The first correlation of women with the healing arts is found in Greek mythology in the person of Aesculapius, who eventually became deified as the God of Healing. One of his children, Hygeia, became the Goddess of Health, and another Panacea (from which comes our word for *cure-all*) became the Restorer of Health. Later most Greek healing centered around shrines in which patients congregated. Attendants were *basket bearers* and those who looked after the sick, somewhat in the manner of nurses. The writings of Hippocrates refer to procedures that would be undertaken in modern hospitals by nurses but do not refer to a nursing vocation as such.

Early Christian Church and Hospitals

The early Christian church and the teachings of Jesus Christ expressed succor to orphans, the poor, travelers, and above all, the sick. The deaconesses of the early church visited the sick, much like modern visiting nurses or home health nurses. They were lay women appointed by the bishops. These appointments were highly esteemed and were given to women of good social standing.

One of the best known deaconesses of the early Christian church was Phoebe, a Greek lady who is also remembered as the bearer of Saint Paul's epistle to the Romans. Visiting nurses soon became an important part of the work of these early deaconesses, and Phoebe is often referred to as the first visiting nurse, as well as the first deaconess.

In addition to being visited in their homes, patients often stayed in the bishops' houses. When this proved impractical, special facilities were set up throughout the Roman Empire through endowments. In Rome the first large hospital was established by Fabiola, a beautiful, wordly woman, who thereby did penance for her second marriage. She administered this hospital so well that her death was mourned by all Rome. Separate hospitals developed for care of lepers, children, the aged, and strangers; these were forerunners of present day specialty institutions. A few centuries later in the Western World the first hospitals immediately under the auspices of the Roman Catholic Church were founded; these still exist. In Lyons the Hotel Dieu was established in 542 AD by Childebert; it is now the hospital with the longest record of continuous service. Detailed records were kept of the Hotel Dieu in Paris, which was founded in 650 AD by Saint Landry, bishop of Paris. It was enlarged in the thirteenth century by Saint Louis and was the prototype of the medieval hospital. The records of this hospital constitute a principal source of information regarding nursing in those days.

Moslem Medicine and Hospitals

During the eighth to the tenth centuries magnificent hospitals were constructed throughout the Moslem world. They were staffed by physicians superior to any in the world because of knowledge gained and preserved from their Greek counterparts. One well-endowed hospital was in Cairo and was especially for *infidels;* it was a prized target that the Crusaders tried very hard to destroy. These Moslem structures were in marked contrast to the rather gloomy Gothic Hotel Dieu in France of a few centuries before. Physiology and hygiene were studied by Arabian scientists and knowledge in *materia medice* was expanded. Surgeons used various drugs as anesthetics, but Moslem belief in the uncleanliness of the dead forbade dissection.

MIDDLE AGES
Influence of the Crusades on Nursing

For 1000 years after Christ there were no attempts to organize nursing. As the Middle Ages advanced, three organizations developed that persisted in some form to the present day or established certain principles still recognized as important. These organizations were the military, regular (religious), and secular orders.

Military Orders. The most spectacular focus of this period was the Crusader, a man who supposedly combined a lofty spirit devoted to the service of God with a fierce belligerent temper and who was ready to fight wherever the infidel was found so that the holy ground on which Christ trod might again belong to His followers. He carried the principles and the glory of knighthood to their fullest as he travelled over the continent of Europe and throughout the Mediterranean basin. When he traveled to the Near East, he learned much from the enemy, including the Arabian idea of the organized hospital. Natural places for the establishment of hospitals were outposts, particularly Jerusalem, where those wounded in battle sought refuge while they recovered. The hospital had to be staffed by physicians and nurses who were members of the regular orders. Men went to battle and then retired to nurse the sick. They were called *night hospitalers.* In later years they devoted themselves entirely to nursing. Two great influences shaped nursing practice during this period—the military and the religious. Gradually the care of the sick was considered more and more a religious duty.

Three nursing orders became preeminent: Knights of St. John, Teutonic Knights, and Knights of Saint Lazarus. Corresponding to these were three orders of women who tended female patients in special hospitals. The Order of Saint John—Italian and highly successful in its mission—originated the entire staff of two major hospitals in Jerusalem. It established an ambulance service and was a major organizer of the International Red Cross, which carries its insignia. This order established customs that remain the heritage of nursing today. Military in character, it was steeped in a tradition of discipline. Modern nursing traces its tradition of obedience to the principles of complete and unquestionable devotion to duty held forth by the Order of Saint John.

Regular Orders. Because of the insecurity of life during the Crusades, people could not be provided nursing care in their homes. Refuge behind moats and walls led to the establishment of monasteries wherein hostels, hotels, and hospices were organized to care for travelers, paupers, and the sick, particularly those with epidemic diseases. As the words *hostels, hotels,* and *hospices* imply, each served a different clientele. It was not until society became better organized and life was more stable that hospitals became separate institutions apart from monasteries.

The early hospital was called a *hotel Dieu*. It was at the Hotel Dieu in Paris that the Augustinian* sisters in charge developed a record keeping system credited with being the most complete of its time.

During the epidemics of this era care of the sick was performed mainly by volunteers who devoted themselves to nursing. One outstanding volunteer was Saint Catherine of Siena (1347-1380). At night her lamp represented to the sick at Siena what Florence Nightingale's lamp came to mean in the Crimea. Catherine received training in her middle-class home, staying at home to help with housework, which was the custom of the day. She later taught herself to read and write. In 1372 the plague came to Siena, and Catherine went to work night and day caring for the sick. She became well known for her work at a hospital in La Scala; it stands as a memorial to her today.

The regular orders were structured so that the sisters advanced from a stage of probationer to wearing the white robe to wearing the hood. In the beginning there was no uniform: nurses wore their regular clothes while on duty. As the Middle Ages advanced, clothes became more gaudy, and because the church secluded itself from the more wordly aspects of life, there was a tendency to adopt a uniform dress, which eventually became standardized.

Secular Orders. The disadvantages of church connections became increasingly apparent. Demands for complete and perpetual devotion to God would not always attract those best suited to care for the sick. Consequently secular orders were developed that were separate lay branches of the regular holy orders but approached regular orders by requiring temporary vows, uniformity in dress, and religious observances. Some of these secular orders include the Third Order of Saint Frances, the Order of Saint Vincent de Paul, and the Sisters of Charity. The Begiunes were active and prolific in West Flanders, the Netherlands, France, and Germany. The Oblates evolved in Italy and the Order of the Holy Ghost, remembered chiefly as a male nursing order, evolved in France.

THE RENAISSANCE

In the early 1300s a great revival of learning and art developed in Italy and spread elsewhere throughout Europe. This period is referred to as *the Renaissance*. Humanists of this time believed that by going back to the classics—literature, history, and philoso-

---

*The first organization of nurses.

phy of ancient Greece and Rome—they could begin a new golden era of culture and human life.

The church played a strong role in the development of this period. There was concern about the large administrative structure of the Roman Catholic church, the weak concern of the church for people, and the increased stress on good works, such as giving to charity, to earn salvation.

The invention of movable type in the mid-1400s helped spread learning through printed books, which resulted in an increased number of laymen (but side church structure) gaining an education.*

Forerunners of the great medical developments of this period are (1) Leonardo da Vinci (1452-1519), whose anatomical studies and sketches remain classical, (2) Andre Vesalius (1514-1564), credited with developing anatomy as a science, and (3) William Harvey (1578-1657), who is credited with founding medical science based on fact rather than tradition. The work of these sixteenth century anatomists enabled physicians to work on a more solid basis. Ambroise Paré (1510-1590), a military surgeon, wrote a book on natural history in general and surgery in particular in which he emphasized that it was necessary to dress wounds with boiling oil and that bleeding could be controlled with ligatures, as well as by red-hot cautery. He also devised artificial limbs for the victims of war. During this period, nursing reached a high level of organization and efficiency in the religious and military orders.

Beginnings of Modern Science

William Harvey discovered circulation of the blood, but contributed something even more important to medicine: he established the principle of the physiological experiment. He received his anatomical training in Padua and returned to Saint Bartholomew's Hospital in London where he served as demonstrator of anatomy at the Physicians' College in Amen Street. Here he completed his discovery, which he communicated in a lecture in 1616. His book was not published until 12 years later. While in Oxford during the reign of Charles I, the city was beseiged during a civil war, his home in London was searched, and all the manuscripts and notes were destroyed. What loss medicine thereby suffered can only be surmised, for some of the titles were of great promise, including "The Practice of Medicine Conformable in the Thesis of the Circulation of the Blood" and "Anatomy in its Application to Medicine."

After several decades of political disturbance, which led to the ultimate beheading of King Charles I in 1649, Harvey returned to London and became a scientific leader. He donated his library to the college of physicians and established a lectureship that has continued to this day and to which is owed, among others, Osler's marvelous oration in 1905 on the founder himself. Harvey exhorted his fellows and members of the college to study the ways of nature by means of experiment.

Thomas Sydenham (1644-1689) was first to set the example of true clinical methodology. His independent and unprejudiced spirit, combined with great powers of observa-

---

*The reference to laymen is literal here, meaning education of men, not women.

tion, made him the prototype of the clinical investigator. Referred to as the *English Hippocrates,* he resurrected the great but simple methods and principles taught by Hippocrates many centuries earlier. He emphasized the need to observe phenomena and let observations logically lead to conclusions. Puritan by birth and outlook, he expounded "We should not imagine or think out, but find out, what nature does or produces." This sounds obvious now but only because Sydenham succeeded to such an extent that his teaching has become commonplace. In his time medical science carried a superstructure of wanton superstitions and theories so complicated and cumbersome that it became deprived of real value. In fact, Sydenham was attacked because he made the practice of medicine too simple and easy. In modern times his name is commonly associated with his description of chorea, although his description of gout was better. His philosophy was to use probability as a guide, thus eliminating fantasies and vagaries that tend to distract the mind.

Sydenham had much in common with his friend John Locke (1632-1704), the physician-philosopher and private physician to Lord Shaftesbury. Locke, a proponent of common sense and straight thinking, was the forerunner of Hume and Kant.

Views that Sydenham held met with great opposition. He did not participate in the activities of the Royal Society of Medicine. Even during his lifetime he was considered one of the great physicians. The true magnitude of his accomplishments, however, was not appreciated for several generations.

During the seventeenth century, London abounded in quackery of all kind. Quacks, mountebanks, chemists, apothecaries, and even surgeons, who in those days were not supposed to treat internal diseases but nevertheless did, joined in exploiting the healing crafts. Druggists copied prescriptions they were supposed to fill and sold the drugs privately over the counter. One was said to have profited a hundred times as much from a simple prescription as did the physician who wrote it. It was thought that there was an overabundance of students graduating in medicine. Whoever wanted to practice in the field accepted being a perpetual slave and servant to the meanest all the days of his life. More than anytime before, increased taxes, polls, large fees for houses, servants, and entertainment were imposed on physicians. In those days, the main requirements for beginning a practice were to have a good understanding with a druggist and to be seen regularly at church (Payne).

People began to ask questions to which they expected rational answers based on facts. The scientific method of inquiry was born. This method of reasoning led to objective observations and to the physical and physiological experiments that form the basis for modern natural sciences. The writings of Locke, Roger Bacon, and Hobbes guided people's thoughts. Gilbert of Rochester assembled knowledge pertaining to magnetism and introduced the word *electricity.* Newton invented calculus, discovered laws governing optics, and the law of gravity; and Boyle introduced atomic theory. Thus, through hundreds of observations and discoveries, which often in the most unexpected way gained practical importance, the foundations for sciences were established. It was the scientific attitude that led to the discovery of steam power and the construction of the steam engine and somewhat later to the discovery of electromagnetism and the construction of the electric motor. Without it, modern engines would not have come into being and the Industrial Revolution would have remained unborn. In the course of time, the scientific attitude laid the foundations for modern medicine; the fundamental work of Harvey and Sydenham was its direct outgrowth. Scientific thinking eventually led to the construction of the engine by which entire lives of subsequent generations were altered.

All these developments had an impact on nursing, perhaps not immediate but in subsequent eras as nursing developed into a science and a profession using these theories as foundation for practice.

THE REFORMATION

The Reformation began in the early 1500s. Martin Luther (1483-1546), a monk and professor of theology, and other scholars of that time developed increasing conflict with the direction in which the church was moving. This began a long struggle in which the teachings of these leaders of the Protestant movement spread through Germany, Switzerland, England, and Scandanavia in particular.

Nursing sank to its lowest levels in the countries in which the Roman Catholic organizations were upset by the Reformation. The state closed churches, monasteries, and hospitals. In England, over a hundred hospitals were closed, and for a while there was little or no provision for the institutional care of the indigent sick. When the demand became too great to be ignored, lay persons were appointed to run the hospitals.

EXAMPLE: St. Bartholomew's Hospital in London, St. Giles in the Fields, and St. Katherine's Hospitals were not run because of the principle of charity but because of a social necessity. There was no honor attached to running a hospital or to being on its staff. At St. George's Hospital a man and his wife were engaged at salaries of L8 and L10 (pounds) per annum to be messenger and matron, respectively. The matron was in charge of the nurses, and a nurse in charge of a ward or a division was called a *sister,* possibly because of the belief that the title might retain some of the devotion and dignity of the old days. However, when deprived of the dignity of the church, nursing somehow lost its social standing.

Nurses were no longer recruited from the respectable classes of the community but from distinctly lower classes. The new Protestant Church abhorred cloisters and religous institutions and did not feel the same responsibility to the sick as had the Roman Catholic Church. Nurses were drawn from discharged patients or from the lower strata of society. Thus followed a dark period in nursing and the social setting dating roughly from the end of the seventeenth to the middle of the nineteenth century.

The Protestant Church advocated religious freedom and freedom of thought, but did not champion freedom for women in the seventeenth and eighteenth centuries and into the Victorian era. The place of the average respectable woman was in the home; a career woman would have been unthinkable around the year 1700. Men performed all teaching, secretarial work, and literary endeavors; work considered unsuitable for men, such as nursing, was entirely unobtainable for the average woman. Women of means hired servants to perform the heavy load of daily housework and gave their efforts entirely to the shallow and superficial life of society. The only profession available to women was acting, and that was not respectable. So women who were faced with the necessity of earning their own living were practically forced to enter domestic service; nursing was considered a not very desirable type of domestic service. The chief duties of a nurse in those days were to take care of the physical needs of the patient, making sure of reasonable cleanliness, although this was not considered essential in early municipal hospitals. Dressings were applied by dressers or by surgeons; the dispensing of medicines was the responsibility of physicians and the apothecary.

Nursing existed in a low and dismal state, without organization and without social standing. Nurses were considered the most menial of servants. They frequently worked 24 or 48 hours at a time and pay was insufficient to support themselves, not to mention dependents. The future for these women looked bleak.

Early American Hospitals

Great discoveries in medicine and the early immigration to America was also the time of the Reformation, which split the European nations into Catholic or Protestant states. The early Spanish and French explorers were Catholic and brought with them Dominicans, Franciscans, Jesuits, and later the nursing orders as missionaries. The care of the sick and wounded among friends and foe in the missions and the wilderness was largely their task. In the Spanish settlements, nursing was the responsibility of the monks, and a high degree of efficiency was never achieved.

American colonies, after the pattern of their homeland, organized institutions for the

---

EARLY AMERICAN HOSPITALS

	Roman Catholic	**Approximate dates**
Mexico City	Established by Cortez	1524
Quebec	Hotel Dieu	1658
New Orleans	Charity Hospital	1737
New Orleans	St Johns Hospital	1737
St Louis	First hospital west of Mississippi River (became DePaul Hospital in 1930)	1830
	Protestant	
Philadelphia	"Old Blockley" (later became Pennsylvania General Hospital)	1734
Philadelphia	Pennsylvania General Hospital	1751
New York	Kings Hospital	1769
Boston	Harvard Medical Center	1773
New York	Bellevue Hospital	1837

care of the sick and the poor, not so much out of Christian charity as for social convenience—something had to be done with the unfortunate. In early days the poorhouses and hospitals were under the same roof. The filth and squalor of some of the early hospitals is well documented and existed in well-known hospitals that remain in existence today, such as Bellevue of New York. Only the utterly destitute went to the hospital. Any who had a home or place to stay remained there when they were sick, and nursing was provided by the mother or grandmother of the home, or in well-to-do homes, by trusted servants. In some areas women gained a reputation in good nursing and were sought for cases of sickness and confinement.

When the great European hospitals were flourishing, American hospitals were just being established. Charity Hospital of New Orleans, established in 1737, may be the oldest hospital still existing in America for the care of the sick. A school of nursing was established there in 1894. The Ursuline Sisters from France made a major contribution to nursing during such major epidemics as yellow fever and smallpox but later went back to teaching, which was their focus, instead of nursing.

During the late 1700s and first decades of the 1800s definite landmarks were established, namely the big "general hospitals" in Pennsylvania, New York, and Massachusetts, as well as Bellevue of New York.

The Philadelphia Dispensary established in 1786 was the forerunner of the modern outpatient department and clinic for ambulatory patients. It was independent of any hospital and supported by civic-minded citizens of Philadelphia. It apparently was so successful that the idea soon spread to other early American cities.

Nursing orders of the 1830s and 1840s established hospitals and practiced high standards of nursing at that time. These were the Sisters of Mercy, the Sisters of the Holy Cross, and the Irish Sisters of Mercy.

American medicine in the eighteenth century was for the most part at a low ebb. Although numerous medical principles and discoveries emerged, there was a great lag between their discovery and application. Medical instruction continued along primitive lines, and physicians persisted in old habits. Benjamin Franklin influenced American medicine not only by inventing bifocal glasses but also by preaching the use of fresh air and by helping in the foundation of the Pennsylvania Hospital. Also, credit is given to the American Medical Association, established much later, for bringing medicine to its present standards.

INDUSTRIAL REVOLUTION TO THE MACHINE AGE
Emancipation of Women

The emancipation of women may be traced to the desire for personal freedom, which was one of the factors in the Industrial Revolution. It is part of the fight for human rights first audibly expressed in the eighteenth century and that became one of the principles of the French Revolution. It is a step that developed nursing from a craft into a profession as it is known today. Therefore the emancipation of women forms part of the background required to understand the evolution of nursing. Many attitudes of Florence Nightingale appear peculiar if one does not appreciate the difference between the social position of women at that time and the present.

Socialism and Social Legislation

Feudalism kept men from realizing their human rights and was a social state that had to be eliminated. Women's suffrage movements developed only after the male population won their rights. Social reformers of the nineteenth century in Europe such as Karl Marx had a resultant impact on the United States as well. The chief enemies of the laboring class were considered to be old age, sickness, exploitation, and unemployment. Protection from these enemies had an indirect, if not direct, impact on nursing. Social legislation was built on the political philosophies that reevaluated human rights and the basic premise that citizens are not chattel, that real power is not in the hands only of people with property or with men. Following this thought to a logical conclusion women became increasingly unwilling to be "property" within the family unit or on the job. They also became less willing to be handmaidens of physicians or property of hospitals.

Before women could advance as a group, they had to be equal with men before the law. The original concept of the family was that of a unit led by a household head; the change in legal concept recognizes members of the family as equivalent members of society. This change is the result of many individual laws, some of which pertain to franchise or occupation; others pertain to the civil standing of women in the community. Some of these changes are listed as follows:

1. Women may acquire and hold property
2. After 1925 a mother in England had the same rights of guardianship of her children as the father did
3. Divorce laws changed in favor of the wife*

Although changing laws give women the same status as men, equal pay and positions lag behind in some fields. The right to vote and the suffragist movement of the 1800s marked a significant move and was accelerated by the antislavery movement. After the Civil War the Abolitionists pushed for a constitutional amendment granting voting rights to all male Americans except slaves. For fear of defeat, feminist leaders such as Elizabeth Stanton interpreted the law to extend voting privileges to women but were unsuccessful in a subsequent election to cast ballots. Susan B. Anthony's arrest and trial aroused widespread public visibility and lent impetus to the feminist movement. Effort was invested at state and federal levels until the first state, Wyoming, granted women the right to vote in 1890. However, it was not until after World War I that the Nineteenth Amendment to the Constitution was ratified and became law. During this period new societies spread everywhere, public demonstrations were held, and militant tactics with parades, heckling of clergy during public appearances, marches, and hunger strikes testify to women's desire to come out of their mold and be recognized.

---

*Reciprocity is increasingly reflected in divorce laws. In some cases customs changed before the law.

Education

When women were recognized equal before the law in decision making (vote) the doors began to open to opportunity for education also. Early in the nineteenth century it was difficult for women to obtain an education except through private tutoring. Such education was expensive and available to only a privileged few. Florence Nightingale was educated by her father and by travel and social contact. At that time there were no colleges where she would have been admitted. If there had been, the evolution of nursing would have been quite different. As it is, the growth of colleges and universities for women has profoundly affected nursing education. Higher educational opportunities for women were available in women's colleges first, among them Oberlin in Ohio (1833), Wheaton at Norton, Massachusetts (1835), and Mount Holyoke (1857). Many others followed in the next 30 or 40 years, outstanding among them is Vassar in New York in 1865.

During the latter part of the century when higher education became more generally recognized, large numbers of institutions all over the country admitted women. Some of them were separate colleges for women; others were established within already existing universities, some coeducational. Tulane University in New Orleans and Western Reserve in Cleveland were the first universities to admit women (1887 and 1888) and soon others followed. The University of Chicago was established in 1893 on the basis of equal admittance to men and women. Not only did the number of women admitted to college increase but the educational standards of institutions admitting them advanced rapidly during this period.

Following the trend of the time, the American Association of University Women was established in 1915. This organization is active in establishing fellowships for the advanced education of women, with the result that an increasing number of women have obtained the degree of doctor of philosophy. Most of these women continue to pursue advanced teaching and research careers although there are signs of more entrepreneurship among women educated at this level.

The participation of the nursing profession as a whole in the development of the education of women will be discussed in subsequent chapters. Note here that a significant number of women seeking professional education go into nursing. Thus the advances made in the education of women form an integral part of the professional evolution of nursing.

It is questionable whether the Industrial Revolution would have extended very far had it not been stimulated by new thought, which may be traced to the Reformation. In addition to the spectacular religious aspects, the new stimulus of thought provided by the freedom that generated from the Reformation transformed ideas regarding government, politics, business, and philosophy. Locke and his concepts of individual perogative, "due process," and privilege to acquire and hold led to the fundamental protestant ethic. Without this the Machine Age of the nineteenth century would have been unthinkable. Unless one understands this, it is impossible to understand subsequent modifications that profoundly influenced the development of nursing.

At the turn of the 20th century, industrialism developed into the Machine Age. Because machines required manpower to operate them, increases in population were welcome and increased family size was an asset. England became the first nation of the factories and the expanding British Empire gave industrialism full support. Now the poverty of feudalism was part of the past because people were no longer occupied simply with obtaining food and other basic commodities. There were ample commodities produced for everyone living under Western civilization if the productive power of the modern industrial structure were at full capacity. In industrial society the two causes of poverty are (1) society fails to provide an adequate distribution of its commodities or (2) the citizens at the bottom of the economic scale lack the capacity or education to acquire a reasonable share of the communal wealth.

Industrialism and the Machine Age resulted in more questions from philosophers regarding the conduct and rights of man. A concern for public health emerged as the new capitalists squeezed the workers and exploited them. Although workers were now free to hold contract and property, starvation wages made them less than free agents and they were unable to achieve a reasonable standard of living. Consequently, with the unhygienic environment of rapidly growing cities the health of the population was jeopardized. The field of public health expanded. Organized health measures required more and better nursing; the Industrial Revolution and its collateral economic, political, and philosophical developments may be considered the soil that nurtered the growth of all the healing arts.

Florence Nightingale

The dominant figure in the development of organized nursing is Florence Nightingale. At the time she made her mark in history, society was generally one in which hospitals seemed amenable to a new profession and there was a realization that the Protestant orders needed some organization similar to Catholic nursing orders with more freedom in various ways.

The training and organization of lay Protestant nurses began before Florence Nightingale made her contribution to nursing, but with her powerful personality, her vision, and her practical organizing ability she took the lead in the movement, placed it on a powerful foundation of organization on sound educational principles and high ethics, and inspired it with an enthusiasm that gave to it an impetus under which it is still progressing. A few years before Miss Nightingale's time there was no professional nursing. At the time of her death nursing was a profession, formerly unthinkable.

However, Florence Nightingale devoted only a part of her life to the advancement of nursing; she also contributed to reforms in the Army, and improved sanitation in India and public health in Great Britain. Her full stature cannot be comprehended unless attention is given also to the following accomplishments.

Early Life and Education

Born in 1820 to Mr and Mrs William Edward Nightingale, Florence was their second daughter and named after the Italian city in which the family then lived. Having considerable wealth, Florence was brought up with good social standing, culture, and the best education available to children of that era. She learned French, German, and Italian and her father personally instructed her in mathematics and the classics.

The Nightingale's permanent home was England, but they traveled extensively. Florence thrived on the many acquaintances and experiences she had as she traveled through France, Italy, and Switzerland. She was expected to enter society when she returned to England but she had expectations of a more satisfying life. Knowing societal attitudes about nursing, her parents discouraged her interest in pursuing such a career. Nevertheless, she persevered and planned to become a nurse at Salisbury Hospital not far from her home.

In 1844, Ms Nightingale met the American philanthropist, Samuel Gridley Howe, and his wife, Julia Ward Howe, who later authored "The Battle Hymn of the Republic." The Lowes stayed at the Nightingale family home and impressed Ms Nightingale with an institution for the blind that Dr Howe had founded in New York. In this facility he planned to make medical and nursing care available without payment to elderly and ill American citizens. At this time Florence explored the possibility of working in English hospitals much as the Catholic sisters did. However, no respectable English woman could expect to pursue such a vocation unless she were to enter the church and Florence's family refused to discuss the matter further.

Until 1845, Florence believed that qualifications such as tenderness, sympathy, goodness, and patience were all that a nurse required. After experience in caring for some members of her family during their illnesses, she recognized that knowledge and skill were also necessary and that acquisition of these required education and training.

After a busy "social summer," Florence returned home to visit close friends of the family. This accomplished a dual purpose: (1) she explored life in a Catholic convent in preparation for nursing (she was not converted to Catholicism although she remained deeply religious throughout her life; by tradition she remained within the Church of England) and (2) she met Mr and Mrs Sidney Herbert through whom she was to go to the Crimea. The Herberts were deeply interested in hospital reform and public opinion was shifting sufficiently to be accepting of Ms Nightingale's expertise regarding hospital reform, a subject which she had collected data about for a long time.

By the age of 28, Ms Nightingale was expected to marry but that did not happen. She continued to travel as opportunities presented themselves, and wherever she went she studied intently what she saw. After a trip to Greece and Egypt she learned about the institution at Kaiserwerth. Through some friends she received the Yearbook of the Institution of Deaconesses at Kaiserwerth in 1846. She studied it carefully and realized that here she could receive the training she wanted. Because the institution was under religious auspices and the character of the deaconesses and pastors beyond reproach, she could go there without the stigma attached to the English hospitals.

Experience at Kaiserwerth

On one of her journeys Florence paid a visit to Kaiserwerth. She followed the visit with the writing of a 32-page pamphlet called the *Institute of Kaiserwerth on the Rhine for the Practical Training of Deaconesses Under the Direction of the Reverend Pastor Flieduer, Embracing the Support and Care of a Hospital, Infant and Industrial Schools, and a Female Penitentiary.* She was impressed with the organization and high purpose of Kaiserwerth but not with the training of nurses.

She assumed several administrative jobs and each time she went back to the task of visiting hospitals and collecting data for reforming conditions for nurses. In the middle of the nineteenth century, social reform was increasingly popular, and people such as the Herberts and their friends became interested in the reform of medical and social institutions. Ms Nightingale realized that nursing reform required the organization of some type of school for the training of reliable qualified nurses. She saw the need for a new type of nurse. One of the administration jobs that Ms Nightingale had was superintendent of nurses at King's College Hospital, thanks to Mr. Bowinan, a well-known surgeon.

The Crimean War

The Crimean war won Ms Nightingale the title of Lady with the Lamp. The British, French, and Turks were fighting the Russians, chiefly near the Black Sea and the Crimean Peninsula. There were serious problems with the handling of sick and wounded soldiers, especially by the British. There was need for a leader to organize an all out effort to save lives of the wounded and sick. Thirty eight nurses were recruited, some of them Roman Catholic sisters, and conditions under which these nurses worked were atrocious. Even the simplest means of healthy living were absent.

At first Ms Nightingale and the nurses did not have the respect and confidence of the physicians but this required time and evidence of what the nurses could do. Florence insisted that the nurses not give help unless they were asked. When large numbers of casualties were present, the nurses were asked for assistance by the physicians. The result was the establishment of a hospital from what had been shambles and by the end of the war there were 125 nurses.

Nursing staff was expected to cooperate and not take charge. A nurse took orders from physicians only. Florence divided her time between administration and personal attention to patients. Her nightly rounds when the day's work supposedly was done are famous. It was during her nightly rounds with her lantern that she made her tour of inspection past the long lines of cots, with a friendly word to some, a smile for others. In all she inspired a feeling of comfort that someone was sympathizing with the patients and striving to make their hard lot a little easier. Of all her activities in Scutari, these nightly rounds are perhaps the most famous; they have been immortalized by Longfellow in his poem *The Lady With the Lamp.*

In addition to being a nurse, Ms Nightingale was a social worker. She was concerned with recreational facilities for soldiers and their families and even developed a type of savings bank through which the soldiers might transmit money to relatives in England.

Toward the end of the war she became ill with Crimean fever (typhoid or typhus) from which she never fully recovered.

At the end of the Crimean War, two figures were prominent: the common British soldier and the nurse. At the beginning of the war most British soldiers were the drunken immoral dregs of society, and the status of women in nursing was not much better. Ms Nightingale's work in the Crimea did much to set the pattern for improvement of conditions for these two groups.

Nightingale Endowment Fund

After the war a public meeting was held in London on November 25, 1855, under the presidency of the Commander-in-Chief, the Duke of Cambridge. The Nightingale Endowment Fund was established for the purpose of furthering nursing education.

In August 1856, Ms Nightingale returned from Scutari, 6 months after the war ended. Her brilliant ambitions were hindered by her lack of physical strength. She did not recover from her malady and her stamina never returned. Some speculate she contracted a neurasthenia. Others believe she suffered from an exhaustion neurosis because she never afforded herself sufficient rest.

In 1856 the result of Ms Nightingale's conference and deliberations was published as *Notes on Matters Affecting the Health, Efficiency and Hospital Administration of the British Army,* a volume of nearly 1000 printed pages. In 1859, she published a small book titled *Notes on Hospitals.*

Around 1860, Ms Nightingale found time to devote to the establishment of a school of nursing financed by the Nightingale Fund. Saint Thomas Hospital was selected, and for many years, Ms Nightingale took an active interest in all details concerning the school. This school was the prototype for others established in the next 30 to 40 years. At the turn of the century, Florence was nearly 80 and spent the last 10 years of her life in a state of decline until she died quietly in her sleep on August 13, 1910. It was proposed she be buried in Westminster Abbey, but according to her wish she was interred in the family burial place at Willows, Hampshire.

Nightingale Pledge

The Nightingale pledge (see box) was taken by many professional nurses who are practicing today. Although recited, it took on a very different meaning from that which it had when it was written.

This pledge reflects Florence Nightingale's philosophy and style. Its tone, at face value, is incongruent with that of contemporary nursing. However, as throughout this text, nurses must acknowledge their past to constructively plan a future that holds the profession and the women and men entering the field in high esteem by our modern society. High moral and ethical standards are expected of professional nurses. The major issue that contemporary nurses may take with the Nightingale oath is the expressed need for more professional partnership with physicians to provide good care from both a nursing and medical standpoint, rather than emphasis on "aiding the physician in his work," i.e., medical care of patients.

THE NIGHTINGALE PLEDGE*

I solemnly pledge myself before God, and in the presence of this assembly, to pass my life in purity and to practice my profession faithfully. I will abstain from whatever is deleterious and mischievous, and will not take or knowingly administer any harmful drug. I will do all in my power to maintain and elevate the standard of my profession, and will hold in confidence all personal matters committed to my keeping and all family affairs coming to my knowledge in the practice of my profession. With loyalty I will endeavor to aid the physician in his work, and devote myself to the welfare of those committed to my care.

---

*This pledge was formulated in 1893 by a committee of which Mrs Lystra E. Gretter, RN, was the chairman. It was first taken by the 1893 graduating class of the Farrand Training School, now the Harper Hospital, Detroit, Michigan.

NURSING MOVES INTO THE TWENTIETH CENTURY
Nursing During the Early American Wars

The Red Cross, developed in Italy in 1859, was inspired by the work of Ms Nightingale during the Crimean War. It was established as an international body by diplomatic conference. In the United States, it was developed by Clara Barton in 1882. During the Spanish-American War, nurses served on both land and sea.

Public health nursing was proposed as a Red Cross program by Lillian D. Wold as early as 1908. It was initially confined to rural nursing, but by 1913 extended to towns having populations as large as 25,000 and became known as the *Town and Country Nursing Service.* In 1915 the first plan for training nurses' aides was proposed, but it did not develop fully until World War I.

Some Americans had heard about the Red Cross and Florence Nightingale's work in the Crimean War. When the Civil War began, little organized information was available. Independent of the previous structure that existed to promote cleanliness and health, the US Sanitary Commission was established in 1861. A branch of this commission opened a bureau in New York for the examination and registration of nurses for war service; about 100 applicants were available as nurses to the federal army at that time.

When the war began, this arrangement was totally inadequate and the Surgeon General agreed to the organization of its own sanitary commission as part of the army. The nurses were supplied by the Roman Catholic orders of the Sisters of Charity, Sisters of Mercy, and the Sisters of Saint Vincent. Protestant nursing orders, including deaconesses, served in the war as well. But all this was not enough. It took women of great strength and insight to move nursing to a new level in a new century.

In the American army, as well as in other armies, two types of nursing developed: (1) a regular army nursing service, which was placed under the direction of Miss Dorothea Dix (1803-1887) and (2) an organization sponsored by private citizens, at first tolerated and later supported by the government. Ms Dix was known for her crusade to improve conditions for the care of the mentally ill. In 1861, she was appointed superintendent of female nurses and proceeded to organize the first nurse corps of the US Army. Ms Dix was rigid in her standards; would accept no nurses under 30 years of age, preferably homely; required no uniform but insisted on black or brown dresses; and paid an allowance of $12 a month to each nurse. She herself served without pay. She found, as did Ms Nightingale before her, that most of the nurses came from religious orders, both Protestant and Roman Catholic.

About 2000 nurses served in the Civil War, a number totally inadequate considering the primitive equipment and hospital conditions. Hygiene was atrocious: the approximately six million medical hospital admissions were mainly from epidemics and contagious diseases; only about 425,000 surgical cases were actual war casualties. In those days, war claimed more victims from disease than from bullets.

The war emphasized, especially in light of Ms Nightingale's work, the desperate need for organized schools of nursing; such schools were accordingly initiated in New York City, Boston, and New Haven.

At the turn of the century when trouble between America and Cuba was imminent, Congress authorized employment of nurses under contract. This was necessary because military nursing had not advanced since the Civil War and because no mechanisms existed by which the surgeon general could find nurses if needed. However, by 1898 when the Spanish-American War began, schools of nursing had been training young women for this profession for about 20 years. More than 500 schools of nursing graduated about 10,000 nurses by the year 1900. In 1900 there were 202 nurses in the nurse corps, and the Army Reorganization Bill presented to Congress in that year provided for a permanent nurse corps as part of the medical department of the army. The Army Nurse Corps, specified as totally female, was created by law in 1901.

Early Nursing Schools

The earliest schools of nursing in America were organized using Nightingale's criteria: (1) they must be independent of hospitals and (2) be administered by boards or committees with power and freedom to develop the school. However, mainly because of lack of endowment, the schools were easily absorbed into the hospitals with which they were connected. Therefore the history of nursing in America is inextricably bound with the growth and development of hospitals; most of the schools were created and conducted by hospitals to serve their needs and the education of the nurse became a by-product of her service to the hospital. Hospitals rapidly discovered that nursing students were a source of free or inexpensive labor under the guise of "practical experience."

Another principle of the early schools was that it be administrated independently with a director of nursing, preferably a nurse with a separate budget from that of the hospital. Finally, students are advisably housed in a separate facility from the hospital.

In 1874, Ms Linda Richard, America's first "trained nurse," instituted the system of keeping written records and orders, which has since become a requirement in all nursing schools. Later, uniforms were introduced. *A Manual of Nursing,* the first text for students, was published in 1876, provided the first formal instruction, and was subsequently improved in other manuals that appeared in subsequent years.

As early as 1909, there were 1105 hospital-based diploma schools of nursing. A developing dialectic force in nursing led to the establishment of the first collegiate school of nursing at the University of Minnesota in that year. In 1917, *A Curriculum Guide for Schools of Nursing* was published and revised in 1927. University standards for nurses were refined and modern nursing began to evolve.

During the 1920s and 1930s, in an effort to eliminate wartime activities, the number of nurses in the army and navy was reduced. These were important years for nursing because during this period, nurses became aware that they were a potent social power and recognized nursing as something far more comphrehensive than taking care of the sick. An equal emphasis was placed on the prevention of illness. Documents by nurses of this period include *Nursing as a Profession,* prepared by Dr Esther Lucille Brown under the auspices of the Russell Sage Foundation, published in 1936, and revised in 1940. In 1936 the National League of Nursing Education published a manual, *Essentials of a Good School of Nursing.* In the same year the division of nursing of the Council of the American Hospital Association and a committee of the league, published *Essentials of Good Hospital Nursing Service.* Although the profession demonstrated a desire to improve education for nurses, a major handicap was lack of trained personnel. The National League for Nursing published a manual in 1933: *The Nursing School Faculty: Duties, Qualifications and Preparation of its Members.*

Professional nursing organizations developed to (1) control conditions of training, work, and compensation, (2) disseminate new knowledge affecting nursing, and (3) maintain communication, such as through alumni associations. Two professional nursing organizations are (1) the American Nurses' Association, which negotiates for improved working conditions and increased economic security, and (2) the National League for Nursing, which concentrates on standards of nursing education, entrance requirements of students, and accreditation of schools of nursing.

Impact of the Great Depression

Wars accelerate the need for nurses and emphasize the necessity for better nursing service, and in nursing the years between World Wars I and II were anything but quiet. The Great Depression began in the United States in 1929 and was followed by a world-wide depression in the 1930s. The New Deal, designed and implemented by President Franklin D. Roosevelt, called for measures to provide relief from the effects of the crashed economy. The Federal Emergency Relief Administration distributed funds to the needy of the nation; this distribution was accomplished at the state level and was a program in which many nurses participated. Other programs involving nurses were the Civilian Conservation Corps, designed to employ young people in reforestation and soil conservation, and the Federal Civil Works Administration, which created jobs for the unemployed. Many nurses worked in government-supported health care. Nursing made a major contribution to society and, during the Great Depression in turn, furthered its own development not only in the United States but internationally.

Before the economic crash, the Rockefeller Foundation, because of its interest in public health and preventive medicine, financed a committee for the study of nursing education. Organized in 1918, this committee's report encompassed a study of the entire field of nursing. It was called the *Goldmark Report,* named after Josephine Goldmark, whose social research skills were used while she was secretary to the committee chairman, Professor C.E.A. Winslow of Yale University.

BEGINNING OF CONTEMPORARY NURSING

Shortly before World War II, curricula in schools of nursing were being readjusted to meet contemporary situations. More emphasis was placed on social sciences. The preventive and social aspects were integrated in the clinical programs, as were mental hygiene and health teaching. More community experiences were recommended for all students. To answer the question of cost for these programs, a study made jointly by a committee of the league and the American Nurses' Association resulted in a pamphlet, *Administrative Cost Analysis for Nursing Service and Nursing Education,* published in 1940. The accrediting program of the league progressed, and collegiate programs increased in number. In 1941 the first list of schools accredited by the National League of Nursing Education was published. In the same year, through the efforts of the National Nursing Council and the Committee on Educational Policies and Resources, and with the cooperation of the US Public Health Service, under the sponsorship of Representative Frances Payne Bolton of Ohio, Public Law 146 was introduced and passed by Congress in 1943. This provided the first government funds for the education of nurses for national defense, and under the terms of the act, 1000 graduate nurses were given postgraduate preparation and 2500 nonpracticing nurses were given refresher courses. The goal was to increase enrollment in over 200 basic schools of nursing.

Early in 1942 a plan introduced the US Cadet Nurse Corps, and in July the bill known as the Bolton Act became a law. The main purpose of this act was to prepare nurses in adequate numbers for the armed forces, government and civilian hospitals, health services, and war industries through appropriations to qualified institutions. The program was supervised by a newly created Department of Nursing Education in the US Public Health Service, with Lucille Petry (Leone), as chief director, responsible to the Surgeon General.

Nursing During World War II

Nursing in World War II differed from nursing in any other war. Tremendous advances in medical science and the widespread activities of a large variety of fighting men presented a challenge and a great responsibility to the Army and Navy Nurse Corps. In World War II the army and navy nurses served in every part of the world. World War II has been described as a *total war,* and as such nurses had to be trained under combat conditions and had to know how to adapt techniques to meet changing conditions. The medical department worked as a team so successfully that 97% of all casualties were saved, and the death rate from diseases was reduced to $1/20$ of what it had been in World

War I. In 1944, full military recognition was given to the nurses of World War II, and they became a permanent part of the regular military force. Colonel Julie O. Flikke, superintendent of the Army Nurse Corps from 1937 to 1942, was the first woman colonel in the US Army. In 1942, she was succeeded by Colonel Florence A. Blanchfield. Training for all military nursing personnel was the responsibility of the Office of the Surgeon General. Direction of the Navy Nurse Corps was under the chief of the Bureau of Medicine and Surgery.

Post World War II Developments

World War II stimulated many new advances in medicine and nursing. Psychiatry and neurology emerged as modern specialty areas. Physiologic research related to the design of protective clothing, and individual equipment was important because soldiers were exposed to extreme climatic conditions. Examples of research in this area include the following:

1. Determination of water requirements in the heat
2. Development of cold weather clothing
3. Description of processes such as acclimatization and physical conditioning
4. Ascertaining the relationship between physical anthropometry to the human engineering of vehicles

Penicillin, discovered and developed by British scientists before World War II, was first used in military campaigns by the Allies in North Africa in 1943. Atomic research led to the development of the atomic bomb and nuclear research. DDT, first synthesized in 1870, was studied by the US Department of Agriculture in 1942 and field-tested by the medical department in Naples in 1943, where it stopped a typhus epidemic. The following year, army malaria control teams introduced DDT to control mosquitoes in the Pacific; DDT is still the primary insecticide for malaria control, although its use is discouraged today because of its toxicity and the crusade against it by environmentalists.

The opportunity to study wounded men, rather than to continue hypothesis based on the use of animal subjects, led to many developments in the understanding of blood replacement, study of shock, and the process of resuscitation. Many men returning from battle with hopes of leading normal productive lives stimulated prosthetic research development, education, and rehabilitation.

The Korean War from 1950 to 1953 prompted studies of frostbite, and correlations made during this time resulted in safer and more functional military and civilian cold-weather living. By the end of the Korean War in 1953, helicopters had developed as a major means of evacuating large numbers of casualties and became widely used as ambulances and rescue vehicles during the Vietnam War and in the civilian world.

Medical care of dependents of military personnel requires an enormous number of health care professionals, many of them nurses. This program was expanded and became the Civilian Health and Medical Program of Uniformed Services (CHAMPUS). A new generation of army hospitals began in 1960 with the construction of ten new facilities in the next 5 years. Restrictions on the promotion of Army Medical Specialists Corps and Army Nurse Corps officers were removed in 1967. In 1968, Congress changed the Army Medical Service back to the earlier Army Medical Department. Colonel Anne Mae V. Hayes, Chief of the Army Nurse Corps, was promoted to the grade of Brigadier General in 1970. She became the first woman general in the US Army. In July, 1975, the Army Medical Department observed its bicentennial anniversary of the beginning of health care for the American soldier.

World War II stimulated the upward mobility of women; for the first time, top ranks were achieved by women in the armed services. The wars after World War II required nursing personnel in hospital evacuation sites, behind battle lines, on ships and aircraft carrying casualties back to the States, and in Veteran's Hospitals providing care to the mentally and physically disabled. This period was the beginning of contemporary nursing. Early leaders who helped move nursing into the twentieth century are listed in the box.

Nursing practice over this period of time developed into the following specialized areas:

1. Private duty nursing
2. Visiting nursing
3. Settlement nursing (work among the poor)
4. School nursing
5. Nurse clinician work
6. Anesthesia
7. Industrial nursing
8. Nurse-midwifery
9. Nursing in the federal government such as in the Armed Services, Veterans Administration, Indian Services, and the US Public Health Service (a department now within the Division of Health and Human Services)

EARLY LEADERS OF NURSING

Isabel Hampton Robb (1860-1910) was one of the founders of *The American Journal of Nursing.*

Lavinia Dock (1858-1956) campaigned against male dominance and its negative impact on the nursing profession.

Mary Mahoney (1845-1926), first professional black nurse in the United States.

Mary Sewell Gardner (1870-1961) is best known for the development of the National Organization for Public Health Nursing.

Annie Goodrich (1876-1955) became a state inspector of schools of nursing, president of the International Council of Nurses from 1912 to 1915, and later, dean of the Army School of Nursing when it was organized in 1918.

Isabel Maitland Stewart (1878-1963) was only recently recognized for her contributions as an educator, writer, organization worker and important figure in international nursing affairs for 40 years.

KNOWLEDGE EXPLOSION, TECHNOLOGY, AND HEALTH CARE

In conclusion, major factors influencing health care and the provision of health services, developments which have come about essentially since World War II, follow.

New Knowledge

A surge of new knowledge occurred within the health sciences. Diagnosis and treatment underwent revolutionary changes as a result of new developments in drugs and equipment and new research findings in psychosocial aspects of health care. Communicable disease control and child welfare programs that reduced the incidence of contagious diseases are now drastically changed. New communicable diseases are threatening the entire population and the statistics regarding infant mortality and morbidity have put the United States to shame, compared with some other nations.

Technological developments refine the quality of care that can be provided but make the administration of that care far more complex. Renal dialysis, heart-lung machines, monitoring devices of numerous kinds, closed-circuit television, computers, and radioactive isotopes preceded artificial organs and organ transplants. All of these developments demand rigorous scientific training of responsible health personnel.

Basic Change in Attitude Toward Health

A basic attitudinal change stems from the philosophy of the World Health Organization (WHO) that thought health is more than the absence of disease; that it is a state of physical, psychological, and social well-being; and that it is a right, not a privilege, to which individuals are entitled—even though the present system in this country does not seem congruent with the philosophy in some cases. Modern mass media has increased public awareness of disease and health problems, even though that awareness is sometimes inaccurate.

Although health care is provided in schools, industries, and public clinics, this is often superficial. Health maintenance organizations have not become a favorite means of obtaining necessary health care for the majority. National health insurance contains inadequacies. Nursing homes have proliferated and can usually provide maintenance and/or skilled nursing care for the chronically ill and elderly; yet workers in this facility often earn minimum wages and the cost to the patient is far beyond personal means or even expenditures of life's savings.

Health Care Personnel Supply and Distribution

President Truman conceptualized a health care team that consisted of physicians, dentists, nurses, and a variety of allied health professionals. He recognized the need for specialization but also acknowledged that increased specialization created a need for allied workers to serve as auxiliary workers, especially in the specialized areas of preventive, psychiatric, and rehabilitative fields.

One difficulty in providing adequate care for everyone in the United States is that health workers and health facilities are located in urban centers. Better distribution of institutions and personnel is a problem that is recognized and studied by medical; nursing; and state, regional, and federal health organizations. Numerous approaches have been tried to deliver health care to the underserved populations. Satellite clinics, mobile units, high-tech communication methods, and rapid means of transportation such as helicopters are used to bring client, patient, and health care professionals together. Rural health teams are an example of the cooperative system of health care delivery in which nurses play a more active part in coordinating efforts and skills of various health care professionals. These nurses specialize and at the same time continue to reflect the needs of the general population that they serve. In this role the nurse is challenged with much more independent practice and responsibility.

Decreased Hospitalization

Incidence of disease has had vast change, and the emphasis has shifted to home care, or early discharge from the hospital when hospitalization is necessary. Follow-up care is provided in clinics or by home health nurses. Long-term illness is managed through outpatient and extended care facilities.

Population Trends

Between 1900 and 1952 the nation's population doubled. After World War II, impetus was given to the family planning movement. Because of new awareness, readily available contraceptive methods, and society's desire to limit the rate of population growth, the population was reduced to zero in 1973. This reversal of the population explosion, partly a result of the continued emancipation of women, resulted in closing of schools, shifting the focus of clinical facilities to care for the older age group, and difficulty of nursing students to obtain clinical obstetric and pediatric clinical experiences.

Increased longevity has changed the health care delivery system. Statistics indicate that the number of persons 65 years of age or more increased from 3 to $11^{1}/_{2}$ million between 1900 and 1952 and by 1960 reached $15^{1}/_{2}$ million. The 1990 census will undoubtedly show even more rapidly increasing numbers, based on estimates made by various polls in recent years.

Changes in morbidity and mortality patterns indicate that today's nurse needs a different type of preparation from that of 50, 25, or even 10 years ago. Heart disease and cancer are leading causes of death. Newly added to the list is AIDS and deaths related to narcotic and drug abuse. Chronic problems associated with the increased incidence of degenerative diseases are more frequent. Alcoholism and other addictions, mental illness, and child and elderly abuse are just some of contemporary society's problems that nurses help prevent and treat.

Prevention and better treatment are replacing custodial care of the mentally ill. However, lack of finances, well-prepared personnel, and adequate facilities are making this change a slow process. Previously reduced maternal and infant mortality is on the rise, related to teen-age pregnancy, lack of prenatal care, and use of drugs and alcohol before and during pregnancy. Chemotherapy has revolutionized the treatment of many severe illnesses but has stimulated new strains of viruses and new diseases such as methicillin-resistant staphylococcus aureus (MRSA) infection. These trends demonstrate the dynamic state of health care and the internal and external pressures on nursing and other health services.

Growth of Junior and Community Colleges

The tremendous growth of junior and community colleges resulted from a population explosion after World War II and the demand of youth for a college education. In addition to this, various studies supported experts in nursing who were urging that all nursing education be placed in institutions of higher learning. With the closure of 3-year diploma and 9- to 12-month licensed practical nurse (LPN) hospital-based schools of nursing, and increased demand for nurses, junior and community college nursing programs came into their own. By 1970, nursing programs of this type increased 445%. Some are only state approved, while others are also NLN* accredited. Junior and community colleges train various other auxiliary health personnel or provide portions of the preprofessional course of study. These institutions usually cost less, so it is financially more feasible for many students to obtain their education this way. These institutions are currently supported and used by health care facilities, especially large medical centers, as an inexpensive means of rapidly manufacturing nursing staff, regardless of quality. Graduates can earn prerequisites necessary to take the basic RN or LPN license examination. Thereby facilities can satisfy minimum requirements in terms of hospital accreditation standards and federal and state criteria for funding and physically staff the various units of the facility. Again the nurse is being manipulated; although on the positive side, it may be a stepping-stone to a better education, independence, and an improved career.

Change takes place slowly and in cycles. This is true throughout the history of nursing also. The negative connotations—lack of good education and conditions on the job—are documented. The task ahead includes better professional preparation, better formal education, and equal standing with other truly professional health care workers. The basic team from the beginning was and remains medicine and nursing. The formation of a true partnership between the two fields is addressed in the text that follows.

Continued Emancipation of Women

Not only are more women entering the labor force, but opportunities for employment in service occupations are also increasing. The predominately female occupation of nursing no longer has first claim on young women. Fewer women are entering this field now compared with the 1950s and 1960s. Meanwhile the small fraction of male students in nursing seems to be increasing; however, the upward mobility of men still remains greater than for women.

Perhaps the early emancipators of women visualized a world in which women and men were equal in all respects of society. However, as long as the family remains the

---

* The National League for Nursing

——————— MAJOR HISTORICAL INFLUENCES ON NURSING ———————	
Event	**Time period**
Crusades	1000 AD-1300
Renaissance	Began 1300s
Reformation	1500s
Industrial Revolution	1800s-early 1900s
Development of modern science and health facilities	Began 1800s-present
World War I	1918-1920s
World War II	1939-1945
Social and basic science research	Began 1945
Social welfare	1960s-1970s
Technology	1980s-present
Equal rights movement	1840s-present

unit of western civilization the larger part of women's efforts will be concerned with homemaking and child rearing. The American reader is aware of the concern about the erosion of the family unit. It is hoped that women, in an effort to gain emancipation and equality in this society, will not be blamed for that erosion.

It has been a long struggle for women nurses to "find their place in the sun."

•   •   •

The twentieth century finds many nurses not only responsible for themselves, but because of social changes, for dependents, usually children or aging parents, but maybe others, as well. The nursing profession has struggled hard to reach its present position. Nurses today find themselves frustrated and eager to plan their futures. The need for nurses is as great as it has always been. Hopefully the rewards will begin to be commensurate with the need.

STUDENT ACTIVITIES

1. During what period in history do you think nursing made its biggest strides toward professionalization?
2. What do you think have been major obstacles in the emancipation of women and subsequent progress in the field of nursing?
3. Based on what you have read and experienced, speculate what nursing will be at the turn of the century.

REFERENCES

A century of nursing; reprints of four historic documents, including Miss Nightingale's letter of September 18, 1872, to the Bellevue School: Foreward by 'Elizabeth M. Stewart and Agnes Galinas, for the National League of Nursing Education, New York, 1950, G. P. Putnam's Sons.

American National Red Cross: The American Red Cross: a brief story, Washington, DC, 1951, American National Red Cross.

Andrews MR: A lost commander: Florence Nightingale, New York, 1938, Doubleday & Co, Inc.

Austin AL and Stewart IM: History of nursing, ed 5, New York, 1962, GP Putnam's Sons.

Banworth C: A living memorial to Florence Nightingale, Am J Nurs 40:491-497, May, 1940.

Barton WE: The life of Clara Barton—founder of the American Red Cross (2 vols), Boston, 1922, Houghton Mifflin Co.

Blackwell E: Pioneer work for women, New York, 1914, EP Dutton & Co, Inc.

Blanchfield FA and Standlee MW: Organized nursing and the army in three wars. Unpublished manuscript on file, Historical Division, Office of the Surgeon General of the Army, Washington, DC.

Brockett LP and Vaughan MC: Women's work in the Civil War: a record of heroism, patriotism and patience, Rochester, New York, 1867.

Chayer ME: School Nursing, New York, 1937, GP Putnam's Sons.

Christy TE: Portrait of a leader: Lavinia Lloyd Dock, Nursing Outlook 17:72-75, June, 1969.

Christy TE: Portrait of a leader: Adelaide Nutting, Nursing Outlook 17:20-24, Jan, 1969.

Christy TE: Portrait of a leader: Isabel Hampton Robb, Nursing Outlook 17:26-29, March, 1969.

Christy TE: Portrait of a leader: Isabel M Stewart, Nursing Outlook 17:44-48, Oct., 1969.

Cook Sir Edward: The life of Florence Nightingale (2 vols in 1), New York, 1942, The Macmillan Co.

DeBarberey H: Elizabeth Seton, New York, 1931, The Macmillan Co.

Dock L et al.: History of American Red Cross nursing, New York, 1922, The Macmillan Co.

Deutsch A: Dorothea Lynde Dix: apostle of the insane, Am J Nurs 36:987-997, Oct., 1936.

Doyle A: Nursing by religious orders in the United States, Am J Nurs 29:775-786, July, 1929 (Part I, 1809-1840); 29:959, 1929 (Part II, 1841-1870); 29:1085, 1929 (Part III, 1871-1928); 29:1197, 1929 (Part IV, Lutheran deaconesses, 1849-1928); 29:1466-1484, Dec. 1929 (Part VI, Episcopal Sisterhoods, 1845-1928).

Dubos RJ: Louis Pasteur: free lance of science, Boston, 1950, Little, Brown & Co.

Dulles FR: The American Red Cross: a history, New York, 1950, Harper & Brothers.

Editorial—Dedication of the American Nurses' Memorial, Florence Nightingale School, Bordeaux France, Am J Nurs 22:799-804, July, 1922.

Editorial—The dedication of the Bordeaux School Building, Am J Nurs 36:491-492, May, 1936.

Extracts from letters from the Crimea, Am J Nurs 32:537-538, 1932.

Epler PH: The life of Clara Barton, New York, 1919, The Macmillan Co.

Engelman RC and Joy RJT: Two hundred years of military medicine, Fort Detrick, Maryland, 1975, The Historical Unit, US Army Medical Department.

Ferguson ED: The evolution of the trained nurses, Am J Nurs 1:463-468, April, 1901; 1:535-538, May, 1901; 1:620-626, June, 1901.

Fishbein M: History of the American Medical Association, Philadelphia, 1947, WB Saunders Co.

Florence Nightingale is placed among mankind's benefactors, Am J Nurs 50:265, 1950.

Frank, Sister CM: Foundations of nursing, ed 2, Philadelphia, 1959, WB Saunders Co.

Gallison M: The ministry of women: one hundred years of women's work at Kaiserwerth, 1836-1936, London, 1954, Butterworth & Co., Ltd.

Hamilton SW: The history of American mental hospitals: one hundred years of American psychiatry, New York, 1944, Columbia University Press.

Hume EE: Medical work of the Knights Hospitallers of Saint John of Jerusalem, Baltimore, 1940, The Johns Hopkins Press.

Jensen DM: History and trends of professional nursing, St. Louis, 1959, The CV Mosby Co.

Jones MC: The training of a nurse, Nov, 1980, Scribner's.

Kernodle, PB: The Red Cross nurse in action, 1882-1948, New York, 1949, Harper Brothers.

Lee, E: A Florence Nightingale collection, Am J Nurs 38:555-561, May, 1938.

Livermore MA: My story of the war, a woman's narrative of the four years' experience as a nurse in the Union Army, Hartford, Conn., 1888, AD Worthington Co.

Marshall, HE: Dorothea Dix, Chapel Hill, 1937, University of North Carolina Press.

McGinley P: Saint-watching, New York, 1969, The Viking Press, Inc.

Noyes CD: American nurses complete fund for Memorial School in France, Am J Nurs 29:1189-1191, Oct. 1929.

Nightingaliana: Am J Nurs 49:288-299, May, 1949.

Nursing and the League of Nations, Am J Nurs 31:1283-1284, Nov., 1931.

Nutting MA: History of nursing (in collaboration with Lavinia L. Dock), vols 1 and 2, New York and London, 1907; vols 3 and 4, 1912.

Payne JF: Thomas Sydenham, New York, 1900, Longmans, Green & Co..

Pavey AE: The story of the growth of nursing, London, 1938, Faber & Faber, Ltd.

Pickett SE: The American National Red Cross, New York, 1924, Century Co.

Robb IH: Educational standards for nurses, Cleveland, Ohio, 1907, EC Koechart.

Roberts MM: Florence Nightingale as a nurse educator, Am J Nurs 37:773-778, July, 1937.

Roberts MM: American nursing: history and interpretation, New York, 1954, The Macmillan Co.

Scovil ER: Florence Nightingale's notes on nursing, Am J Nurs 27:355-357, May, 1927.

Seymer L: St. Thomas' Hospital and the Nightingale Training School, Int Nurs Rev 11:340-344, 1937.

Sharp EE: Nursing during the pre-Christian era, Am J Nurs 19:675-678, June, 1919.

Stephen B: Florence Nightingale's home, Int Nurs Rev 11:331-334, 1937.

Strachey L: Eminent Victorians, New York, 1963, GP Putnam's Sons.

The American National Red Cross: Jane A Delano: a biography, ARC 781, Washington, D.C. 1952.

The A.N.A. and you, New York, 1941, American Nurses' Association. p 2.

Tiffany F: Life of Dorothea Lynde Dix, Boston, 1890, Houghton Mifflin Co.

Transactions of the American Hospital Association, p. 91, 1913.

Trevelyan GM: History of England, London, 1928, Longmans, Green & Co, Ltd.

Whittaker EW and Olesen VL: Why Florence Nightingale? Am J Nurs 67:2338-2341, Nov., 1967.

Williams BC: Clara Barton, daughter of destiny, Philadelphia, 1941, JB Lippincott Co.

Vreeland EM: Fifty Years of Nursing in the Federal Government Nursing Services, Am J Nurs 50:626, Oct, 1950.

Wald LD: Windows on Henry Street, Boston, 1934, Little, Brown & Co.

Woodham-Smith C: Florence Nightingale, New York, 1951, McGraw-Hill Book Co, Inc.

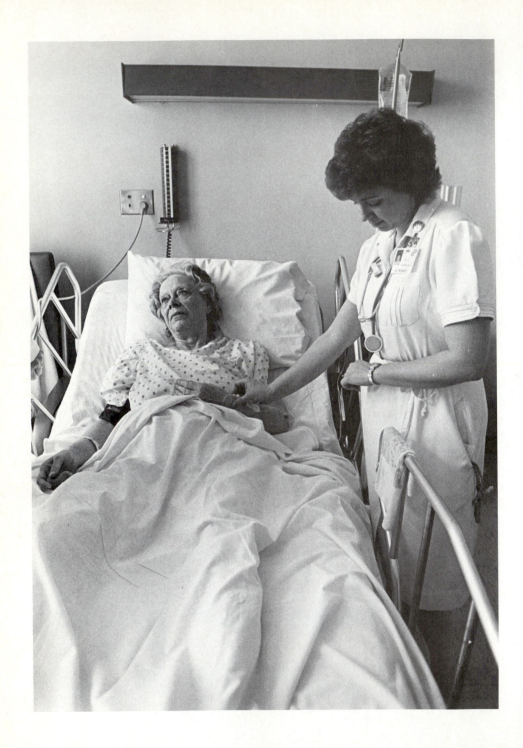

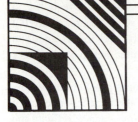

C H A P T E R **2**

THE EVOLUTION OF NURSING SCIENCE AND PRACTICE

Janet W. Kenney

OBJECTIVES

After completing this chapter the reader should be able to:

* Discuss what is meant by the statement that nursing is an art and a science

* Describe how nursing practice has changed over the past 40 years

* Relate historic events, reports, and studies that have had an impact on nursing education and practice

* List the currently accepted components of the nursing process

* Describe what is meant by a nursing model

* Discuss what is meant by nursing theory

* Name six or more contemporary nursing theorists who have made a contribution to the scientific body of nursing knowledge

 During the past four decades the nursing profession made significant progress toward developing a body of scientific knowledge and establishing the credibility of nursing science. This body of knowledge grows as nurses are educated to critically study nursing practice, develop theories and conceptual models of nursing, conduct nursing research, and test nursing theory. Concurrently, nursing practice changed in response to societal needs and the developing body of nursing knowledge. Consumers' changing health care needs, their demands for accessibility, accountability and involvement in decision-making, and escalating health care costs have all contributed to the evolution of professional nursing.

This chapter describes the evolution of nursing as a science and a practice discipline. It begins with a discussion of the development of knowledge and the interdependence of nursing practice, theory, and research. The development of nursing science reflects the ongoing struggle with various philosophical and methodological issues. These are presented as historical background, followed by a brief summary of major societal changes that affect nursing practice and nursing theory development. The evolution of the nursing process and theory development is described through historical events, publications, and contributions of nursing leaders. Nurse scholars and leaders who have shaped the nursing profession are acknowledged and their contributions emphasized. Current views of nurse leaders and their projections of the future of nursing practice, theory, and research are presented. The chapter concludes with suggestions for the continuing advancement of professional nursing.

EVOLUTION OF NURSING KNOWLEDGE: WAYS OF KNOWING

During the past 40 years, nursing was depicted as a series of tasks; a caring, comprehensive service; a process involving cognitive, psychomotor, and interpersonal skills; and an art and science of human health and behavioral responses.[22] In their quest to achieve the status of a science for professional nursing, nurse leaders and scholars have sought answers to the following questions:

What is a science?
How does a science evolve?
What is the purpose of science?
What are the characteristics of science?

What is a Science?

As early as 1959, Johnson[30] wrote about the science of nursing, citing several definitions. Johnson noted that professional disciplines usually represent applied sciences rather than basic sciences. Their goals are to use knowledge in practice. Johnson believes that nursing should be a body of knowledge with the following goals:

1. Prevent illness
2. Promote and maintain health
3. Provide comprehensive care

Figure 2-1 illustrates the development of a nursing science.

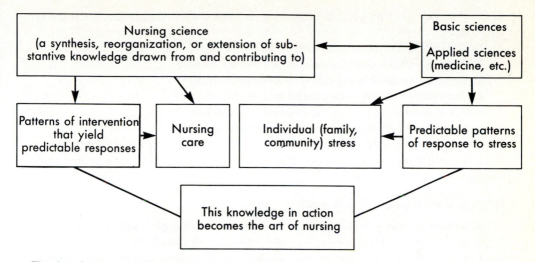

Fig. 2-1 Schematic presentation of the knowledge in nursing care.
(From Johnson DE: The nature of a science of nursing, Nursing Outlook 7(5):291-294, 1959. Copyright American Journal of Nursing Co. Used with permission. All rights reserved.)

In 1969, Abdullah[1] described nursing science as "a body of cumulative scientific knowledge, drawn from the physical, biological, and behavioral sciences, that is uniquely nursing." She explained the need for nursing to develop a highly organized and specialized field of knowledge and listed steps to achieve a nursing science. Abdullah emphasized the need for concept identification and nursing research to clarify nursing theory.

The question "what is science?" was adeptly addressed by Jacox[27] in 1974. She described science as a *process* (research and inquiry) and a *product* (body of knowledge). She (1) emphasized the importance of empirical knowledge, which can be perceived and verified through the senses by others, and (2) described how knowledge accumulates through examination of phenomena, concept identification, model building, and theory testing. Jacobs and Huether[26] support the viewpoint that "science is a product created by a process" that is directly related. They assert that the major aim of science is to develop theory to explain, predict, and control nursing practice. The purpose of nursing science—to develop theory and knowledge for its own sake (basic), rather than for direct application in practice (applied)—was challenged again.

How Does a Science Evolve?

Johnson[29] wrote that each science emerged from the study of different phenomena or a unique perspective of observation and interpretation of a specific field. Silva[53] described the development of a science as the need to categorize and structure different fields of knowledge. She listed the following six principles of science that are still relevant today:

1. Science must show a certain coherence
2. Science is concerned with definite fields of knowledge
3. Science is preferably expressed in universal statements
4. The statements of science must be true or probably true
5. The statements of science must be logically ordered
6. Science must explain its investigations and arguments

These six principles must be applied for science to be a body of knowledge (product) and a research methodology (process). Nursing, as a profession, is striving to meet these principles today.

What is the Purpose of Science?

In addressing the purpose of science, nurses have struggled with several issues. Many nurse scholars cite Kerlinger,[32] a noted authority, who firmly believes that the purpose of science is to describe, explain, predict, and ultimately control natural events. That is, science is the development of *basic* knowledge through research. Other nurse authors believe the aim of nursing science is *applied* research and knowledge to guide nursing practice. A third contingent supports the need for both basic and applied knowledge.

Meleis[37] wrote that nursing knowledge is based on its evolving philosophy and former practice, as well as emerging ideas, theory, and research. She concludes that the nursing domain consists of the following four major elements:

1. Major concepts and problems of nursing
2. Processes for assessment, diagnosis, and intervention
3. Tools to assess, diagnose, and intervene
4. Research designs and methods congruent with nursing knowledge

If an emerging discipline establishes its major concepts and identifies the problems to be addressed, the other three elements will gradually evolve. Nursing continues to make dramatic progress in each of these areas.

As an evolving discipline, nursing is developing an organized body of knowledge, composed of specialized concepts and terminology, and interrelated beliefs, facts, principles, theories, and methodologies, that is used in education, research, and practice. Each discipline defines specific areas of study and methods of determining its body of knowledge. The discipline identifies credible research methods, acceptable standards of practice, and criteria for educating practitioners in the field.

During its evolution, nursing sought professional status by establishing a scientific base for its practice and emerging theories. The search for empirical knowledge became predominant and was based on observable, objective, logical data and rational thought. Other forms of knowledge were considered less acceptable. However, empirical knowledge alone provides a narrow view of reality.

In 1978, Carper[10] described four basic patterns of knowledge that are used in nursing and many other disciplines. Each pattern is an equally necessary component of nursing and has its own method for determining credibility of knowledge in each field. The four patterns of knowledge are described as follows:

1. Empirical knowledge: based on objective evidence obtained by the senses and requires validation and verification by others
2. Ethical knowledge: examines the philosophical premises of justice and seeks credibility through logical justification
3. Esthetics: judges creativity, form, structure, and beauty through criticism of the meaning of the creative process and product
4. Personal knowledge: integrates and analyzes the current interpersonal situation with past experience and knowledge

A discipline's body of knowledge would be incomplete if it relied exclusively on one form of knowledge. Most disciplines, including nursing, integrate all four patterns of knowing to form a more complete picture of reality.

Nurses are beginning to recognize the value and validity of different ways of knowing and to realize that no single form of knowledge is superior. Peggy Chinn[11] wrote extensively in support of Carper's patterns of knowing. She refuted the superiority of empirical knowledge as the only relevant science. With assistance from members of the Nursing Theory Think Tank, Chinn and Jacobs[12] clarified the patterns of knowing as follows:

1. Empirics: scientific theory, models, and linguistic descriptions of observable reality
2. Ethics: standards, codes, and normative theory
3. Esthetics: expressed in an art or act
4. Personal knowing: expressed in the authentic self

They also developed a process for determining the credibility of knowledge (see Table 2-1). As more nurses recognize the value, credibility, and necessity of *all* patterns of knowing, the science of nursing will continue to advance.

INTERDEPENDENCE OF PRACTICE, THEORY AND RESEARCH

Historically, nursing practice was based on apprenticeship and the performance of technical skills, with little consideration for a knowledge base. As nursing education shifted from hospital programs to academic institutions, there was a gradual increase in emphasis on developing a body of nursing knowledge that could be applied in practice.

Although the movement of nursing education from hospitals to academic institutions was a positive move, it created several problems. Nurse educators and scholars were isolated from practice and had difficulty identifying appropriate questions, developing relevant nursing practice models and theories, and applying nursing theory and new knowledge to nursing practice.

Ideally, nursing theory, research, and practice are interrelated. From observations in nursing practice, questions arise and conceptual models are formulated. This may lead to

Table 2-1 Process for determining credibility of knowledge

Pattern	Ethics	Esthetics	Personal	Empirics
Form of expression	Standards Codes	Art/act	Authentic self	Scientific theory
	Normative/ ethical theory			Models Factual descriptions
Critical question	Is this just? Is this respon-sible?	What does this mean?	Do I know what I do and do I do what I know?	What is it and how does it function?
Method for determining credibility	Justification	Criticism	Reflection	Validation
Social/ political context	Dialogue	Empathy consensus	Response	Replication

From Chinn PJ & Jacobs M: Theory and nursing: a systematic approach. ed 2, St. Louis, 1987, The CV Mosby Co.

theory development and testing through research. Although theory is used primarily to guide research, it also interacts with and guides nursing practice. Research validates and modifies theory, which then changes nursing practice.

Nursing models and theories serve many purposes in practice. They can assist the nurse to understand the client's health/illness situation. Theories and models provide a framework for deciding which nursing actions are appropriate and effective in achieving the desired client outcomes. Nursing practice provides the necessary observations and experiences for nurses to develop and test theory. As theories evolve, nurses gain greater control over practice because the rationales for their actions are based on tested theory.

The application of nursing models and theories in practice is difficult and requires advanced education, critical analysis, and creativity. Several major problems have hindered progress in this area. Many nursing programs do not include knowledge and application of nursing theories or models in their curriculum, and therefore graduates are not prepared to use them in practice. Some nurse leaders contend that nursing models and theory are not sufficiently developed to apply in practice.[26,65] Since 1980, however, several textbooks have been written that explain how to apply nursing models in the nursing process.[13,49]

Walker[56] believes that to apply abstract nursing models to practice, the nurse must have the following:

1. A solid understanding of relevant theories
2. Knowledge of contextual factors affecting the client

3. Creativity to synthesize theory within the situational constraints
4. The ability to apply theory to a unique client situation

That is, the nurse must consider and synthesize the major concepts of a theory, the client's health/illness variables and uniqueness, and the constraints and variables of the employing agency. The ability to synthesize all of these variables in practice requires previous learning and practice in critically analyzing each individual factor. Nurse educators who know and value nursing models and theories can teach students to apply these models appropriately by considering all the variables. In practice settings, the incorporation of theory and research is an evolutionary process that is just beginning. It requires a nursing staff that asks questions, seeks answers, and looks for new ways to handle old problems.

The link between nursing practice and research has been under scrutiny and discussion for years. With the growing cadre of nurse researchers and the increasing number of nurses who understand research and can translate findings into practice, there is a stronger link between research and practice. Gradually more nurses, in both practice and academic settings, are involved in nursing research. Findings from their studies are reported in nursing journals and presented at various conferences. As knowledge from studies is disseminated, many practitioners welcome the opportunity to creatively implement it in practice to test the findings. Reports of the effectiveness on client outcomes in practice settings support the theorist's and researcher's work. Reports of ineffective or negative results lead to modification of their theories and research.

The following major factors have facilitated the integration of research in nursing practice:

1. More nurses are knowledgeable about the research process and recognize the value of applying research in practice
2. More nurses are conducting research
3. Nursing journals and conferences are disseminating information about research studies and implications for findings in practice
4. Health care agencies are encouraging nurses to attend both in-service education programs and conferences to improve and update their knowledge based on research
5. Some nursing administrators in health delivery settings are encouraging and supporting research by clinicians and practitioners

Discussion of the interdependence of nursing practice, theory, and research is incomplete without a model depicting the interaction. Doris Block, at the Nursing Research Branch of the Division of Nursing, US Department of Health and Human Services, developed an excellent model, shown in Figure 2-2. Block's[6] model depicts a process in which research questions focusing on human responses and professionals in health care systems are generated in the practice setting.

In nursing education, fundamental research questions may also arise about student learning and faculty teaching. These questions lead to fundamental research in practice or education. Specific research in specialized areas of nursing practice, delivery of nurs-

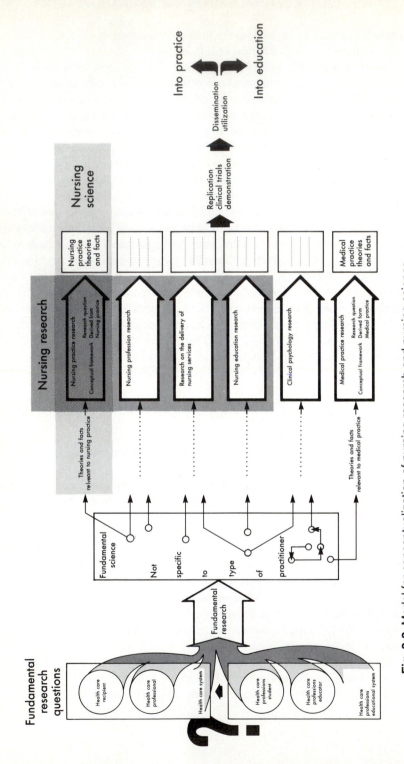

Fig. 2-2 Model for conceptualization of nursing research and nursing science.
(Developed by Doris Block, 1985. In McCloskey JC and Grace HK, eds: Current issues in nursing, ed 2, Boston, 1985, Blackwell Scientific Publications.)

ing care, and nursing education follow. Research tests nursing models and theories, and generates nursing theory, which forms the base for the growing body of knowledge essential to nursing science. With continued testing and replication of studies and clinical trials, theories are modified, refined, and disseminated through the literature and at conferences. New knowledge of supported theories and models can then be applied in practice and education.

Block's model emphasizes the inseparability of nursing practice, theory, and research in the development of nursing science. Both basic and applied (practice) research are important to the translation of nursing interventions into practice.[6] Sometimes the importance of applying theory *in practice* is overemphasized, underestimating the value and usefulness of developing theory *from practice*. Theory guides practice, but the theoretical concepts in nursing are formed from practice.[14] Most nurse scholars agree with this model, which supports the basic goals of theory development and research to generate knowledge for the improvement of nursing practice and education.

• • •

Nursing practice, theory, and research may be viewed as separate components that are intrinsically interrelated. To paraphrase Firlit[20] nursing theory is generated from practice, tested in research, and returns to explain or direct nursing practice. This leads to further refinement or expansion of theory. Although current nursing theories and models need further development, nurses are applying theoretical concepts to practice and validating theories through research. As theory acquires continued support, the body of knowledge in nursing science grows.

PROFESSIONAL NURSING'S RESPONSE TO SOCIAL CHANGE

Professional nursing evolves in response to major trends in society and to changing health care needs. The following three major trends continue to influence nursing today:

1. The scientific era emphasizes empirical research, logical reasoning, sound judgment, and advanced technology
2. Escalating costs of health services generate government involvement and the need for increased financial accountability, cost-containment, and quality assurance
3. Changing needs and attitudes of the consumer population lead to changes in nursing needs and attitudes

These major trends interact with and influence other trends. Within each trend are many complex issues that involve economic, social, political, cultural, and ethical considerations, which provides an important contextual background for subsequent discussions of the nursing process and theory evolution. Discussion of economic, social, political, cultural, and ethical aspects are presented in greater depth in subsequent chapters.

The Scientific Era

In the 1950s, a second scientific explosion marked the age of Sputnik, television, computers, and future spaceships. Science was a way of discovering, organizing, and controlling the world. It was thought that knowledge discovered by logical, systematic empirical research would pave the way to the control of nature and destiny. Research, considered the most extensive investigative process of science, would lead scientists to discover new facts, theories or applications, and revise old ones. Science would provide new technology and the power to conquer new worlds and disease. In this era, medical scientists made significant discoveries that have controlled many diseases and dramatically extended life.

With the scientific explosion and rapid advancement of knowledge in every field, it is estimated that cumulative knowledge doubles every 2 years. Today's discoveries make yesterday's knowledge obsolete. Major scientific revelations are rapidly disseminated to the public with the assistance of high-technology communication. Present society constantly seeks "the best scientific evidence" with religious fervor and welcomes each new major development with new questions raised about its effect on humans. Each new development must be considered for its risks, benefits, consequences, and impact on the environment.

Nursing responded to the scientific era by developing ways to incorporate the scientific process into nursing. This integration began in the 1950s as nurse leaders encouraged practitioners to search for objective data and to diagnose human responses. In 1973, the American Nurses' Association (ANA) wrote the Standards for Nursing Practice,[3] which incorporated the scientific method into the nursing process and were soon adopted by the profession. The Standards remain the major guidelines for general practice today, and have been modified and accepted by most clinical specialties.

In this age of scientific advancement, nurses seek advanced education in various disciplines that rely on research and empirical methods. Although initial experiences in research are limited to theses and dissertations, they recognize the value of nursing research in establishing the credibility of nursing as a profession. Nursing research assists the profession to develop nursing theories and to describe, explain, predict, and control nursing actions. As research and theories evolve, nursing accumulates a specific body of knowledge and moves toward becoming a science. In the last two decades, the number of nursing research studies increased substantially in clinical practice, administration, education, and theory. The quality of these studies has improved tremendously as a result of competition for federal and state grants to support the research. Several research conferences are held each month throughout the United States to disseminate the results of nursing research studies. The science of nursing is gradually evolving as nursing theories are generated and tested, and knowledge unique to nursing expands.

Technology and Use of Computers. Scientific discoveries in the medical disciplines have influenced nursing practice, education, and research. Advanced medical technology includes new high-tech devices such as cardiac, respiratory, and oxygen monitors; pulmonary artery and central venous pressure catheters; fetal monitors; and mechanical ventilators. Advanced technology requires highly skilled nurses. Hospitals employ over 70% of the practicing nurses,[23] and acute-care patients occupy the majority of hospital beds. Consequently, because nursing has changed to provide expert care to acutely ill patients, this care often involves the use of high-tech equipment. Nurses receive specialized education to operate, monitor, and use these devices. Life and death decisions are based on the nurses' interpretation of the information provided by high-tech equipment. Unfortunately, the cost of scientific advances surpasses economic resources, and the application of advanced technology may not be available to everyone.

As the number and types of technological equipment to diagnose, monitor, and treat patients grow, nursing roles change. Some nurses are skilled technicians in acute intensive care settings. Others study the impact of these new devices on the patient's needs, and the evolving role of the nurse. They are also examining the effect on nurses who use high-tech devices and work in intensive care units. Nurse educators are exploring effective and efficient methods to teach students about new technology and nurses' roles.

Computer technology rapidly developed with medical technology. The silicon chip boosted the computer's capacity for infinite scientific discoveries and technological innovations. Computers automate and consolidate information and increase the speed and efficiency of data processing, which improves control over patient data, including costs, diagnoses, order, plans and outcomes. Some schools of nursing offer computer courses that soon may be required as a "second language." Most health care institutions and agencies use computers; a few hospitals have a computer at every patient's bedside. At some hospitals, nurses use computers to enter patient data, check nursing or medical orders, and order services from other hospital departments. New computer programs have tremendous flexibility, with integration of word processing, data processing, spreadsheets, and graphics. In this scientific era of rapid knowledge explosion, nurses' roles are changing. They now include rapid processing of multicomplex data, which affects the client, the nurse, and the health care delivery system.

Escalating Health Care Costs

The rising cost of health care is a major problem in the United States today and is discussed in detail in Chapter 3. Professional nursing responses to escalating health care costs include the following:

1. Establishing ANA Standards of Nursing Practice
2. Defining the nursing Code of Ethics
3. Establishing the nursing process
4. Promoting utilization of nursing research
5. Encouraging nursing autonomy and accountability
6. Developing nurse-managed health centers and independent practice
7. Seeking federal financial support for nursing education and research
8. Clarifying nursing roles in state nurse practice acts
9. Studying ways to further improve effectiveness and efficiency in health care delivery

10. Establishing standards and mechanisms for accrediting academic nursing programs
11. Developing guidelines for peer review and quality assurance programs
12. Identifying ways health care institutions achieve excellence and effcency

Many of these topics are addressed in subsequent chapters; however, they are dynamic and interact with each other and have multiple ramifications.

The effects of rising hospital costs produced some major changes in nursing practice and education. Hospitals attempted to control expenses by curtailing nurses' salaries or reducing the nursing staff. In response, nurses organized to form labor unions, often represented by the ANA. The unions negotiated with the hospitals to improve staffing levels, wages, and schedules.

Consumer's Changing Health Care Needs

In the past 2 decades, consumer health care needs changed and problems arose in the health care delivery system. Some of these problems are listed as follows:

1. Increase in chronic illness and the number of elderly
2. Inequitable distribution of health care services and funding to low socioeconomic groups
3. Lack of consumer participation in health care decisions

As consumer needs change, the nurse's role as consultant, counselor, caretaker, and collaborator evolves and a partnership is formed.[13]

In the 1970s, the women's movement and other activist groups began to assert their rights in health care, and several versions of a "Patient's Bill of Rights" appeared. In response to consumer demands for greater participation in determining health policies at the state and local level, consumer health care advocates were frequently appointed to serve on various advisory boards. Nurses in this role provide information that clients seek; assist them to examine values, beliefs, and goals; and help them to evaluate and choose from available courses of action.[21]

•　　•　　•

Nurses can appropriately respond to societal changes by improving their knowledge base, expanding services, and adopting new roles. These areas are covered in greater detail in subsequent chapters.

Evolution of the Nursing Process
Early Nursing Practice: 1920 to 1950

In the early 1900s, nurses' training was accomplished through hospital apprenticeship. The emphasis was on experience, with little concern for education. The educational needs of nursing students were often sacrificed to meet hospital demands for service. Nurses were trained to fulfill physicians' orders, which usually consisted of simple treatments, and to provide comfort and hygiene measures to the ill.

In 1926, the Goldmark Report on Nursing and Nursing Education in the United States criticized the educational inadequacies of hospital nursing schools and recommended raising the standards of nursing education. This report was the first to recommend nursing education in a university setting. In 1927, the National League for Nursing published its curriculum for schools of nursing, which also addressed the quality of nursing education. And, after a 5-year study of nursing and nursing education, the ANA Committee on Grading of Nurses issued a similar recommendation to upgrade nursing education and practice.[65]

After these reports were released, inferior hospital schools were closed. However, with the advent of World War II and the increased need for military service, hospitals soon faced a critical shortage of nurses. To augment the supply of nurses, Congress passed the Bolton Bill in 1943. This bill provided free nursing education. Then in 1948, Brown's classic book, *Nursing for the Future,* was published.[8] Brown recommended that nursing education be moved from hospital schools to universities, where nurses could receive education comparable to other professionals.[65]

Impact of the Scientific Era: 1950 to 1970

After World War II, the United States and Russia competed for technological and nuclear supremacy. The competition for world power spearheaded the emphasis on scientific advancement in all major fields, including medicine and nursing.

Initially, nurses adopted the medical approach to science. This method, currently called *logical positivism,* emphasizes examination of separate parts of the body through empirical scientific research. Scientific discovery focuses on identifying and classifying mutually exclusive and exhaustive categories. Logical positivism is prevalent in nursing today and represents a major world view of how science should be conducted.

In response to the growing scientific perspective, nursing recognized the need for new knowledge, skills, and techniques. In an effort to define nursing, Peplau[47] described nursing as an *interpersonal process* between the patient and the nurse. Peplau's classic work was deemed one of the first models in nursing. Yura and Walsh[62] credit Lydia Hall with first naming nursing a *process* in 1955. The term *nursing process* also appeared in Orlando's text (1961), *The Dynamic Nurse-Patient Relationship.* Orlando[44] describes the nursing process as the interaction between the client's behavior, the nurse's action, and the nurse's reaction. She emphasizes that nurses must deliberate and validate patient needs, rather than respond intuitively.

In the early 1960s, nurse leaders suggested that nursing was a dynamic process that changed as the patient's health changed. Nurses were encouraged to collect information about the patient. Kelly[31] describes the data available for nursing assessment as: patient's physical signs and symptoms, medical history and diagnosis, social history and cultural background, and environmental factors. Knowles (1967) identifies the importance of discovery, delving, deciding, doing, and discriminating in nursing, linking nursing with the scientific process. Systematically collecting data and rigorously analyzing it is stressed by Johnson.[28] Nursing diagnosis was defined at that time as *determining the etiology of a symptom.* This same year, Yura and Walsh[63] published the first comprehensive book describing the nursing process as four components: assessing, planning, implementing, and evaluating. These authors emphasize the intellectual, interpersonal, and technical skills of nursing practice.

Defining the Nursing Process: 1970s to the Present

Nurse educators originally developed the nursing process as a teaching tool to guide students in learning the scientific approach to nursing practice. In 1973 the ANA adopted, and thereby legitimized, the components of the nursing process in the ANA Standards of Nursing Practice. The ANA Standards consist of eight specific nursing activities that describe the nursing process. However, most nurse educators taught the nursing process as a four-step method during the 1970s. Since 1975 most states revised their Nurse Practice Acts to reflect changes in nursing practice, including use of the nursing process. In 1982, the National Council State Board of Examination was revised, and currently tests knowledge of the five phases of the nursing process.

The components in the nursing process often developed independently as different nurse scholars focused on a specific step. Many nurses describe relevant aspects and important factors to consider in nursing **assessment.** Numerous tools to assess the client, family, and community appeared in the nursing literature in the 1980s. The amount of assessment data available expanded considerably. Recently, the application of nursing models and theories in assessment is emphasized.[25,49]

In the mid-1970s, several nurses described nursing **diagnosis** as separate from the assessment or planning steps.[4,7,38] Other writers combined data collection, analysis, and diagnosis with nursing assessment.[9,34] The First National Conference on the classification of nursing diagnosis was held in 1973. The conference group met again in 1975, 1982, 1984, and most recently, in 1990. Thirty-seven nursing diagnosis labels were approved at the second conference. Additional diagnoses were approved at subsequent conferences. In 1982, The National Conference Group for classification of nursing diagnoses became the North American Nursing Diagnosis Association (NANDA). The accepted list of nursing diagnoses describes the phenomena that nurses treat and provides a common language to assist nursing practice. These diagnoses differentiate nursing from medicine and serve as a framework for future nursing research.

Nursing diagnosis gradually evolved into a separate component of the nursing process in the early 1980s.[25] In 1980 the ANA refined their definition of nursing to read: "Nursing is the diagnosis and treatment of human responses to actual or potential health problems."[2]

The **planning** component of the nursing process evolved over the years through the contributions of many nurses.[9,36] Planning is separated into several sequences: prioritizing nursing diagnoses, establishing goals and objectives, developing strategies, and writing nursing orders.[13]

Evaluation in the nursing process was addressed by other nurses and include establishing criteria and describing the differences between structure, process, and outcome evaluation.[48,59] Quality assurance mechanisms were occasionally integrated in the evaluation component.

The nursing process components were originally depicted as logical sequential steps, beginning with assessment and ending with evaluation. More recently, the five components are viewed as an open system, with an interacting network of smaller units.[49] Christensen[13] developed a feedback model, in which each component interacts with all the other components to varying degrees. This model is illustrated in Figure 2-3.

Currently Accepted Components of the Nursing Process

The nursing process is a systematic approach to nursing practice that leads to sound judgments and actions. Nurses use a comprehensive knowledge base to assess the client's health status; make judicious decisions and diagnoses; and plan, implement, and evaluate appropriate nursing actions. As the core of nursing practice, the nursing process provides the structure for nursing care. Five interacting (not linear) components, with various steps, comprise the nursing process (see Figure 2-3 and Table 2-2).

The nursing process model (see Figure 2-3) depicts the usual flow of information by the dark lines and heavy arrows clockwise from assessment to diagnosis, planning, implementation, evaluation, and back to assessment. The small arrows in the opposite direction show that information from the succeeding components affects the previous ones by providing feedback. The lighter lines intersecting with the nurse-client relationship show that this relationship affects each component of the nursing process and that each component is interdependent with all other components.

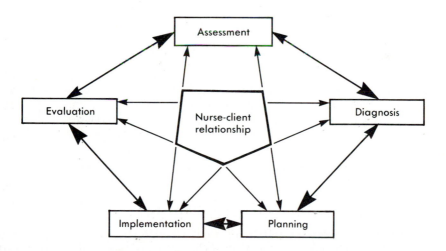

Fig. 2-3 Nursing process: feedback system.
(Developed by PJ Christenson. From Christenson PJ and Kenney J: Nursing process: application of theories, frameworks, and models, ed 3, St. Louis, 1990, Mosby-Year Book, Inc.)

Table 2-2 Components, definitions, and activities in the nursing process

Components	Definitions	Activities
Assessment	Ongoing process of data collection to determine client strengths and health concerns	Data Collection: Interview History Examination Review records
Diagnosis	Analysis/synthesis of data to identify patterns, and compare with norms and models	Data analysis and synthesis: Identify gaps Categorize Recognize patterns Compare to norms and models
	Clear, concise statement of client health status and concerns appropriate for nursing intervention	Diagnostic statements: Actual concerns Potential concerns Etiology
Planning	Determining how to assist client in resolving concerns related to restoration, maintenance, or promotion of health	Establish priorities: Set goals/objectives Select strategies Write nursing orders Describe rationale
Implementation	Client and nurse carry out the plan of care	Perform interventions: Collaborate Ongoing assessment Update/revise plan Document responses
Evaluation	Systematic, continuous process of comparing client response with written goals/objectives	Compare responses to objectives/ goals Determine progress Revise plan of care

Christensen P & Kenney J, eds: Nursing process: application of theories, frameworks and models, ed 3, St. Louis, 1990, The CV Mosby Co.

Each component of the nursing process has several steps or phases; the number and types of steps in each component varies in the nursing literature. The following description of each component and the various steps represents a synthesis of the current literature as described by Christensen and Kenney.[13]

Assessment. Assessment is a continuous process of collecting data about client responses, health status, strengths, and concerns. Data are comprehensive and multifocal, reflecting historical and current data from a variety of sources. Interview, direct observation, and measurement are used to gather data. Data are subjective or objective, and can be based on personal knowledge, experience, or clinical knowledge. Subjective data are obtained from the individual family, and/or community. These data consist of clients' signs, symptoms, feelings, and perceptions of health concerns and how they managed those concerns. Objective data are more measurable and include physical assessment and examination data, results of laboratory tests, records and reports in the client's chart, and stated observations of health team members. Information is systematically recorded and serves as the data base for all other components in the nursing process. Data collection continues throughout the nursing process.

Diagnosis. Nursing diagnosis involves two steps. First, data are sorted into appropriate categories to identify behavioral patterns. Client behavioral patterns include signs and symptoms, which are compared with a nursing model, health standards, and scientific or developmental norms to identify health concerns, strengths, and resources. The underlying etiology of client behavioral patterns and health concerns are identified, forming the basis for the nursing diagnosis. Each diagnosis is validated with the client or with other health care professionals to verify the accuracy of the data interpretation.

The second step is to write the nursing diagnostic statements in clear concise language. Each diagnosis should be client-centered, specific, and accurate. Each should include an etiological or descriptive statement. Nursing diagnoses reflect only health concerns that can be treated by nurses. They provide direction for nursing interventions. The list of nursing diagnoses accepted by NANDA may assist the nurse.

Planning. Planning occurs when the client and nurse identify activities to prevent, reduce, or correct the nursing diagnoses. The steps in planning are to: prioritize nursing diagnoses, establish client goals and objectives, identify strategies, determine nursing orders and scientific rationale, and write the nursing care plan. The setting of the nurse-client interaction, whether it is the emergency room, clinic, hospital unit, home, or another site directly influences planning. Goals and objectives describe the client's expected behavioral outcomes. Goals are usually broad, long-term statements; whereas objectives are discrete, short-term steps leading to the achievement of a specific goal. Each goal is based on a specific nursing diagnosis and reflects realistic resolution of the diagnosis. Goals are within the client's capabilities and limitations. Usually several objectives are written to achieve each goal. Objectives are client-focused and reflect mutual planning with the client. They include specific criteria to measure client behavior and are written in the sequence in which they will be performed.

The nurse identifies which nursing strategies will effectively achieve the objectives and goals. Strategies are designed to prevent, reduce, or correct a nursing diagnosis. The choice of strategy is based on: anticipated effectiveness in achieving the client's outcomes; the benefits and risks for the client; and the available resources, including people, equipment, time, finances, and facilities.

Nursing orders are written to describe strategies and specify who will do what within a given time period. They state client and nursing objectives. Nursing orders are stated in concise, specific terms and are listed in the appropriate sequence. They may include maintenance, promotion, and restorative aspects of care, as well as coordination and collaboration with other health team members. Nursing orders support the medical regimen of care and are kept current, revised, and describe alternate plans as necessary.

Scientific rationale explains the scientific basis for planning. The reason for each nursing order is clearly identified. The rationale may include principles, theory, research findings, and current literature.

Implementation. Nursing orders designated in the plan are performed by the client, nurse, or others. Implementation may include ongoing assessment and collaboration with other health care providers in performing responsibilities. Nursing actions and client reactions or behaviors are recorded to verify that the plan was implemented and to evaluate the effectiveness of the plan.

Evaluation. Evaluation involves comparing client health status with stated objectives and goals and determining client progress toward goal achievement. Evaluation is a process that continues during ongoing assessment and implementation of nursing care.

The purpose of the nursing process is to provide a systematic framework for nursing practice. As such, it unifies, standardizes, and directs nursing practice. The nurse's roles and functions are defined, and communication, collaboration, and synchronization of health team members is enhanced by the nursing process. Equal emphasis is given to health prevention, maintenance, restoration, or peaceful death.

The nursing process includes the following seven major characteristics:

1. Goal-directed, to provide quality client-centered health care
2. Systematic, provides organized logical approach to nursing care
3. Dynamic, because it involves an ongoing process focused on the changing responses of the client
4. Applicable, to individuals, families, and community groups at any point on the health-illness continuum
5. Adaptable, to any practice setting or specialization and the components may be used sequentially or concurrently
6. Interpersonal, based on nurse-client relationship
7. Useful, with any type of model, especially nursing[13]

Future Trends in the Nursing Process

The nursing process is an integral and essential part of the curriculum in nursing education today. It is the basis for learning nursing practice and for making decisions about nursing care. However, as nurses acquire advanced knowledge and experience, they internalize this thinking process and develop an intuitive grasp of the client's situation.[5] From her study of different ways practicing nurses think, Benner[5] identified five levels of nursing proficiency. The first level (novice or student) relies on a set of rules or guidelines such as the nursing process. With increasing experience, nurses attain a proficient or expert level of practice in which they perceive the client situation as a gestalt, and initiate actions without separately analyzing each factor. Benner's research suggests that as nurses develop proficiency, they use a more holistic approach and can visualize future possibilities for their clients. Reliance on the structured nursing process by proficient nurses may reduce their creative approaches to nursing practice.

Some baccalaureate nursing programs introduce the application and integration of nursing models into the nursing process. These models provide a framework that defines the nurse's role, the client, and the meaning of health. There are several models that nurses use to guide their practice, some of which include Maslow's[35] Hierarchy of Needs, Erikson's[18] Stages of Man's Development, Orem's[43] Self-care Model, or Roy's[51] Adaptation Model. Nursing models can direct each component of nursing practice and assist nurses to:

Collect, organize, and classify data

Understand, analyze, and interpret the client's health situation

Plan, implement, and evaluate nursing care

Explain nursing actions

As more nurses learn about nursing models and theories and their application in practice, the commitment in the nursing profession for theory-based nursing practice will grow.

In the future, the five components of the nursing process will be further refined. An "essential data set" will be identified for nursing assessment, as well as newer assessment tools to obtain client data specific to clinical areas. Additional nursing diagnostic classifications will evolve that may generate studies to determine costs for nursing based on diagnostic-related groups (DRGs). Standardized nursing care plans based on nursing diagnoses may be transferred to the client's computerized chart. Nursing interventions or strategies will be refined and modified after replicative research studies. Evaluation tools and methodologies will be developed to use with clients' computerized charts.

In summary, the nursing process as it is known today evolved over a 40 year span as the result of the nursing profession's response to societal needs. Many nurse leaders contributed to its development and refinement. As consensus was reached by the profession, the ANA formulated the Standards of Nursing Practice, and clinical specialty groups adopted modified versions. State Board Examinations were changed to reflect the five components of the nursing process and most state nurse practice acts were revised to reflect the current scope of nursing practice and the use of the nursing process.

THEORY DEVELOPMENT IN NURSING
The System of Theory Development

Nursing theory develops through a process of four sequential interacting phases. These phases are considered a *system* because each phase influences preceding and succeeding phases. Although each phase may be viewed as discrete, it is continuously interacting with other phases. Theory development is a process and a product. *Process* includes the activities in each phase. *Product* of these activities is represented by the level of theory development, as shown in Table 2-3.

Initially, theorists examine beliefs, values, and assumptions about what nurses do, for whom and where. This is expressed as their philosophy of nursing. The major concepts are identified, analyzed, and defined. Then, the relationship between some concepts is constructed by stating propositions or relational statements. This is considered *descrip-*

Table 2-3   Theory development system

Process	Activities	Product
Identify values, beliefs, and assumptions	What do nurses do (actions, skills), for whom (individuals, families, community) When (under what conditions) Where (in what settings) How (roles, i.e., practitioner, research)	Philosophy of nursing
Concept analysis	Define and describe major concepts Nursing (action, interactions, process) Clients (individual, family, community) Health (maintenance, prevention, restoration) Environment (hospital, community, clinic)	Concept identification
Construct relationships	Descriptive theory Describes relationships between concepts, but the relationship is not clearly defined between *all* concepts	Conceptual model
Test relationships	Explanatory theory Explains the interrelationship between major concepts; however, logical and empirical adequacy of relationships requires further explication	Theoretical framework
Validate relationships in practice	Predictive and prescriptive theory Provides a set of interrelated concepts and relational statements that are logical and amenable to empirical testing, and explain or predict phenomena	Theory

tive theory, with a conceptual model being the product. Because all of the concepts are interrelated through the construction of relational statements, a theoretical framework emerges. However, further refinement of the relational statements is required before testing. This level of theory development may be considered *explanatory theory.* A theorist's work is considered a theory when it provides a set of interrelated concepts and logical relational statements that are amenable to testing the relationships. However, the theory must be tested and validated in a variety of practice situations to be supported and accepted. The activities and products of theory development are described as follows:

1. Philosophy—a theorist's viewpoint, i.e., what the theorist assumes, believes, or holds to be true. The theorist examines: what is nursing, what does the nurse do, how, and for whom? Each of the well-known nursing theorists has unique views about the nature of nursing, which will be discussed later.

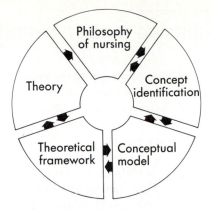

2. Concept—an abstract word that conveys a mental image. Concepts are names, labels, or categories for objects, persons, or events. Each individual interprets a concept based on past experiences and perception of its present use. Concepts must be specifically defined within a contextual statement if they are to have meaning. Alone, concepts are useless. For example, the concept "nurse" has different meanings for everyone. In theory development, the theorist identifies the major concepts, then analyzes and describes what each concept means.

3. Conceptual model—a group of related concepts, but the relationship is not explicit.[13] In nursing, the difference between a conceptual model, theoretical framework, and theory continues to be debated. What one writer considers a conceptual model, another writer calls a theory. Conceptual models attempt to represent the real world, but they are not reality. The concepts symbolize meanings, but the relationships between the concepts are obscure and subject to many different interpretations.

4. Theoretical frameworks—a set of defined concepts and some relational statements linking them. A relational statement is a proposition stating how the concepts interact: their positive or negative association, or cause-effect relationship. A theoretical framework requires explication of the specific relationships between *all* major concepts before it may be considered a "true" theory. The relationships that are clearly specified may be tested for empirical adequacy.

5. Theory—a set of clearly defined, interrelated concepts and relational statements that systematically represent a portion of reality. The term *theory* is very complex, with many arbitrary meanings and little agreement among the disciplines. For some, theory includes ideas or hunches. Others argue that a theory must be rigorously tested and can be accepted only on consensual agreement with a discipline. A theory symbolically represents reality. It is abstract and tentative. The level of abstraction varies with the types of concepts and relational statements in the theory. Theory is considered tentative until it is repeatedly tested and validated in practice.

EVOLUTION OF NURSING THEORY: CHRONOLOGY OF DEVELOPMENT

Many nurse scholars cite Florence Nightingale as the first nurse theorist. In her *Notes on Nursing,* Nightingale[42] describes her view of the nature of nursing practice. She emphasizes the importance of observation and the recording of observations, as well as her concerns about cleanliness and the ward environment. Nightingale's book describes her philosophy of nursing and was an inspiration for later theorists.

With the exception of Nightingale's work, nursing theory development had its initial beginnings in the 1950s with the publication of Peplau's book: *Interpersonal Relations in Nursing,* (1952). Peplau[47] described nursing as an interpersonal process between the nurse and patient, leading to further discussion on the nature of the nurse's role.

In this same decade, the federal government initiated two programs to assist nurses with graduate education. In 1955, the US Public Health Services (NIH) offered special predoctoral research fellowships. These were awarded directly to students to finance doctoral study. In addition, the Nurse Scientist Training programs offered grants to schools of nursing to support doctoral education of faculty. Many nurses were assisted by these grants. They later developed doctoral programs in nursing and promoted the need for nursing theory and science. Many nurses seeking doctoral education studied behavioral sciences such as sociology, psychology, and education until well into the 1980s. Even in the 1980s lack of access to doctoral programs in nursing still leads many nurses to seek the doctoral degree in these fields. Having been grounded in disciplines, nurses eventually developed theories derived from the social sciences.[52] By the 1960s, four universities offered doctoral programs in nursing: Teachers College at Columbia University, New York University, Boston University, and the University of Pittsburgh. These programs were small and the few students attending were challenged to identify what made nursing unique from other disciplines.

With the emergence of the scientific era in the 1960s, nurse scholars criticized uneducated intuitive nursing practice. The nature of practice was debated during this decade as nursing leaders recognized the need to define nursing practice, develop nursing theory and create a substantive body of knowledge. Several nurse leaders, including Abdellah, Orlando, Weidenbach, Hall, Henderson, and Levine developed and published descriptions of nursing. Their work evolved from personal, professional, and educational experiences, and reflected their perception of 'ideal' nursing practice.

Table 2-4 lists the nurse leaders who made scholarly contributions to the development of nursing theory. These theorists described nursing as an interpersonal process, meeting clients' needs, and/or providing care. A brief overview of their work follows:

1. 1960. Faye Abdellah published the first of her three textbooks on patient-centered approaches. She advised nurses to use a problem-solving approach in resolving 21 nursing problems related to individual health needs.
2. 1961. Ida Jean Orlando described nursing as a dynamic interaction between the nurse and patient. She described the nursing process as the nurse's perception of

the patient's thoughts, feelings, and actions, and the nurse's actions to meet the needs of ill patients.

3. 1964. Ernestine Wiedenbach delineated four components of nursing: philosophy, purpose, practice, and art. She defined nursing as helping patients through identification, ministration, validation, and coordination.

4. 1964. Lydia Hall described nursing practice at the Loeb Center for Nursing at Montefiore Hospital. She viewed nursing as three interacting circles: the core, the care, and the cure. The *core* represents application of the biological sciences and therapeutic use of self by the nurse; the *care* reflects intimate bodily care and nurturing; and the *cure* is based on understanding and implementing the physician's orders.

5. 1966. Virginia Henderson's major contribution was a concise definition of nursing. She described nursing as assisting individuals, sick or well, to regain independence. She listed 14 components of basic nursing care.

6. 1967. Myra Levine defined nursing as supportive and therapeutic interventions based on scientific or therapeutic knowledge. She believed that all nursing actions are based on four principles: conservation of energy, structural integrity, personal integrity and social integrity.

The work of nurse-theorists, from Peplau through the 1960s, focused on defining the nurse's role and nursing actions to assist patients toward healthy outcomes. After the 1960s, several nurse theorists expanded the earlier models in different directions.

In the early 1960s, Lucille Notter became editor of the journal *Nursing Research*. Under her guidance, the articles published and the topics they addressed encouraged open discussion of the nature of nursing and theory development. Another important influence on nursing theory development was the federal financial support given to nursing schools to sponsor conferences on the nature and development of nursing science. Three landmark conferences were held in the late 1960's. These conferences were:

Theory Development in Nursing at Case Western Reserve, 1967

The Nature of Science and Nursing at the University of Colorado, 1968

The Nature of Science in Nursing at the University of Colorado, 1969

After careful peer review, the proceedings were published in *Nursing Research* (see Table 2-4).

The purpose of these conferences was to gather nurse scientists together to discuss the nature of nursing, the development of basic and applied research, and ways to develop a nursing science. These conferences provided a forum for discussion and synthesizing knowledge from a variety of disciplines. Nurses developed a commitment to regular conferences for nursing research, theory, and practice.

Dickoff and James[16] presented their position paper, "A Theory of Theories," at the first conference. They introduced the idea that significant nursing theory must be "situation producing"; i.e., nursing must develop theories that prescribe nursing actions for predictable patient outcomes. Their controversial position has been debated for many years.

In 1969, the First Nursing Theory Conference was held in Kansas City, with the sec-

Table 2-4   **History of nursing theory development**

Events	Year	Nurse theorist
	1860	Florence Nightingale Described nursing and environment
	1952	Hildegard E. Peplau Nursing as an interpersonal process Patients with felt needs
Scientific era: nurses questioned purpose of nursing	1960	Faye Abdellah (also 1965, 1973) Patient-centered approaches
	1961	Ida Jean Orlando Nurse-patient relationship Deliberate nursing approach
Process of theory development dis- cussed among professional nurses	1964	Ernestine Wiedenbach (also 1970, 1977) Nursing: philosophy, purpose, practice, and art Patient with needs
	1966	Lydia E. Hall Core (patient), care (body), cure (disease)
	1966	Virginia Henderson (also 1972, 1978) Nursing assists patients with 14 essential functions toward independence
Symposium: theory development in nursing	1967	Myra Estrin Levine (also 1973) Four conservation principles of nursing
Symposium: nature of science and nursing	1968	
Dickoff, James, and Wiedenbach wrote "Theory in a Practice Discipline" in *Nursing Research*		
Symposium: theory development in nursing		
First nursing theory conference: the nature of science in nursing	1969	
Second nursing theory conference	1970	Martha E. Rogers (also 1980) Science of unitary man: energy fields, openness, pattern, and organization
Consensus on nursing concepts: nurse/ nursing, health, client/patient/ individual, society/environment	1971	Dorthea E. Orem (also 1980, 1985) Nursing facilities patient self-care
Discussion on what is theory, its elements, criteria, types and levels, and its relation to research	1971	Imogene King (also 1975, 1981) Theory of goal attainment through nurse- client transactions
NLN required conceptual frameworks in nursing education	1973	
Borrowed theories from other disciplines Expanded theories from other disciplines	1974	Sister Callista Roy (also 1976, 1980, 1984) Roy's adaptation model: nurse adjusts patient's stimuli (focal, contextual, or residual)

Table 2-4   **History of nursing theory development—cont'd**

Events	Year	Nurse theorist
Recognized problems in practice and developed theories to test and use in practice	1976	Josephine Paterson and L. Zderad Humanistic nursing
Nurse educator conference on nursing theory	1977	Madeline Leininger (also 1980, 1981)
Articles on theory development appeared in *ANS, Nursing Research, and Image*	1978	Transcultural nursing Caring nursing
	1979	Jean Watson (also 1985) Philosophy and science of caring Humanistic nursing
Books were written for nurses on how to critique theory, how to develop theory, and described application of nursing theories	1980	Dorothy E. Johnson Behavioral system model for nursing
Graduate schools of nursing developed courses in how to analyze and apply nursing theories		Betty Neuman Health-care systems model: a total person approach
Research studies in nursing identified nursing theories as framework for study	1981	Rosemarie Rizzo Parse (also 1987) Man-living-health: a theory of nursing
	1982-present	Numerous books published on analysis, application, evaluation, and/or development of nursing theories

ond conference the following year. These conferences brought nurse theorists and scholars together to debate the issues of the purpose of nursing theory and science, how theory can be developed, and what types of theory are needed in nursing.

By the 1970s, there were numerous publications on the development of nursing theory and nursing science. However, the 1970 report by the Joint Commission on Nursing Theory and Nursing Education noted the absence of nursing theory and research in practice. The report indicated that the commission believed this omission hindered the development of nursing. As more nurses received doctoral education in nursing and other disciplines, they recognized the value of theory in explaining nursing actions and in developing a science of nursing. Nurses also became aware that theories developed in other disciplines were insufficient to describe nursing. They concluded that nurses needed to develop their own theories. Dickoff and Wiedenbach[17] stimulated this trend by describing how theory is developed for a practice discipline. Although their approach to theory development was debated, it sparked a growing commitment by nurses to develop their own models and theories.

In 1972, Newman[40] described the following three approaches that nurses used to develop nursing models:

1. Theories "borrowed" from related disciplines and integrated into a science of nursing
2. Nursing practice situations analyzed to identify theoretical underpinnings
3. Conceptual models of nursing from which theories could be derived were created

Newman's classification of the evolution of nursing theory provided one view. In reality, many nurse theorists combined several approaches in developing nursing models. New models in the 1970s often expanded the work of earlier theorists. One theorist would pick up where another left off, adding insight to a missing piece. The nursing models that evolved in the 1970s were a product of accretion rather than accumulation.[41]

CURRENT NURSING MODELS: CONTEMPOARY THEORISTS

The work of early nurse theorists contributed to the development of the central concepts in nursing. In the 1970s a consensus among nursing leaders included the following major concepts[19]:
1. Nursing—roles and actions of nurses
2. Client—recipient of nursing care
3. Health—client's place on the health-illness continuum
4. Environment—context for nurse-client interactions

These four concepts and their interrelationships were accepted as the bases for nursing models and theories, which would become a science of nursing. For several years, nurse leaders debated whether there should be one model or theory to describe nursing, or several models to describe the relationships between the four concepts.

Since 1970, ten nurse theorists published books describing their models. Each nursing model or theory represents the theorist's unique view of each of the four major concepts. In addition to describing the major concepts, each theorist developed several subconcepts, which describe the interaction between the nurse and client, or further clarify the activities or role of the nurse.

The essence of the work of these ten contemporary nurse-theorists is presented in chronological order (see box). For a thorough understanding of each theorist's viewpoint, the literature includes numerous primary and secondary sources.

Categories of Nursing Models

Nursing models may be categorized in the following ways:
1. Underlying theoretical base
2. Level of theory development
3. Level of abstraction

These categorizations provide a different way of looking at the theorist's work. The three categorizations are explained below.

Underlying Theoretical Base. Although each nursing theorist's model is unique, some similarities exist. Each model is based on one or two theoretical premises that ultimately influence the overall work. Three theoretical themes evolved in nursing since the 1970s. The first predominant theme was introduced in the early "interactional" models of Peplau, Orlando, and King, and focused on the interpersonal nurse-patient process. Peplau[47] integrated theories from psychiatry to help nurses analyze nurse-patient interactions. Orlando[44] used psychiatric and communications theory to describe the nurse's

——————————— CONTEMPORARY NURSE THEORISTS ———————————

Rogers' Science of Unitary Human Beings (1970)

Nursing: A science and art to facilitate and promote symphonic interaction between human beings and their environment

Client: Any human being or individual and their environment

Health: An expression of the life process characterized by behaviors emerging from mutual simultaneous interaction between human beings and their environment; a continuum based on value judgments

Environment: A four-dimensional negentropic energy field identified by pattern and organization, and encompassing all that is outside any given human field; any setting worldwide where nurse and client meet

Orem's Self-care Model (1971)

Nursing: A service of deliberately selected and performed actions to assist individuals or groups to maintain self-care, including structural integrity, functioning and development

Client: An individual who is unable to continuously maintain self-care in sustaining life and health, in recovering from disease or injury, or in coping with their effects

Health: An individual's ability to meet self-care demands that contributes to the maintenance and promotion of structural integrity, functioning, and development

Environment: Any setting in which a client has unmet self-care needs and a nurse is present

King's Model—A Theory of Goal Attainment (1971)

Nursing: An interaction process between client and nurse in which transactions occur and goals are achieved as a result of perceiving a need, setting goals, and acting on them

Client: An individual (personal system) or group (interpersonal system) who is unable to cope with an event or a health problem while interacting with the environment

Health: An ability to perform the activities of daily living in one's usual social roles. A dynamic life experience of continuous adjustment to environmental stressors through optimum use of resources

Environment: Any *social system* in society; social systems are dynamic forces that influence social interaction, perception, and health, and include hospitals, clinics, community agencies, schools, and industry

Roy's Adaptation Model (1974)

Nursing: Uses the nursing process to promote client adaptation in the four modes to enhance health

Client: A person, family, group, or community with unusual stresses or ineffective coping mechanisms

Health: A state and process of being and becoming an integrated and whole person

Environment: All conditions, circumstances, and influences surrounding and affecting the development and behavior of persons or groups; any health-related situation is implied as the setting.

Paterson and Zderad's Humanistic Nursing (1976)

Nursing: An existential experience of being and doing with another person to respond to their fundamental needs

Continued.

CONTEMPORARY NURSE THEORISTS—cont'd

Client: A unique individual who is struggling to know about self and others

Health: A state in which basic needs are addressed by another to assist growth of awareness and make responsible choices

Environment: Any situation whereby nurse and client seek awareness of the experience by responding to the client's needs

Leininger's Transcultural Nursing Model (1978)

Nursing: A humanistic and scientific mode of helping a client, through specific cultural *caring* processes, (cultural values, beliefs, and practices) to improve or maintain a health condition for life or death

Client: An individual, family, group, society, or community with possible physical, psychological, or social needs within the context of their culture.

Health: defined by the specific culture; technology-dependent cultures view health and health care differently from nontechnology dependent societies

Environment: Any culture or society in which ethnocaring is practiced by nurses assisting clients

Watson's Model of Human Caring (1985)

Nursing: A transpersonal process of caring that enables the client to find meaning in wellness, gain self-knowledge and control, and restore inner harmony for self-healing

Client: Any individual who enters into a transpersonal caring process with a nurse

Health: Unity and harmony within the mind, body, and soul, which is associated with the degree of congruence between the self as perceived and the self as experienced

Environment: The setting is undefined, but any situation in which the nurse interacts with a client is implied

Johnson's Behavioral System Model (1980)

Nursing: Regulates external forces to stabilize client's behavioral system, and restore, maintain, or attain balance

Client: A behavioral system (person) threatened or potentially threatened by illness (imbalance) and/or hospitalization

Health: An efficient and effectively functioning behavioral system (person) that is in balance/stable as a result of adapting/adjusting to outside forces

Environment: No specific setting identified

Neuman's Health-Care Systems Model (1980)

Nursing: Assists clients to reduce stress factors and adverse conditions that affect optimal functioning

Client: Individual, family, or group with an identified or suspected stressor that may disrupt harmony and balance

Health: A level of wellness in which all needs are met and more energy is built and stored than is expended

Environment: Includes internal and external forces surrounding the client; nurse-client settings are not described

---

CONTEMPORARY NURSE THEORISTS—cont'd

Parse's Man-Living-Health Model (1981)

Nursing: Guiding of individuals and families to share and uncover personal meaning of their living-health situation

Client: Person or family concerned with their quality of life situation; man is viewed as an open whole being, influenced by past and present lived experiences, who interchanges with the environment through choices and responsibility for those choices

Health: A process of unfolding, continuously changing, lived experiences, including a synthesis of values and a way of living

Environment: Setting is undefined, but any health-related setting is implied

---

deliberative approach of analyzing the patient's behavior, actions, and reactions. Building on these theories, King[33] described the transactional process of goal attainment in the nurse-patient relationship. She added systems theory to expand the patient's environment to include the family and community social systems.

Subsequent theoretical approaches that emerged in nursing include the following:

1. Systems theory—serves as the basis for the models developed by King, Johnson, and Neuman. Neuman's model was an outgrowth of systems theory used in organizational behavior theory.[15] The client is viewed as a system interacting with and adjusting to other systems, such as the family, community, or environment.

2. Stress-adaptation theory—used in the models developed by Roy, Johnson, and Neuman. These theorists believe the client experiences stress, which leads to disequilibrium. The nurse's role is to restore equilibrium and facilitate adaptation.

3. Existential-phenomenological view—the theoretical basis for the work of Rogers, Paterson and Zderad, Parse, and Watson. The existential component refers to human transactions that transcend body and mind, and include the spiritual and higher sense of self. The phenomenological component refers to the client's complex past, present, and future as perceived and experienced in relation to the here and now in all spheres. This emerging theme is a major shift that is difficult to comprehend, yet is receiving growth support among scholarly nurses. Previously, nurses accepted a reductionistic, mechanistic view of humans as composed of separate parts. This new world view recognizes the transactional, metaphysical, humanistic nature of humans and their environment.

From the mid-1960s, professional nursing attempted to define nursing and differentiate nursing practice from medical care. Henderson's (1966) definition of nursing as "do for the patient what he cannot do for himself to promote independence," was widely accepted. In a similar theme, Orem[43] proposed a model delineating three roles for nurses to promote the patient's self-care. Johnson's (1980) behavioral systems model describes nursing as assisting patients to regain stability or equilibrium. Roy's[51] adaptation model describes nursing as reducing the patient's stimuli and promoting adaptation. These theorists viewed patients as somewhat incapacitated within the health-illness continuum. The nurse's role was to help the patient regain independence and equilibrium, or perform self-care activities.[39] The various philosophical schools of thought are discussed in Chapter 7.

The existential approach began with Rogers[50] at New York University. Based on her knowledge of physics, quantum theory, and the law of thermodynamics, she emphasized the inseparable interaction of man and environment. Nursing, according to Rogers, promotes symphonic interaction between man and environment, which is dynamically evolving during the life process. The work of Parse and Watson extends Roger's work in slightly different directions.

Level of Theory Development. Classification of nursing models according to the level of theory development was first described by Stevens.[55] She classified nursing theory as descriptive, explanatory, or predictive, as shown in Table 2-3. Descriptive theory is the first level of development. Major concepts such as client, nursing, and health are identified and described by the theorist. The relationship between concepts, however, is not described. Explanatory theory attempts to describe how or why the major concepts are related. The theorist explains the relationship between some concepts. However, further clarification of the logical and empirical adequacy of the relationships is needed for testing. Predictive theory is achieved when the conditions under which concepts are related is stated and the relational statements consistently describe future outcomes. This highest level of theory development permits repeated testing of the theory for validation. In nursing and the social sciences, it is generally accepted that predictive theories are actively being pursued, but presently do not exist.

Level of Abstraction. Walker and Avant[58] classified nursing theory according to the level of abstraction. They identify the following four levels:

1. Meta-theory—highest level of abstraction; focuses on broad philosophical and methodological issues related to theory development; at this level, nurse scholars analyze the purpose and type of theory nursing needed, propose sources for theory development, and examine criteria for evaluating theory in nursing
2. Grand nursing theories—provide global conceptual frameworks for nursing practice and education; broad abstract descriptions of the nurse's actions or roles
3. Middle-range theories—more limited in the scope of nursing practice than grand theories; also provide more direction for practice and research
4. Practice theory—first described by Dickoff and James;[16] specifies the goal and the nursing actions necessary to achieve the goal; can be tested in practice; nursing is moving in this direction

Acceptance of Nursing Models

The publication of nurse theorists' work in journals and textbooks has sparked a growing interest among nurses to understand, analyze, apply, test, and evaluate their models. As nurse educators became familiar with the theorists models, a few were taught in some nursing programs, notably Roy's stress-adaptation model and Orem's self-care model. In the mid-1970s several nurse theorists expanded and revised their earlier work in attempts to describe their theories within the framework of logical empiricism. Orem, King, Roy, and Rogers published more explicit definitions of their concepts and relational statements and tried to show the logical adequacy of their theories. Some nurse scholars describe the application of selected models in practice, and others describe research studies based on a nurse theorist's framework. This growing body of literature contributes to the gradual acceptance of several theorists' models. In addition, the theorists presented their models at national conferences where nurse educators sought an understanding of how to apply the models in practice.

Acceptance of a theorist's model by the nursing profession is contingent on numerous factors. First, the theorist's work must be a substantial publication, well disseminated, and widely read. The model must be sufficiently described and clearly explained for nurses to grasp the ideas and comprehend their application in nursing. There must also be a cadre of educated nurses who thoroughly understand the theorist's work, can teach it to others, apply it in practice, and test it in research. Martha Rogers taught her theory at New York University in the master and doctoral programs in the 1970s. Many of her graduate students wrote their dissertations based on her theoretical work, and some have continued to conduct research based on her work. Rogers' proteges include Margaret Newman, Jacqueline Fawcett, and Rosemarie Parse. The work of Rogers, and those of her followers, continues to strongly influence nursing practice, theory, and research. The nursing diagnostic conference group is well represented by Roger's proteges, who have influenced the list of accepted diagnostic categories. The nursing models by Parse[45] and Watson[60] reflect the strong influence of Rogers' work.

By the 1980s, most graduate nursing programs included a core course in theory development, which provided an overview of nursing theorists' work. Concurrently, various nurse scholars continue to debate how theory is constructed and what evaluation criteria must be achieved for a theorist's work to be called a theory. At this time, most nurse scholars believed that the purpose of theory was the description, explanation, and prediction of phenomena. A strong commitment to logical empiricism is reflected in the writings of Chinn and Jacobs,[12] Fawcett,[19] and Walker and Avant.[58] It was believed that rigorous and logically structured theory, with operational definitions of the concepts, was necessary for theory testing and validation—the ultimate criteria of a theory. In the late 1970s, nurse scholars recognized the limits of logical empiricism and quantitative research in dealing with nursing phenomena. As nursing began to emphasize humanism and holism, scholars sought more meaningful and creative ways to describe nursing theory and research.[54] By the mid-1980s, there was a gradual shift, from acceptance of empirical scientific knowledge as the sole way of knowing, to a broader view of knowledge, based on the inclusion of ethical, esthetic, and personal knowledge. This shifting viewpoint reflects a syntheses of the influences of Rogers (1970), Carper (1978), Parse (1981), Benner (1984), and Chinn and Jacobs (1987).

Future Trends in Theory Development

Nursing, like any scientific discipline, will continue to experience shifts and new trends in its evolution. Nursing theory will continue to respond to the dynamic changes occurring through social change and science—the evolution of humans and their environment. As the body of nursing science grows, older models and theories will be replaced by newer ones that more completely explain nursing. Nurse practitioners and researchers will continue to apply and test nursing models in practice settings. Nurse theorists will continue to develop, refine, and test their models and theories. Practice theories may be constructed and tested in specific clinical situations.

The nurse scholars in education will establish closer working relationships with practitioners, researchers, and theorists to keep abreast of changes in society and in nursing practice. Collaboration in theory construction among these professionals, and cooperation in testing theory through conducting research in practice settings and disseminating findings, will advance the science of nursing.

PROFESSIONAL NURSING PRACTICE

In the future, professional nursing practice will continue to respond to the changing needs of society in new and unique ways. Allegiance to the medical profession and health delivery systems is diminishing as nurses struggle for increasing autonomy. Professional nurses' autonomy will grow with the development of a body of knowledge and nursing science. As nurses acquire the necessary education, apply nursing models creatively in practice, conduct research to test theories, and expand their personal knowledge nursing science will mature.

The professional nurse will want to be knowledgeable about current nursing research and to creatively apply valid findings in practice. To accomplish this task, practitioners must visualize possibilities beyond the common clinical constraints. They must recognize the impact and application of changing world views, scientific discoveries, and shifts in nursing models and theories.

EXAMPLE: The shift from a mechanistic empirical view of knowledge to a holistic and humanistic view may inspire the professional nurse to study the meaning of "quality of life" for a specific target population. This type of study would likely incorporate phenomenological and qualitative research methods. Initially, such a study may be viewed as unscientific by one's peers. However, there is a growing acceptance of esthetic, ethical, and personal knowledge in the profession. Professional nurses will take risks and seek creative challenges.

Having internalized the nursing process, professional nurses will see the client's situation as a gestalt and creatively apply appropriate nursing models. With experience, professional nurses will identify common patterns in client situations, raising new questions. Some of these questions, such as, Would this nursing action or another action be more effective in assisting the client? are worthy of further pursuit. The nurse may discuss these questions with peers, search the literature for answers, initiate a research study, or develop clinical impressions for publication. The professional nurse always looks for new meanings in nursing phenomena. The ability to see new relationships in human behaviors or new patterns of response leads to more questions about nursing actions. Rather than revert to lock-step thinking, where if X happens, then Y is the appropriate nursing action, the professional nurse critically analyzes multiple factors and examines all feasible possibilities. Experience in practice, a broad knowledge base, and continuous updating of research and theory stimulates the professional nurse to raise new questions about practice and seek greater knowledge. It is in the practice arena that theories are generated and tested. New questions and problems lead to continuing refinement of theory and development of new theories. Like other disciplines, nursing knowledge and science will never be static. As trends and shifts occur in technology, economics, politics, and culture the professional nurse seeks an understanding of these changes by raising questions and searching for answers in theory, research, and practice. The continuous search for answers to new questions is what stimulates the development of new knowledge and contributes to the growing body of nursing science.

● ● ●

The evolution of nursing science has made great strides in the last 40 years. During the scientific age, the emphasis on empirical knowledge stimulated the profession to develop and refine the nursing process. By the 1980s, the five components of the nursing process were legitimized in the Standards of Nursing Practice and the National Council Licensure Examination.

Efforts to achieve professional status were augmented by nurses who sought doctoral degrees in other disciplines. Nurses then developed doctoral programs in nursing. Some of the nurses described their conceptual models for practice and initiated research studies to test their models and theories. The profession reached consensus on four major concepts in the nursing domain. Although a dichotomy continues to exist between nursing practice and nursing theorists and researchers, there is a growing commitment toward integration of theories, research and practice. Nursing science and research are moving toward acceptance of other ways of knowing, such as ethical, esthetic, and personal knowledge.

New approaches in practice, theory development, and research will be developed to expand nurses' understanding of humans and their health care needs. The future will bring stronger collaboration between practitioners, scholar-theorists, and researchers to improve nursing science. In this way, the nursing profession can best respond to the ever changing social forces of our time and to the impact that these major social forces have on the health care needs of individuals, groups, and society.

STUDENT ACTIVITIES

1. How well do you feel that nursing as a profession is responding to the knowledge explosion and rising health care costs?
2. To what extent do you feel that nursing theory is influencing nursing practice?

3. Which of the various nursing models and theories do you personally find most adaptable to your nursing practice? Why?

REFERENCES

1. Abdellah FG: The nature of nursing science, Nurs Res 18(5):393-399, 1969.
2. American Nurses' Association: Nursing: a social policy statement, ANA Publication Code: NP-63, 35M, December 1980.
3. American Nurses' Association: Standards of nursing practice, Kansas City, Mo, 1973, American Nurses' Association.
4. Aspinal MJ: Nursing diagnosis: the weak link, Nurs Outlook 24(7):433, 1976.
5. Benner P: From novice to expert, Menlo Park, Calif, 1984, Addison-Wesley.
6. Block D: A conceptualization of nursing research and nursing science. In McCloskey JC and Grace HK, eds: Current issues in nursing, ed 2, Boston, 1985, Blackwell Scientific Publications.
7. Block D: Some crucial terms in nursing: what do they mean? Nurs Outlook 22(11):689, 1974.
8. Brown MI: Research in the development of nursing theory: the importance of a theoretical framework in nursing research, Nurs Res 13(2):109-112, 1964.
9. Carnevali D: Nursing care planning: diagnosis and management, ed 3, Philadelphia, 1983, JB Lippincott.
10. Carper B: Fundamental patterns of knowing in nursing, ANS, 1(1):13-23, 1978.
11. Chinn P: Debunking myths in nursing theory and research, Image 17(2):45-59, 1985.
12. Chinn P and Jacobs M: Theory and nursing: a systematic approach, ed 2, St. Louis, 1987, the CV Mosby Co.
13. Christensen PJ and Kenney JW, eds: Nursing process: application of theories, frameworks, and models, ed 3, St. Louis, 1990, the CV Mosby Co.
14. Conant LH: Closing the practice-theory gap, Am J Nurs 15(11):37-39, 1967.
15. Deloughery et al.: Consultation and community organization in community mental health nursing, 1971, Williams and Wilkins.
16. Dickoff J and James P: A theory of theories: a position paper, Nurs Res 17(3):197-203, 1968.
17. Dickoff J et al.: Theory in a practice discipline, Part I: practice oriented theory, Am J Nurs 17(5):415-535, 1968.
18. Erikson E: Childhood and society, ed 2, New York, 1963, WW Norton & Co.
19. Fawcett J: The "What" of theory development, National League for Nursing, Theory development: what, why, how? New York, 1978, National League for Nursing.
20. Firlet SI: Nursing theory and nursing practice: separate or linked? In McCloskey JC and Grace HK, eds: Current issues in nursing, ed 2, Boston, 1985, Blackwell Scientific Publications.
21. Gadow S: Basis for nursing ethics: paternalism, consumerism, or advocacy, Hosp Progr 64(10):62-67, 78, 1983.
22. Gortner SR: The history and philosophy of nursing science and research, ANS 5(2):1-8, 1983.
23. Grace HK: Can health care costs be contained? Nursing's responsibility. In McCloskey JC and Grace HK, eds: Current issues in nursing, ed 2, Boston, 1985, Blackwell Scientific Publications.
24. Griffith-Kenney J: Contemporary women's health: a nursing advocacy approach, Menlo Park, Calif, 1986, Addison-Wesley.
25. Griffith-Kenney JW and Christensen PJ: Nursing process: application of theories, frameworks and models, ed 2, St. Louis, 1986, the CV Mosby Co.
26. Jacobs MK and Huether SE: Nursing science: the theory-practice linkage, ANS 1(1):63-73, 1978.
27. Jacox AK: Theory construction in nursing: an overview, Nurs Res 23(1):4-13, 1974.
28. Johnson D: Professional practice in nursing. In the shifting scene: directions for practice, NLN Pub. No. 15-1252, New York, 1967, National League for Nursing.
29. Johnson DE: Development of theory: a requisite for nursing as a primary health profession, Nurs Res 23(5):372-377, 1974.
30. Johnson DE: The nature of a science of nursing, Nurs Outlook 7(5):291-294, 1959.

31. Kelly K: Clinical inference in nursing, Nurs Res 15(1):23, 1966.
32. Kerlinger F: Foundations of behavioral research, New York, 1973, Holt, Rinehart, and Winston.
33. King I: Toward a theory for nursing, New York, 1971, John Wiley and Sons, Inc.
34. Little DE and Carnevali DL: Nursing care plans, ed 2, Philadelphia, 1976, JB Lippincott.
35. Maslow A: Motivation and personality, ed 2, New York, 1970, Harper & Row Publishers.
36. Mayers J: A systematic approach to the nursing care plan, ed 3, New York, 1983, Appleton-Century-Crofts.
37. Meleis AI: Theoretical nursing: development and process, Philadelphia, 1985, JB Lippincott.
38. Mundinger MO and Jauron GD: Developing a nursing diagnosis, Nurs Outlook 23(2):94, 1975.
39. Neuman B: The Neuman systems model, New York, 1982, Appleton-Century-Crofts.
40. Newman MA: Nursing's theoretical evolution, Am J Nurs 20(7):449-453, 1972.
41. Newman MA: The continuing revolution: a history of nursing science. In Chaska NL: The nursing profession: a time to speak, New York, 1983, McGraw-Hill Book Co.
42. Nightingale F: Notes on nursing, 1869.
43. Orem DE: Nursing: concepts of practice, ed 2, New York, 1980, McGraw-Hill Book Co.
44. Orlando IJ: The dynamic nurse-patient relationship, New York, 1961, GP Putnam's Sons.
45. Parse RR: Man-living-health: a theory of nursing, Philadelphia, 1981, John Wiley and Sons.
46. Paterson JG and Zderad LT: Humanistic nursing, New York, 1976, John Wiley and Sons.
47. Peplau HE: Interpersonal relations in nursing, New York, 1952, GP Putnam's Sons.
48. Phaneuf M: The nursing audit: profile for excellence, New York, 1972, Appleton-Century-Crofts.
49. Pinnell NN and deMeneses M: The nursing process: theory, application and related processes, Norwalk, Conn, 1986, Appeton-Century-Crofts.
50. Rogers M : Science of unitary human beings, 1970.
51. Roy C Sr: Introduction to nursing: an adaptation model, ed 2, Englewood Cliffs, NJ, 1984, Prentice-Hall, Inc.
52. Schmidt M: The current status of practice theories in nursing. In Woodridge PJ et al: behavioral science and nursing theory, St. Louis, 1983, the CV Mosby Co.
53. Silva MC: Philosophy, science, theory: interrelationships and implications for nursing research, Image 9(3):59-63, 1977.
54. Silva MC and Rothbart D: An analysis of changing trends in philosophies of science on nursing theory development and testing, ANS 6(2):1-13, 1984.
55. Stevens BJ: Nursing theory: analysis, application, evaluation, Boston, 1978, Little Brown & Co.
56. Walker LO: Theory and research in the development of nursing as a discipline: retrospect and prospect, In Chaska N, ed: The nursing profession: a time to speak, New York, 1983, McGraw-Hill Book Co.
57. Walker LO: Toward a clearer understanding of the concept of nursing theory, Nurs Res 20(5):428-435, 1974.
58. Walker LO and Avant KC: Strategies for theory construction in nursing, Norwalk, Conn, 1983, Appleton-Century-Crofts.
59. Wandelt MA and Ager JW: Quality patient care scale, New York, 1974, Appleton-Century-Crofts.
60. Watson J: The philosophy and science of caring, Boston, 1979, Little, Brown and Co.
61. Watson J: Nursing: human science and human care: a theory of nursing, Norwalk, Conn, 1985, Appleton-Century-Crofts.
62. Yura H and Walsh MB: The nursing process: assessing, planning, implementing, evaluating, ed 2, 1973, Appleton-Century-Crofts.
63. Yura H and Walsh MB: The nursing process: assessing, planning, implementing, evaluating, New York, 1967, Appleton-Century-Crofts.
64. Zeluskas BA et al.: Bridging the gap: theory to practice, research application, Nurs Man 19(9):50-52, 1988.
65. Ziegler SM et al.: Nursing process, nursing diagnoses, nursing knowledge: avenues to autonomy, Norwalk, Conn, 1986, Appleton-Century-Crofts

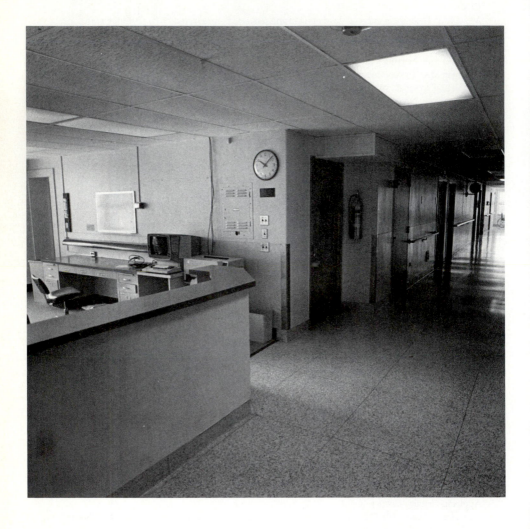

3

ECONOMICS OF HEALTH CARE

Philip Jacobs
Grace L. Deloughery

OBJECTIVES

After completing this chapter the reader should be able to:

- Describe the curve/relationship between the amount spent on health care and health status

- Define Medicare, identify its basic provisions, and describe current problems with its program

- Define Medicaid, identify its basic provisions, and describe current problems with its program

- Describe what is meant by an economic flow analysis

- Identify the various ways in which a household may cover health care costs

- Define Supplemental Medical Insurance

- Describe the government's role as intermediary, insurer, and reimburser of health care

- Define DRGs and briefly describe how they function

- Define HMOs and briefly describe how they function

- Define PPOs and briefly describe how they function

- Describe direct and indirect costs of illness and health care costs

- Explain the concept of incentives in health care

Economics is the discipline that deals with the analysis of behavior when scarcity exists. In the health care field scarcity has always existed in the sense that the resources devoted to health care could have been used in other ways. Since at least 1966, when the two large governmental health insurance programs, Medicare and Medicaid, were instituted the proportion of the total production of *all* goods and services that was devoted to medical care has risen somewhat dramatically. National expenditures on medical care have risen from 5.9% of the nation's gross national product (i.e., production of all final goods and services) in 1966 to 11.2% in 1987[5] (Figure 3-1).

What is striking about this statistic is that it represents a *share* of the total economic pie, not merely a dollar amount. But is this increasing share, dramatic as it is, bad per se? In itself, this would not necessarily constitute an economic problem if the benefits from these expenditures were readily apparent.

Central to the economic problem in health care is the belief that in many instances the benefits are *not* there. The hypothesis was forwarded that medical care is subject to "diminishing returns." This means that as more and more dollars are spent on medical care, the effectiveness or impact on health of the additional expenditures is somewhat diminished. Such a relationship between health and medical care is very difficult to measure and it certainly would not hold for all types of medical care under all circumstances. The essential question is whether it holds true in general. If it does, then the case for a careful examination of medical care expenditures is all the more compelling.

This hypothesized relationship between health and medical care is presented pictorially with a famous curve. Figure 3-2 shows the population's health status on the vertical

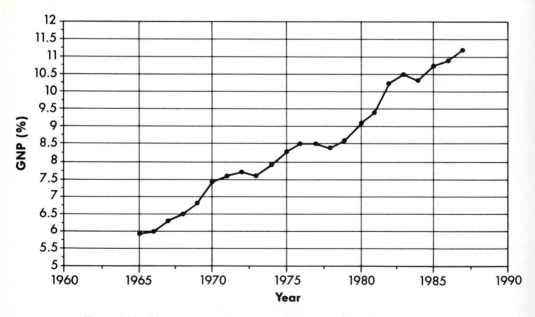

Fig. 3-1 Health care expenses as percentage of GNP, 1965 to 1987.

axis and the quantity of medical care on the horizontal axis. Note how, at low amounts of medical care, the level of health rises quickly; at these levels of care, medical care is effective. However, additional amounts of medical care, while still effective, are not as effective as when the population had less care. And farther along, the curve becomes almost flat, i.e., with more medical care there is very little net addition to health. This position on the curve is termed *flat of the curve* medicine. Paying for additional care, in effect, yields very little benefit! A growing number of commentators are suggesting that we have reached this level of medical care in America.

Numerous examples of waste or potential waste have been suggested to pinpoint areas that are contributing to this phenomenon. These include intensive care expenditures for patients who will never recover,[8] excessive use of lab tests and ultrasound,[1] and use of cesarean section, as opposed to normal deliveries.[4] If flat of the curve medicine is a reality, substantial savings could be made by paying more attention to the economic aspects of health care dellivery, and selected cutbacks could be initiated with little, if any, resulting loss of health: this is where the overall importance of health care economics lies.

This chapter will provide an introduction to the topic of health care economics, demonstrate a few of the more important techniques in the field, and show how they can be applied. The reader will readily see that one can improve understanding of many economic policies and events with only a few very basic economic concepts.

Medicare policies will be examined and used to illustrate the use of our principles. Medicare is the federal program of health care insurance primarily for residents over 65

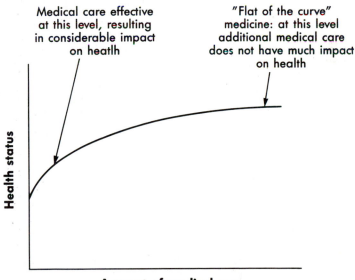

Medical care effective at this level, resulting in considerable impact on heatlh

"Flat of the curve" medicine: at this level additional medical care does not have much impact on health

Health status

Amount of medical care

Fig. 3-2 Hypothesized relationship between medical care and health.

years of age; it should be distinguished from Medicaid, a joint federal-state program primarily for lower income groups. These two programs form over one half of all national health care expenditures. Many of the problems of these programs are reflections of national health care problems, and thus they form excellent examples of how economics can be used to analyze issues of the health care delivery system.

The following basic economic topics that will be presented are:

1. Tracing economic flows in the system
2. Measurement of costs of various activities in the system
3. Analysis of incentives to the system
4. Understanding incentives using cost analysis and how they impact on economic behavior
5. Using these concepts to examine several different types of economic organizations

---

ECONOMIC FLOWS IN THE HEALTH CARE SYSTEM

Economic flow analysis is a very simple tool that is enormously useful in understanding economic systems.[12] It involves identifying various financing, spending, and consuming bodies within the system, and tracing flows of money and services between these groups. This is simply a *descriptive* task, i.e., there is no explanation of what caused the behavior, simply a description of what happened. Although it is limited, this task is nevertheless one of considerable importance. One must understand the flows in any economic system before one can understand the economic relationships in the system.

As a partially simplified beginning, a picture of the flows in the traditional American health care system is presented, circa 1980. Many of the relationships in the first example still exist, although the scene has become more complicated since that date. Figure 3-3 illustrates that money flows from the ultimate payors for medical care to two key groups of providers—physicians and hospitals. These flows are described with arrows; note that not all participating groups in the systems are included (for instance, nursing homes) and not all of the possible flows have been drawn. This is to keep the illustration simple.

Households: Consumers and Insurees

The ultimate payors for medical care are consumers (households) and employers (business firms). Households pay for medical care in the following three major ways:

1. Purchase of insurance from health insurance companies. The payments for these purchases are called *premiums*. In return for premiums, the insurance companies insure households, i.e., when some member of the household receives medical care, the insurance company pays part or all of the bill (depending on amount of coverage).
2. Direct or out-of-pocket payments. An extremely important form of payment, these are direct payments made by households to providers. These payments may

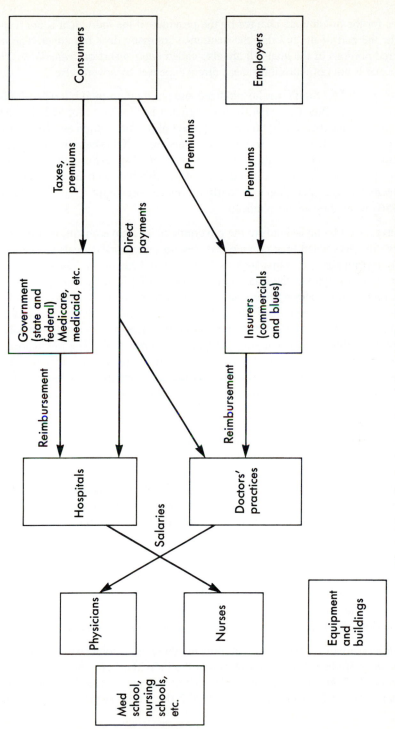

Fig. 3-3 Simplified presentation of financial flows in the health care system.

be for the full amount charged by the provider (if the individual is not insured) or for the part of the bill that the insurance company does not cover. The noncovered portions of the total bill are also called *copayments* or *deductibles*. The consumer is not reimbursed for these direct expenses by anyone else.

EXAMPLE: Mrs Smith was hospitalized and her total hospital bill was $4000. Her husband has Blue Cross family coverage that he purchased for $1200 a year. He pays a deductible of $200 for each episode of hospitalization and Blue Cross covers the rest. Thus the Smith's premiums are $1200. Their direct cost of hospitalization is $200 (what they pay out-of-pocket). The rest is paid by the insurer. As an example of the size of a deductible, individuals who are covered by Medicare will, according to recently introduced regulations, have a deductible of $564 when they are hospitalized.

3. Taxes, paid by households to the government. The government, in turn, reimburses providers when they provide services for certain individuals who are covered by government programs such as Medicare and Medicaid. These taxes can take many forms (part of the general income tax, social security taxes, etc.).

To put these flows in perspective, in 1985 consumers directly paid 9.3% of their hospital bills and 26.3% of their doctor bills. Of course, this is just an average figure for the nation and hides the enormous distributions of payment between different classes of users. Medicare direct payments, for example, are considerable. The Medicare program was instituted on July 1, 1966 by the federal government to cover high medical expenses for people over 65 years of age (its current coverage is somewhat broader and includes disabled individuals and those with end stage renal disease). Medicare is designed in two parts. Its compulsory component (with zero enrollment premiums for beneficiaries) is called *hospitalization insurance* (HI) and covers hospital expenses and some extended care benefits as well. Initially, HI was designed with limited out-of-pocket payments by the beneficiaries, but because hospital expenses rose rapidly throughout the period since Medicare was instituted, direct user fees were raised annually. By 1987 the out-of-pocket deductible for HI was $520 in total for the first 60 days of hosptalization. In addition, if the individual required over 60 days hospitalization during a year, there was a co-payment of $130 a day, up to 90 days. The individual had a lifetime reserve of 90 days in addition, and could dip into this reserve if the 90 days in a year were exceeded; the copayment for this was $260 per day. Beyond this, no coverage was provided.

EXAMPLE: Mrs Rubin, 66 years old, was hospitalized at City General Hospital for 10 days in 1987. Her total payment was the deductible, or $520. If she was hospitalized five times in 1987 and was in the hospital for a total of 65 days, she would have to pay the deductible (just once) and an additional $130 for each day over 60 days.

In addition to the compulsory component, there is a voluntary component called *Supplementary Medical Insurance* (SMI) that the individual can obtain with payment of a premium of $17.90 per month (in 1987). SMI covers physicians' fees and other outpatient benefits. In 1987 it had a deductible of $75 (i.e., the first $75 of expenses incurred by the individual were paid out-of-pocket by the individual) and a co-payment of 20% of expenses beyond that.

EXAMPLE: If Mr Hall was 70 years old in 1987, he could purchase SMI for $17.90 a month. If a physician treated him on an outpatient basis for a stomach disorder and the treatment required five visits, the physician's bill would be $25 a visit, or $125 total. Mr Hall would pay the first $75 out of pocket, and then he would have to pay 20% of the remaining $50 ($10). Medicare would pay $40. If Mr Hall needed additional physicians' care during the year, he would pay 20% of the bill.

As medical care costs have increased over the years, so have the out-of-pocket expenses of the Medicare beneficiaries. In 1962, before the institution of Medicare, the average elderly person spent about 8% of household income on medical care. By 1985, this figure had risen to 15%.[11] The poor elderly spend even larger proportions of their income on medical care. Because of the growing burden of out-of-pocket medical expenses by the elderly, which has occurred in spite of Medicare, the Medicare program has been revamped by the Catastrophic Health Bill of 1988. From 1989 catastrophic (i.e., large expenditure) coverage is provided for those individuals with very large out-of-pocket expenditures. Coverage includes 365 zero-copayment days after a $564 deductible, and out-of-pocket SMI costs will be limited to $1370 a year. The increased coverage will be partly financed by higher SMI premiums ($4 monthly in 1989 for all beneficiaries plus an income-related premium).

Premium Payers: Businesses

Business firms are involved as payors because the bulk of nongovernment health insurance in America is provided through employers. The internal revenue tax code currently exempts the benefits received by workers in the form of health insurance premiums from employees' income tax. This means that a nurse in a hospital receiving a salary of $20,000 yearly will pay a tax based on that salary. However, if the hospital additionally provides health insurance coverage by paying an insurance company a premium of, say, $800, there will be no tax on these benefits. This makes benefits such as health insurance coverage a very attractive form of compensation, because otherwise health insurance is quite costly. Many companies pay only part of the premium for health care and the employee pays the rest. Businesses, of course, also pay taxes, some of which support government health care programs.

Intermediaries: Governments and Insurers

The next group involved in the flows of the health care system are called *intermediaries,* because they act as insurers and reimbursers. Intermediaries include Blue Cross (for hospitalization) and Blue Shield (for insurance of physicians' services) and the "commercials," a euphemism for all other health insurance companies, including such well-known insurers as John Hancock, Aetna, and Prudential. They receive premiums from individuals and employees, and when the insured individuals require medical care, they reimburse the providers on a specific contractual basis. Remember, they may or may not pay the entire bill, depending on whether they require a copayment on the consumer's part.

EXAMPLE: Blue Cross may have 3000 subscribers that it insures; its premium rate might be $1000 annually for each subscriber. Blue Cross's total receipts, its premiums, are $3 million. Its payments are its reimbursements to hospitals (e.g., $2.5 million) and its other expenses such as salaries (e.g., $.3 million). Blue Cross is left with a surplus of $.2 million.

The other intermediary is the government. The government receives payment in taxes, and sometimes premiums, and reimburses the providers for covered care. Two important government programs already mentioned are Medicare and Medicaid. Medicare's hospitalization insurance plan is administered through the HI Trust Fund. Government receipts for this fund come almost exclusively from a flat rate tax on taxable income, called an *employment tax*. In 1966 this tax amounted to about one third of 1% of taxable income from each employee and the employer (two thirds of 1% of taxable income in total). By 1983 this increased to 2.6%, and by 1988 it was 2.9%. This tax rate, like all tax rates, can be changed by law, but not without a good deal of opposition. Note that government receipts from the tax depend on the tax rate and the number of employees.

The HI Trust Fund's expenses are primarily reimbursements to hospitals; in addition the government wants to keep an additional reserve in the fund. The expenditures of the fund are determined by hospital expenses (reimbursements) per beneficiary and the number of beneficiaries hospitalized.

As the population ages and hospital costs increase, reimbursements to hospitals increase. In fact, the increase in expenditures paid out by the fund have grown much more rapidly than the increase in receipts from the employment tax. Although in the mid-1980s receipts from the tax were less than the expenses, conservative projections based on the growth of hospital expenditures and the use of hospital services by the aged forecast a narrowing of receipts-expenditures gap, and by the mid-1990s the projections indicate a deficit of the Trust Fund[3] (Figure 3-4). Projected expenditures and receipts of the HI Trust Fund are expressed as a percentage of taxable income. Note the crossover point between 1989 and 1990. At that point, hospital expenditures from the Trust Fund are about 2.9% of taxable payroll income, which is what the tax rate would be. The deficit occurs a little later because there are still reserves in the system at that time. This projected deficit causes alarm in policy circles. Any search for a solution has to recognize that (1) further increases in taxation are limited and (2) the population will continue to age (and thus hospitalization will continue to grow). A solution to this deficit problem has to control hospital expenditures per beneficiary, which means containing the reimbursements per unit of hospitalization. This leads to dramatic policy shifts in hospital reimbursement, discussed next.

Medicare's voluntary program, the SMI program, has also experienced increased economic pressures. This program's revenues come from two sources: a premium for enrollees and receipts from government general tax revenues. The fact that nonpremium

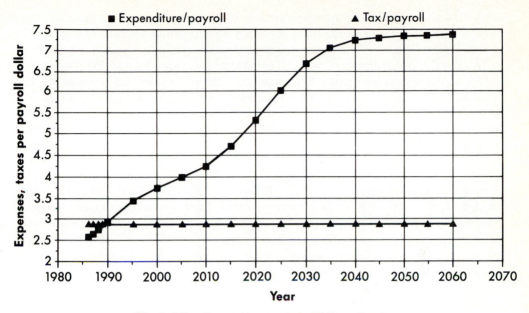

Fig. 3-4 Receipts and payouts in HI Trust Fund.

receipts come from general revenues means that the SMI Trust Fund is not nearly as constrained in its revenue sources; projected deficits can be met by additional appropriations. The SMI program's expenditures are primarily for Medicare's share of reimbursement for physician care and outpatient services. Remember that the copayment and deductible under SMI (i.e., the beneficiary's share) is significant.

Providers: Recipients of Funds

The next stage of the flow system is the reimbursement of the providers by the payors (households, governments, and insurers). Hospital reimbursement has taken several different forms in recent years. Before 1983, Medicare and Medicaid reimbursed hospitals on the basis of the costs that they had already incurred. This basis of payment is termed *retrospective reimbursement.* What it means is that if the hospital spends $1200 for treating a Medicare patient, medicare will base its reimbursement on that $1200. The reimbursement may not be exactly $1200 because the intermediary may make certain adjustments, such as discounts. This form of reimbursement does not foster efficiency, in that hospitals are reimbursed more if they spend more (see Incentives, p. 83).

Private insurers generally reimburse hospitals on the basis of what they charge (i.e., their prices). Prices are usually greater than costs because hospitals add a "mark-up" to their costs to set their rates. For example, if the mark-up is 20%, the charges associated with the Medicare patient discussed previously would have been $1200 (the costs incurred plus 20%, or $1440). Private insurers would have had to pay that amount for their insured patients.

In 1983 a revolution occurred in hospital reimbursement. Induced by the projected deficits in the HI Trust Fund, Medicare began paying hospitals on the basis of diagnosis-related groups (DRGs), which means that each Medicare patient is assigned to a category based on his or her diagnosis, age, and procedure. There are a total of 468 DRG categories, and each category supposedly contains patients with similar cost experiences. As a result, a prospective price is set for each category and this is what the hospital is paid. The reimbursement rate for each patient within a DRG category is based on two numbers: a relative weight for the particular DRG category and an overall rate applied to the weighted figure.

EXAMPLE: The relative weight set by Medicare for DRG 159 (hernia procedures for persons over 69 years of age) is .9297; if the DRG rate is $3000, then the hospital will receive $2789 (.9297 × $3000) for each case it treats. There is considerable controversy over the particular weights for specific DRGs, as well as the setting of the overall rate. One objection relating to weights is that they are not good reflections of economic costs; e.g., it is claimed that actual nursing costs vary considerably from DRG weights, and in setting the weights more attention should be paid to nursing input.

Note that this payment is prospective: i.e., the price is set before the patient is treated and the hospital knows what the price is. This form of reimbursement (discussed later) dramatically changed the incentive system in hospital reimbursement; in this case, and unlike the retrospective case, if the hospitals spent more they *didn't* get any more reimbursement.

Physicians traditionally were reimbursed on a fee-for-service basis, i.e., for each service performed, a separate charge was made.

EXAMPLE: For each initial check-up, physicians in Alberta receive a payment of $29.75. Each visit to a physician can result in several procedures being performed and billed. A visit for a check-up can result in a complete examination ($29.75), a chest x-ray ($16), a blood test ($9.80), and an electrocardiogram ($8.60). The total billings are greater than for a simple examination.

In the past, physicians set these fees themselves. Recent changes suggest a greater involvement in the setting of fees by insurers, based on factors such as the average fee level for all physicians in an area. Fee-for-service reimbursement has a built in incentive for the physician to perform more services, and for this reason an alternative form of reimbursement, called *prepayment,* has been promoted by payors. This important development will be discussed later.

The providers, physicians, and hospitals in the simplified example must spend some of their receipts on expenses, such as nurses' salaries, supplies, and drugs. The remainder is retained in surpluses, or profits, for themselves. Thus if Naragannset Community Hospital receives $2 million in reimbursement from Blue Cross, $1 million from self-pay sources, and $4 million from Medicaid and Medicare, its total receipts are $7 million. Naragannset's expenditures are $4 million for nurses' salaries, $1 million for supplies, and $1.5 million for other expenses. Its surplus, what it has left over, is a half million dollars.

Inputs

The complete picture of the flow of funds in the medical marketplace includes groups who produce the inputs (physicians, nurses, etc.). These input-producing groups include medical schools, nursing schools, and drug companies. Nursing school revenues are students' fees and government funds. Nursing schools graduate nurses to work in the system.

The simplified picture of the flows in the health care system is now complete. It is designed to provide an understanding of the prime factors in the health care system and how money flows between them. Although not all the factors, or flows, are identified in this presentation, it presents an idea of where things fit. The picture just drawn is one of the traditional system that was predominant around 1980. Since then, a number of changes have been made. One in particular is the emergence of several new types of factors on the scene: the Health Maintenance Organization (HMO) and the Preferred Provider Organization (PPO).

HMOs

Figure 3-5 illustrates a modified version of the flow diagram (see Figure 3-3) that incorporates the HMO. From a funds flow view, the essential point about the HMO is that it is both an insurer and a provider. That is, the consumer, employer, or government pays annual premiums to the HMO; in return the HMO directly assumes the responsibility of providing care—basic medical, hospital, and drugs, among others. Note the difference between this form of "prepaid" care and traditional care, as previously outlined. Under traditional care, premiums are paid to the insurer who reimburses the physicians and hospitals for the care they provide to the insured patient. Under prepayment, the HMO assumes responsibility for the provision of care, and must cover its costs out of its premiums.

The HMO thus incorporates insurance functions and provider functions within its organization. Figure 3-5 illustrates this by incorporating the participating components of the HMO in a dotted line area. Note, however, that an HMO need not have the physicians, hospitals, and insurers all in the same institution. An HMO can take the form of a contractual arrangement, with insurers, hospitals, and physicians independent of one another, but each contracting to provide the agreed upon service.

EXAMPLE: The Coosa River Textile Company has 1000 employees. It decides to provide them with HMO health insurance coverage as an employment benefit. It contracts with Blue Ridge HMO for $1000 an employee. For this fee, Blue Ridge agrees to provide all medical, hospital, and drug care for the 1000 employees and their dependents. Blue Ridge receives $1 million in premiums. Because it has agreed to provide medical care for the 1000 employees and their dependents, it must make some arrangements to do so. The arrangements that Blue Ridge can make are numerous. It can purchase its own hospitals, hire its own (salaried) physicians, and be a provider; or it can contract

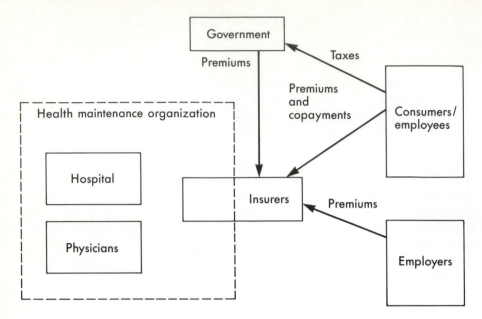

Fig. 3-5 Flow presentation of the health maintenance organization.

with physicians and hospitals to provide care for its members. In the latter case, Blue Ridge becomes a reimburser of care, but what distinguishes it from a traditional insurer is the fact that it is responsible for providing the care (or seeing that care is provided). Under HMO membership the member must be treated by the HMO's selected providers. Under traditional care, the consumer is free to select the providers. This gives the HMO a greater degree of control over the providers. It can select providers with "conservative" practice patterns, and thus reduce the degree of hospitalization of its members. The traditional insurer has no such control over its insurees' providers.

Note that the HMO premium is a fixed prepaid amount (e.g., $1000) per employee. The HMO, as *insurer,* receives this sum as its receipts. But the HMO is also a *provider,* or a contractee for providers, and as a provider it receives a fixed sum per member. Unlike a hospital or a physician providing traditional care, the more care an HMO provides, the more it costs the HMO, but *it doesn't get reimbursed any additional amount for providing more care.* It receives only the fixed prepaid amount ($1000). As will be shown, the HMO operates under radically different incentives from the provider under traditional insurance.

Membership in HMOs has grown dramatically in recent years. In 1971 there were 3.6 million subscribers nationally. By 1986 this number had grown to 28 million.[6]

PPOs

The PPO is not an insurer, nor is it a provider, although it may have links to both. It is a true "middleman," a result of the competitive marketplace. To illustrate what a PPO

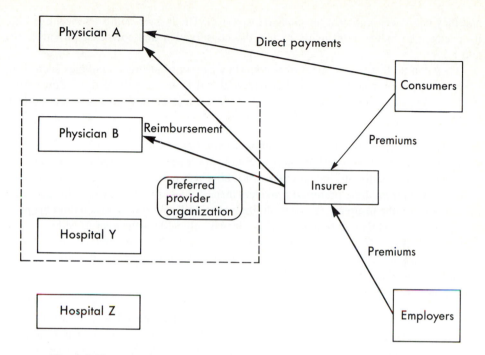

Fig. 3-6 Financial flows and the Preferred Provider Organization (PPO).

does, the flows diagram is again slightly redrawn (Figure 3-6). The illustration shows two competing physicians and two competing hospitals (more could be added but would complicate the diagram). Each physician and each hospital is vying for patients. The problem for them, in a competitive environment, is how to sign up patients. One possibility is to attract them with favorable prices.

The insurer is also part of this picture. The insurer wants to keep premiums down so it can attract the business of employers who will contract with it to insure its employees. The prime way that the insurer can keep rates down is to contain reimbursements to physicians and hospitals. If the insurer can contain the reimbursement rates that it pays to these providers, as well as the number of times the consumers are hospitalized, it can succeed in lowering its costs, and also its premiums.

The PPO is an intermediary that tries to develop a favorable package of physician and hospital care and sell it to insurers. First, the PPO signs up physicians with conservative practice patterns and hospitals with low charges. It then develops a system of reviewing the use of potential clients so that the utilization will be kept low. Because of the favorable utilization experience of consumers, as well as reasonable rates, the PPO will have a favorable package, which it can promote at reasonable premium rates. The problem is to induce consumers to use the "preferred" providers. PPO arrangements, similar to traditional insurance, allow consumers free choice of providers. They can select physicians with nonconservative practice patterns (Physician *A* in our diagram), and they can select high cost hospitals (Hospital Z). The insurer builds an incentive into its package to induce consumers to use the conservative and low cost providers (B and Y).

They can do this in a number of ways. They can write insurance policies such that, when the consumers go to preferred providers B and Y, they pay little or no direct payments. When they go to the nonmember providers A and Z, they have to make a direct payment.

EXAMPLE: The Green Hills Insurance Company can offer employers a preferred package consisting of a specified list of physicians, Smith and Jones, and a specified hospital, Gander County Memorial. The premium is $1200 a year per employee. If the employees seek treatment from these preferred providers there is no additional payment (as per agreement with the insurers). If, however, they go to M.D. Brown, who is not on the preferred list, Green Hills will reimburse M.D. Brown only $20 for the visit. If M.D. Brown's bill is $50, the consumers who choose to go to M.D. Brown will pay the additional $30 directly. Thus there is a penalty to consumers for using nonpreferred providers. Note that unlike other HMO arrangements, under a PPO system the consumer can use nonmember providers. There is a penalty for doing so, however.

The PPO can be operated by providers, insurers, or independent contractors. The essential ingredient in the PPO is that it contracts with providers and manages the care they provide. In performing this monitoring function, the PPO can offer a group of services at reduced rates. The PPO is not directly an insurer or a provider; it does not collect or pay out funds. It performs a flow-through function, and tries to reduce the funds flowing through. The PPO might, therefore, be reimbursed on a commission basis, and thus it gains a portion of any savings it creates.

COSTS

Cost is a fundamental economic concept that refers to the size of a resource commitment. An activity is measured by its cost, which refers to the quantity of resources that have gone into that activity. Often costs are associated with dollar expenditures.

EXAMPLE: Mrs White becomes ill and needs $800 in treatment costs (measured by physicians' fees and drug costs). In addition, Mrs White loses three days' wages ($60 a day) from her part-time factory job as a ballpoint pen assembler. Her husband has insurance coverage with some deductibles, resulting in Mrs White paying $200 of the $800, with the insurance company paying $600. What is the expense of Mrs White's medical care? And what are her illness costs?

To identify the true expenditures, cost must be defined and the definition used as a guide to measuring costs. There must also be a clear definition of the activity to be measured. In this case there are two activities to measure: the cost of medical care and the cost of illness. The cost of medical care refers to the size of resource commitment (in dollar terms) resulting from the use of medical services. This is measured by the flow of money received by the providers (as well as the administrative costs of the intermediaries) (see Figure 3-4). In Mrs Smith's example, this is $800. The cost of illness refers to the size of the resource commitment in dollar terms resulting from the illness. This is a broader concept; it incorporates medical care costs and costs from any other resources resulting from the illness. Mrs Smith lost three days of work, resulting in an additional cost of $180. The total illness cost was thus $980 and the medical care cost was $800. Medical care costs are referred to as *direct costs* and foregone costs are referred to as *indirect costs*. In this case, $800 of the total costs of $980 was direct and $180 was indirect.

There may be an objection at this point that the $180 was not a true cost because Mrs Smith never had the $180. This would be a mistaken notion of cost. The cost of a nursing education includes fees (say $2000 a year) and books and supplies (say $1000). But what about time expenditure? If not a nursing student, one could be working full time. For example, a sales clerk may make $15,000 a year. This $15,000 is a cost to the nursing student, and even though it hasn't come directly out of pocket, it is as real as if it did. The student has, in fact, *given up* this $15,000 by going to nursing school. Therefore in the true meaning of the term *cost* (the amount of resources committed) the total costs to the nursing student are $18,000 per year.

Total illness costs can also be categorized by who bears the burden of the costs. In our example, Mrs Smith bore $380 of the total burden of $980; $180 was borne indirectly and $800 directly. $200 of the $800 in direct medical care costs was borne by Mrs Smith (Figure 3-7).

Note that the $600 in costs that is reimbursed by intermediaries ultimately is paid by individuals. As discussed in the previous section, insurers' revenues come from premiums and government revenues come from taxes. Premiums and taxes are paid by individuals. At times it is difficult to determine exactly who pays. An employer's health insurance premiums are made at the expense of employees' money wages, though the employees may not fully recognize this. And Medicare's receipts for Part A come out of social security taxes, although, again, the payers may not fully recognize this. Nevertheless, *all* costs are borne by someone. When Mrs Smith receives $800 in medical care for $200, she may believe she is getting a bargain, but Mrs Smith's husband pays health insurance premiums, as does his coworkers, and the $800 comes out of their premiums.

The concept of costs explains the waste incurred by "flat of the curve" medicine, mentioned at the beginning of this chapter. A cost benefit analysis is a comparison of the costs of a particular activity with its benefits. Medical care's goal is to improve health. The benefits of health can be measured in dollar terms as the dollar savings from reduced illness. Without medical care, Mrs Smith may have been incapacitated for 10 days. The medical care she received created benefits of 7 extra days of good health. The dollar value of these benefits can be roughly stated at $60 a day, or $420 total.

Because the costs of medical care were $800, the benefit cost ratio is 420/800 or about 0.52 to 1. A ratio of less than one signifies that benefits were less than costs, and

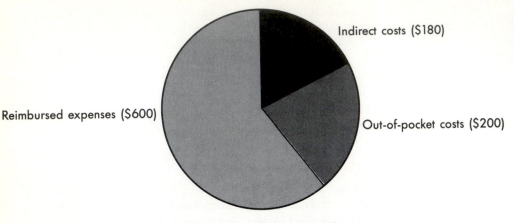

Fig. 3-7 Breakdown of Mrs Smith's total illness costs.

the activity was not worth it from a strict dollar standpoint. This illustrates the wastage arising from flat of the curve medicine. If additional medical care is costly and little additional health results from it, then the benefit cost ratio will be very low. It is not that flat of the curve medical care is of *no* value, but that the benefits it creates, though positive, are less than the costs.

One particularly difficult problem arises in this analysis. A private viewpoint of the cost benefit ratio, that of Mrs Smith's, is different from the public viewpoint. Mrs Smith's private benefit cost ratio, the ratio of her private or out-of-pocket costs to benefits is $420 to $200 or 2.1 to 1. The lower her out-of-pocket costs (because of heavier insurance coverage) the more beneficial the ratio. A social standpoint, however, presents a different picture. It costs "society" (everyone, including Mrs Smith) $800 to secure $420 in benefits. Clearly, this is not cost beneficial. When analyzing costs and benefits, it is important to distinguish the point of view.

There is an additional important reminder relating to benefit calculations. In many instances there are no good estimates of benefits. Employment benefits such as Mrs Smith's are of limited use for calculating the benefits of those who are not currently employed, such as the retired, the unemployed, and the very young.

EXAMPLE: A 70-year-old grandmother suddenly gets pneumonia. Hospitalization will make her well, but the cost is $3000. Because she does not work, the dollar value of employment benefits are zero. Is the benefit cost ratio zero? Total money benefits are clearly greater than employment benefits; however, if there are no employment benefits and dollar values are attributed to improved health from those who are not working, many problems are encountered. This is one area of economics in which satisfactory solutions do not exist. Still, the resources are scarce and have alternative uses. Using resources in one way results in taking them away from another valuable use. Not having a sound measure of benefits merely makes the decision making all the more difficult.

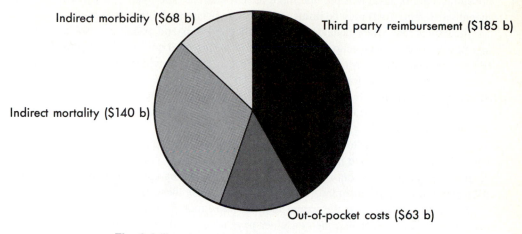

Fig. 3-8 Illness cost breakdown, United States, 1980.

Compared with Figure 3-7, what is the actual breakdown of costs in the United States? An analysis similar to that in Figure 3-7 for the United States, 1980, is shown in Figure 3-8. As illustrated, direct out-of-pocket costs in 1980 were about one quarter of all payments to all providers (institutions and practitioners). That is, the total costs, which are generated when individuals receive medical care, are four times those that individuals directly experience. Further, indirect illness costs were roughly the same order of magnitude as were medical care costs. The burden on the economy of illness is much greater than that resulting from the provision of medical care alone.[7,9]

INCENTIVES IN HEALTH CARE

A dean of medicine in a large medical school once remarked that it wouldn't make any difference if a hospital was given a lump sum of $40 million to operate, or if it was paid $4000 a patient and limited to reimbursement of 10,000 patients. The total cost in either case would be the same. He was correct in observing that the total cost would be the same. But, he was not correct in saying that it wouldn't make any difference to the outcome. The incentive systems under the two types of reimbursement are radically different, and the outcomes will be different as well. Indeed, one of the most important lessons to be learned from economics is that an incentive system can radically affect the output of the system.

Output refers to the outcome of economic behavior by the consumer or provider. For the consumer, economic behavior refers to the quantity of medical care demanded. For the provider, it refers to the quantity and quality of medical care provided. When it is said that incentives influence output, it means that these groups will behave differently—will consume more or less, will provide more or less quantity and quality, depending on the incentive system. Costs may be influenced by these behavioral differences as well.

Incentives that affect behavior consist of the rewards and penalties associated with any particular course of action. Every course of action by a consumer and provider has rewards and penalties associated with it. The consumer or provider will assess these and choose the course of action with the greatest net rewards (rewards minus penalties). It is in this way that costs enter the picture. Costs to a consumer or provider are penalties. If a consumer or provider bears more costs for a particular course of action, then that course of action is less appealing.

Now the concept of flows and the concept of costs with the idea of incentives can be tied together. As discussed in the flow section of this chapter, one of the key flows in the health care system is the out-of-pocket costs paid directly by consumers to the provider. Alternative policy and insurance arrangements can alter these flows, in that the copayment can be increased (to the extent that the consumer pays the full cost of care) or decreased (to the extent that the consumer pays no cost). They key point in behavioral economics is, *it matters which option is chosen.* If the consumer bears a greater portion of the costs directly, the penalty for using medical care will be greater. Therefore the consumer will use as little medical care as possible.

EXAMPLE: If Mrs Smith has full insurance coverage, she might visit the physician four or five times for a particular episode of illness. The rewards are there (improved health) but the penalties are not (no out-of-pocket costs). But if the out-of-pocket cost to Mrs Smith is raised to $20 a visit, the rewards from treatment are unchanged and the penalties are increased. Mrs Smith now finds going to the physician costly, and she will cut down on her visits. The result is, *the incentive system has changed her behavior.*

The analysis just described is the basic demand analysis of economics. It states that individuals will demand more of any commodity if the direct price falls. Note that it is not the total cost which governs individual behavior, but the out-of-pocket cost. It is this cost that the patient reacts to. The service can be very costly (e.g., intensive care), but if the service is insured or subsidized, the individual will behave as if it were inexpensive.

As previously discussed, incentives can work on the demand side. They can also influence providers in terms of the quantity and quality of services they are willing to provide. To illustrate that various incentive schemes will cause very different behaviors on the part of the providers, an example of provider behavior in nursing education follows.

EXAMPLE: Not long ago the health economics course at Faber College of Nursing, a well-respected midwestern institution, was taught in a staid, routine manner by a part-time lecturer who had been teaching the course since 1969. The lecturer was paid $2000 to teach the course, and he was given a modest budget for course-related expenses such as supplies, travel, and honorariums for visiting speakers. His average cost summary for the years 1985 to 1987 are shown in the box; these figures are close to what they were in 1969. In fact, everything about the course was similar to what it was in 1969.

This lack of dynamism in the course surfaced in 1987 when the college's nursing administration program was reviewed for accreditation. As part of the accreditation process, a review of the program's courses was made by an external body of experts. The health economics course did not fare well in that review. The review team discovered that the teacher had used the same lecture notes since 1969, and still (in 1987) referred to the "new" Medicare and Medicaid programs, as well as the need for regulation to curb hospital cost inflation. Students who were interviewed professed to being bored by the lectures, although they praised the fact that the exams were easy because they were the same from year to year.

The review team concluded that the course was *stagnant* and cited the *reimbursement* system as a major cause of the inertia. They asserted that there were no incentives for the professor to improve or update the course, and that there were no sufficient resources to support updating.

The dean at Faber, whose objective included providing the very highest quality of education, took the criticisms seriously, although she questioned the means recommended by the committee to attain these ends. Being a full-time academic, she believed that academics were motivated solely by the pursuit of truth, just as lawyers are motivated solely by the pursuit of justice and physicians solely by the pursuit of their patients' health. The dean argued that a good teacher will teach well under any payment system. Still, despite her reservations, she acquiesced and, with the help of a hospital administrator, designed a new reimbursement system for the health economics course.

The new reimbursement system was called *cost plus* (which, because it was designed by a hospital administrator, resembled the pre-1983 formula used by Medicare and Medicaid to reimburse hospitals). According to this system the college would reimburse the lecturer for education-related expenses plus a percentage of costs to cover the professor's salary. Because the ratio of educational costs to salary for the 1985 to 1987 period

---

SUMMARY OF EXPENSES FOR HEALTH ECONOMICS COURSE
ORIGINAL PAYMENT METHOD

Item	Expense ($)
Photocopying	400
Field trips (Saint Ives Hospital)	150
Honorarium for guest speakers:	
Mr Jack Spratt, Administrator, Fat City General Hospital	200
Miss M. Muffett, Director of Nursing, Tuffet Memorial Hospital	200
Computer time	150
Expense total	1,100
Instructor's salary	2,000
Total course expense	3,100

was about 1 to 2, the dean decided that this figure would be used in the formula. The final formula, then, was that the professor would be reimbursed for education costs such as speakers, supplies, and travel, plus an amount equal to twice these educational costs for his lecturing fee.

The system was initiated, and at the end of the semester, the dean was presented with a bill (see box) of $117,000—one third of which was for course expenses. She immediately called a conference with the health economics professor and protested. The professor explained each item and tried to explain that he was trying to provide the students in Nurs Adm 103 with the very highest quality of education, and was grateful to the education system for allowing him to do so. He explained that the two super-quality VCRs were purchased ($1500 each) so that the students could view the PBS special series on the health care system tapes ($1000). He explained that his trip to the British Museum ($1600) was expressly made to research the life and times of Florence Nightingale, which perked up the students' interest in emergency care nursing. He defended his trip to the US Public Health Service (NIH) library in Bethesda ($800) on the grounds that, only there, could he obtain materials pertinent to his lecture on the role of the federal government in nursing. When questioned about the relevance of the outside speakers, the professor stated that if one wanted to provide current and high quality education, second rate speakers would simply not do. Thus, Oliver North was invited to speak on nursing

---

EXPENSES FOR HEALTH ECONOMICS COURSE
COST-BASED REIMBURSEMENT FORMULA

Item	Expense ($)
1 set VCR tapes: "Health Care in the US"	1,000
2 super deluxe VCRs	3,000
Library trip to British Museum to research Florence Nightingale papers	1,600
1 slide projector system w/sound	800
Slide production	900
Supplies (Cross pens, etc.)	1,100
Trip to Bethesda, NIH Library to research nursing administration collection	800
Speaker: Bill Cosby on nursing and the family	11,000
Speaker: Henry Kissinger on nursing economics and international affairs today	8,000
Speaker: Col. Oliver North on nursing economics and the Contra affair	5,000
Speaker: Governor Dukakis on nursing management and liberalism	2,000
Speaker: Erma Bombeck on the lighter side of nursing management	4,000
Total direct expenses	39,200
Total salary (direct expenses × 2)	78,400
Total reimbursed	117,600

administration and the Contras, Bill Cosby on nursing economics and the family, and Governor Dukakis on nursing economics and liberalism. If one wanted the best expert on nursing management and international affairs, who better to speak than Henry Kissinger? Or Erma Bombeck on a lighter side of nursing economics? Although the point was well made the dean felt that Faber's budget could not support such extravagance and she sought a new funding formula.

The formula that followed in the spring of 1988 was based on a simple fee schedule. A new instructor was presented with a basic fee schedule (see box), which specified a price for each "procedure" that the professor performed. This was similar to a physician's fee schedule. For a short lecture (under 30 minutes) the professor was reimbursed $10, regardless of size of the class. A longer (over 30 minutes) lecture was funded $15. A separate fee was set for each student examined, with a $4 fee set for each student examined on a multiple-choice basis. In addition, fees were set for tutorials, beginning with $6 for a minor clarification, $9 for a major clarification, and $20 for a tutorial in which the student exhibited a major incomprehension.

The dean at Faber expected efficiency and she got it. Lectures were generally short—very short, in fact, lasting 10 minutes each. There was a multiple choice exam after each class. In spite of this, there were many major incomprehensions, and the students were continually lined up outside the professor's door for remedial tutorials. In fact, each student in the 14 week course averaged 21 multiple-choice tests and over 30 major incomprehensions. Again, the dean's preconception that truth would prevail was borne out, but the *manner* in which the professor taught the truth varied. This variation was due to the fee schedule, or incentive system.

It can be hypothesized that had the fee schedule differed, the behavior of the professor would have differed as well. For example, if the fee had been $5 for a short lecture and $30 for a long one, there would have been more long lectures. Or had a multiple-

---

FEE SCHEDULE FOR TEACHING "PROCEDURES"
HEALTH ECONOMICS

Item	Fee ($)
Lecture (less than 30 min)	10.00
Lecture (over 30 min)	15.00
Exam, multiple choice	4.00
Exam, short answer, under 200 words per question	5.00
Exam, essay, over 200 words per question and over 4 questions	6.00
Term paper, less than 10 pages	12.00
Term paper, more than 10 pages and 50 item bibliography	16.00
Tutorial for minor clarification	6.00
Tutorial for major clarification	9.00
Tutorial for total miscomprehension	20.00

choice test's fee been 25 cents and the fee for a long essay $10, there would have been more long essays and not as many multiple-choice tests. All of this would have been accomplished in the search for truth and high quality education! (It is not the goal that would change with the reimbursement method, but how that goal was sought.)

Regardless, the dean was unhappy with the results, and again, in the summer session of 1988 the reimbursement system was changed (as was the professor). This time, the new professor was reimbursed on a prepaid, per student basis. This type of payment was similar to that of the HMO. For each student taught, the professor was paid $40. If the professor brought in outside speakers such as Bill Cosby or Jim McMahon, he had to bear the cost himself. Unlike cost plus reimbursement, the penalty for incurring higher costs fell on the professor. As one might expect, instructional costs fell dramatically (see box), but the professor's promotional budget soared, with beer bashes, propellor beanies with the insignia "Nursing Adm 103 is A-OK," and advertisements on the college radio station. The dean was less concerned, however, because these expenses were paid from the professor's per capita payment.

As expected, enrollment in Nurs Adm 103 initially skyrocketed. But what of the quality of education? Did it remain the same? There will always be those who will say that quality deteriorated. But there are some who will say that the students learned more this way because every one got an A in the course.

However, enrollment began falling on other courses. To counter the falling enrollments, instructors in the other courses began clamoring for per capita payments as well. Those that got them began to promote their courses. Soon the campus was filled with promotional signs for courses such as NursAdm 222 and Psych 239. And in early

---

EXPENSE SUMMARY FOR PER CAPITA REIMBURSEMENT HEALTH ECONOMICS	
Instructional	**Expense ($)**
2 pieces of chalk (first broke)	.16
1 pencil to record names	.11
1 paper pad	.89
Student recruitment	
1 recruitment session at Porky's	289.98
Color ad in Phi Kappa Theta News	99.00
20-30 second spots on WROK-1330	60.00
1000 propeller beanies with insignia "For an A-bsolutely A-ssured A-experience-Take NursAdm 103"	500.00
Distribution of beanies by Greek Society	125.00
Total expenses	1,075.14

September, just before fall registration, meeting rooms at the local Jeffrey Amber Pub were booked solid by professors who were holding course orientation meetings.

Once again, the outcome changed. Although the professor was still pursuing the same goal of quality education, each time the incentive system changed, the manner in which the course was taught changed as well. That is, the professors in charge of resources used them in different ways. By this time, the dean was a believer that the reward-penalty system would affect resource use decisions.

Remember the query of the dean of a medical school who wondered what difference it would make if a hospital was paid a flat sum of $40 million or if it was paid $4000 per patient up to a maximum of 10,000 patients. The lesson of this section is, that it would make a great deal of difference. Just as they worked at Faber, the various reimbursement schemes in the health care field work to influence delivery patterns. Depending on the specific rewards and penalties associated with a particular reimbursement system, health care providers will alter their delivery patterns accordingly.

Note that it is not necessarily due to greed of the providers that outcomes are determined in this way. A change in the incentive system makes it more costly to do things in a certain way, and discourages providers from behaving in certain ways. For example, providng a myriad of lab tests and x-rays is not necessarily bad (even if it is costly). It represents one way of providing health care, and if this manner of provision is rewarded (as it is under the cost-based and fee-for-service reimbursement systems) then it will be continued. Under prepayment, resource intensive care results in the provider bearing the costs more directly and thus being penalized for providing resource intensive care. The provider will choose a less intensive mode of care under per capita payment. It is another question, and an open one, as to which type of care will be more effective in promoting health. Certainly, this issue is also part of the evaluation of the various types of delivery, as is cost.

ECONOMIC ORGANIZATION OF MEDICAL CARE

Since 1966 the US health care system has gone through three distinct phases, each of which is associated with specific economic characteristics. In this section the focus is on the use of concepts that were developed previously in this chapter to understand the functioning and *performance* of these three phases. Central to our understanding of system performance, then, are the various incentives that have been adopted by the system.

Performance of a health care system refers to the operation of the system in the light of specific criteria, standards, or goals. As shown in Figure 3-9, performance has two sides to it: (1) setting of the standards themselves, by which the system's activities are evaluated and (2) behavior (often called *conduct*) of the entities in the system, which, as discussed previously, are significantly influenced by economic incentives. Performance refers to comparison of actual conduct with the established standards. Note that in evaluating economic conduct the incentives that influence it are being evaluated also.

Remember that the economic conduct was influenced by these incentives in the first place, although there may be variables other than incentives that affect behavior. To influence behavioral changes, incentives must be high.

The first step in evaluating the function of the economic organization of a health care system then, is to specify the social goals or objectives that are being assessed. The following three important criteria used to gauge a system's performance are:

1. Total cost—comprises the efficiency with which providers deliver care (the unit cost of care) and the number of units of care provided. The goal of reducing cost is desirable for a number of reasons, just one of which is that lower costs help the government reduce the budget deficit.

2. Consumer access to care—refers to the availability of care to consumers. Access has a number of economic characteristics, including the out-of-pocket price (which reduces access when this price is increased) and waiting and travel costs (which increase when availability or supply is reduced). Although access is a desirable trait, remember there is a "flat of the curve" possibility beyond which more care is not desirable. Also, total cost and access may at times be conflicting goals. Availability is increased by increasing supply and hence costs, resulting in a trade-off between these objectives, and the choice must be made as to how much of each is preferred.

3. Quality of care—quality is a very elusive term and can refer to a number of characteristics. It usually is associated with resource intensiveness of care, but even that may not be accurate if resource intensiveness does not lead to improved outcomes (better health). Quality is defined as relating to improved health outcomes, but these are hard to measure in practice. To the extent that quality and resource intensiveness go hand in hand, quality is a costly goal and again results in a trade-off of quality for costs. Because quality and cost conflict with one another, the highest quality of care may not be feasible; it may simply be too costly.

The following is an examination of three stages of the US health care system since 1966, focusing on the role that incentives play in these systems. When Medicaid and Medicare were instituted in 1966, the reimbursement systems established by Congress included fee-for-service payment for physicians and cost-based reimbursement for hospitals. Direct payments (i.e., copayments and deductibles) for Medicare beneficiaries were reasonably low (the deductible for hospital care was $40—low by current standards), and premiums for those who chose the optional medical benefits (SMI) coverage were also comparatively reasonable. As previously discussed, low copayments, cost-based reimbursement for hospitals, and fee-for-service reimbursement for physicians

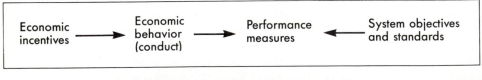

Fig. 3-9 Conceptual elements in an evaluation.

encourage increased use and costs of the health care system. Conclusions are summarized in Figure 3-10, with reference to economic goals, which shows that the incentives of the post-1966 system were such that they encouraged greater costs, greater access, and greater quality. Of course, more of everything is not always better; greater accessibility and quality are achieved at the expense of greater costs, and greater costs are not well appreciated by those who bear them, primarily insurance premium payers and taxpayers. Also, there may be limits to how much access is desirable; if flat of the curve medicine is indeed a reality, then at some point increased access to *health care* adds little to *health*.

Shortly after these incentives were implemented, their inflationary tendencies were recognized. Although there was little disagreement about the effects that these financial arrangements were having, there was considerable disagreement about how to curb their inflationary effects. Introducing different incentives, such as higher out-of-pocket costs (deductibles or copayments) would curb demand pressures, but this would mean compromising on the goal of access. And cutting back on payments to providers (e.g., hospitals) would mean less resources available for patient care, which would compromise the quality goal. Initially, Congress was not willing to compromise on either goal. Instead it introduced a series of regulations that were attempts to directly impose restrictions on providers to contain costs.

Regulation refers to direct attempts on the part of an authority to control the behavior of organizations. It is conducted by a government-appointed agency, i.e., given the

System	Characteristics	System goals		
		Costs	Access	Quality
Pre-1970	Low direct consumer prices; cost base and fee for service reimbursement	↑	↑	↑
1970s	Same as above but with regulatory controls	↑	↑	↑
1980s	Increasing direct prices, prospective reimbursement, per capita (HMOs) increasing	↓	↓	?

Fig. 3-10 Overview of economic characteristics of health care system in three periods and their influence on goals of the system.

authority by the legislature to monitor and control specific aspects of economic behavior of the regulated providers. For example, a regulatory agency may be given the authority to control the amount that hospitals spend on new equipment. The agency reviews all new equipment spending plans and approves the projects that fall within its guidelines. By setting very strict guidelines, the agency may curtail new spending on equipment.

Note that there is nothing in the regulatory process that changes how much the providers want to spend. Regulation by itself does nothing to change the incentives of the providers. If the incentives encourage spending, imposing regulations will not discourage the desire for providers to spend more. What the regulation will do is disallow providers from spending as much as they want to. However, depending on the incentives, the providers may seek ways of circumventing the regulations.

One type of regulation introduced to curb rising health care costs is capital expenditure review. This type of regulation provides a regulatory body in charge of reviewing all new hospital expenditures for major equipment purchased and additions or renovations to the facility. Approval of the expenditures by the agency results in the issuance of a "certificate of need," certifying that the hospital's plans are in accordance with the regulatory agency's guidelines. The rationale behind this type of regulation is the belief that increases in hospital operating expenses are fueled by new equipment and plant. Thus one way to curb operating costs is to curb new equipment and facilities. Certificate of need regulation first appeared in New York State in 1964, but it was the mid-1970s before a full-scale effort at capital expenditure planning was begun, with the passage of the National Health Planning and Resources Development Act of 1974. This act established regional Health Systems Agencies to review all large-scale hospital capital expenditures.

Establishment of these agencies represented one additional step in a history of regulating the economic behavior of health care providers. But by the late 1970s, the role of economic regulation in general was being questioned, and the effectiveness of capital expenditure review did not escape the growing scrutiny of the effectiveness of regulation. A study undertaken late in the 1970s by Salkever and Bice raised considerable doubt about the effectiveness of certificate of need regulations in controlling capital expenditures in existing facilities. Federal funds for the national health planning effort were reduced, and the national certificate of need effort was curtailed, with a host of other regulatory efforts in diverse industries such as trucking and air travel. It remained with the states to determine whether they would continue the certificate of need regulations.

From the nursing perspective, the key point should be re-emphasized. Certificate of need regulation did nothing to change incentives that hospitals used to increase their operating costs. Throughout the 1970s, hospitals were reimbursed on the basis of their costs; therefore they had incentives to expand these costs. The imposition of capital expenditure regulations simply amounted to the parachuting of an outside body to control a system that retained its inflationary tendencies. This is like trying to contain the size of an expanding balloon by pushing in one of its sides. The balloon will keep expanding around the surface that is contained. In the same way, hospital administrators found ways around certificate of need regulations, thus reducing the attempts to contain hospital costs through regulation alone. As a result, in terms of the system goals in Figure 3-10, there was no difference in the performance of the pre-1970 unregulated system and the post-1970 regulated system *because the incentives were unchanged.*

The growing disillusionment with regulation as a mechanism to control health care costs resulted in an increasing interest in the role of incentives. Provider reimbursement schemes were receiving increased attention. In addition, the role of income tax regulations were gaining greater recognition. Income tax rules allowed health insurance premiums paid by employers as nontaxable benefits, and allowed individuals to deduct premiums they paid from their income. It was contended that these income tax regulations were too lax, and encouraged over-insurance for health care expenditures. With low direct prices, people sought care to the extent where they were on the flat of the curve. It was contended that, with the failure of regulations to remedy the inflationary situation, incentives would have to be introduced.

Proposed incentive changes in the early 1980s included the limitation of tax-free insurance premium benefits[2] in the belief that, if consumers had to directly bear a greater portion of the costs of health care insurance, they would look for less costly alternatives. Health maintenance organizations offered lower cost alternatives, and a rationale for this proposal was that if consumers had to pay a greater share of their health insurance premiums, they would switch to lower-cost forms of insurance. At about the same time, faced with lower profits from recessionary times and foreign competition, US businesses were also examining ways to lower their health insurance benefit costs.

Limited tax-free health insurance benefits never materialized, but because of increasing deficits, several other policy initiatives were proposed. Medicare sought to enroll at least some of its beneficiaries in HMOs and, in an attempt to contain its hospital expenditures, it initiated the prospective payment system by introducing hospital payment by DRGs in 1983. These initiatives, especially the latter, helped reduce medicare's costs, but several new issues arose. First, there was a growing concern that, with the incentive to curtail resource use, hospitals also contained quality of care. The degree to which this occurred is difficult to measure and is largely unknown (the ? in Figure 3-10). Second, in their efforts to contain costs, hospitals were less willing to treat non-paying patients, those who had no insurance coverage from any source (roughly 37 million persons in 1985) and who could not afford to pay for the high cost of hospitalization.* This problem is known as the *indigent problem* and is a major issue in the health care sector today.

Note that being *uninsured* does not mean being *untreated*. Most hospitals provide free or heavily subsidized care for those in need, but there are indications that some hospitals are doing so with increased resistance. Therefore conditions under which the indi-

---

*From the General Accounting Office, 1988.

gent population receive care may be less than optimal. Reduced access is a price a person pays for tightening fiscal constraints.

• • •

Health care costs continue to increase in spite of various approaches to curb them. Health care costs are a major concern of Americans today. No easy solutions seem to be forthcoming in the near future. In fact, the challenges and threats to finding solutions appear at times to overshadow what little progress is made. It remains to be seen how health care issues, delivery systems, and economic aspects of providing health care will evolve in the coming decade.

STUDY ACTIVITIES

1. As a nurse in everyday practice, list as many ways as possible to cut health care costs for patients and clients.
2. List ways that health care costs to society can be decreased.
3. Recalling senior adults for which the reader has provided nursing care, explore what they are paying individually for supplemental health insurance and out of pocket.
4. What was the author's point in the example of various reimbursement systems *costing the same* but *being different?*

REFERENCES

1. Angell M: Cost containment and the physician, J Am Med Assoc 254(9):1203-1207, 1985.
2. Enthoven A: Health plan, Boston, 1980, Addison Wesley.
3. Federal Hospital Insurance Trust Fund, 1986 Annual Report. Washington, DC, 1986, Health Care Financing Administration, Office of the Actuary.
4. Goldfarb M: Who receives cesareans? Patient and hospital characteristics, HCUP research note 4, National Center for Health Services Research, Sept 1983, DHHS Publication (PHS) 84-3345.
5. Health Care Financing Administration, Division of Health Cost Estimates: National health expenditures, 1986-2000, Health Care Financing Review, 8(4):1-36, 1987.
6. Health Insurance Association of America: 1986-1987 source book of health insurance data, Washington, DC, 1987, Health Insurance Association of America.
7. Lazenby H, Levit KR, and Waldo DR: National health expenditures, 1985, Health Care Financing Administration Publication 03232, No. 6, Sept 1986.
8. Noseworthy TW: Resource allocation of adult intensive care, Annals Royal College of Physicians and Surgeons of Canada, 21(3):199-203, May 1988.
9. Rice DP, Hodgson TA, and Kopstein A: The economic cost of illness: a replication and update, Health Care Financing Review 7(1), 1985.
10. Schwartz WB: The regulation strategy for controlling hospital costs, N Engl J Med 305(21):1249-1255, 1981.
11. Smeeding TM and Straub L: Health care financing among the elderly: who really pays the bills? J Health Polit Policy Law 12(1):35-52, 1987.
12. Sutcliffe EM: The social accounting of health. In Hauser MM, ed: The economics of medical care, London, 1972, George Allen and Unwin.

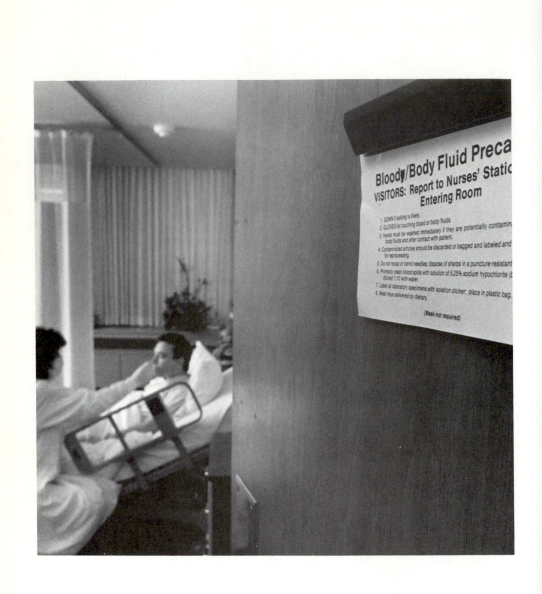

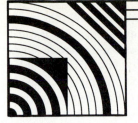

CHAPTER 4

SOCIAL POLICY AND HEALTH CARE DELIVERY

Barbara Talento

OBJECTIVES

After completing this chapter the reader will be able to:

- Discuss what is meant by the question "Is health care a universal right or a privilege?"

- Explain what is meant by "the greatest good for the greatest number"

- Discuss the pros and cons of national health insurance, and where (in what countries) national health insurance is/is not mandatory

- Discuss health insurance in the United States, who can and cannot pay, and how health care is paid when persons are uninsured and financially unable

- List population groups that have special health care needs and how nurses can improve their skills to provide access to health care as needed

- Describe the rule of the legislative, executive, and judicial branches of government as it relates to delivery of health care

ACCESS TO HEALTH CARE

Access to health care in America has been a problem and will continue to be so until the decision is made whether health care is a universal right or a privilege. Today, it is neither. Therefore some Americans have the best care that medicine and technology can provide and others can't afford the medicine that would be prescribed if they could afford the physician's office visit. If one believes in the ethical canon, "The greatest good for the greatest number," then every citizen should have basic minimum levels of health care. But who defines what is basic and minimum? A second question should be, "How fair is a system that allows everyone the basics, and access to high technology such as transplants, dialysis, and by-pass surgery only to the rich?" Can the nation afford to supply everyone with the level of care each individual may want? If not, who should be given access to the health care delivery system, who should decide, and how will this nation pay for that care?

Table 4-1 shows what percentage of the Gross National Product of various nations is spent on health care. The United States and South Africa are the only industrialized nations without national health insurance. Yet one of the biggest buyers of health care is the US government. The United States spent 10.7% of its Gross Domestic Budget (GDP) in 1984 on health care, higher than 20 other developed countries that average less than 7.5% of their GDP on health care. Unlike the United States, these other countries provided health care coverage for all ages, and many for long-term services as well. However, statistics indicate that the federal government pays more for health care for the middle class and the rich than it spends on care for the poor because tax deductions for health insurance cost the government 29 billion dollars, whereas the bill for Medicaid comes to 20.3 billion dollars. In 1985 the US government spent $425 billion on health care, yet it is fragmented and uncoordinated.

There are 35 million Americans, about 15% of the population, without any form of health insurance. Some are underemployed or work seasonally, some are between jobs, and some are excluded from health insurance policies. The greatest majority of uninsured are the working poor, people who work but have incomes below the poverty level. The working poor earn monthly incomes averaging about $500.00, which makes them

Table 4-1   Total health expenditure 1987

Gross National Product	(%)	Health expenditure (%)
Australia	7.1	71.8
Austria	8.4	67.6
Belgium	7.2	76.9
Canada	8.6	74.8
Denmark	6.0	85.5
France	8.6	78.3
Germany	8.2	77.0
Japan	6.8	73.2
Norway	7.5	97.6
Sweden	9.0	90.6
United Kingdom	6.1	86.6
United States	11.2	41.4

Source: Organization for Economic Cooperation and Development, Health Data Bank.

ineligible for welfare. The US Census Bureau[32] estimates that 9 million adults work full-time but earn less than $11,203, the poverty level. Two out of three of these workers have no employer- or union-subsidized health insurance. Of the underemployed and the unemployed almost 60% are not covered by private or public insurance.

In addition to the working poor, there are the unemployed who rely on Medicaid for their health needs. Cuts in the Medicaid budget and redefinition of eligibility reduced the numbers of indigent families who qualified for assistance. The federal government gave more authority to the individual states in the form of block grants. The states could then set limits on the amount of money or the types of services for which they would pay. The majority of these changes were under the 1981 Omnibus Budget Reconciliation Act (US PL 97-35). Overall the result of the block grants, limitation of eligibility, and consolidation of various programs resulted in an 18% reduction of funding from the federal to the state government, with concomitant reductions to the recipients of these funds. These barriers to access to health care affect diverse populations such as women, children, and the elderly in multiple ways.

Prenatal Care

Budget cuts continue to threaten the Women, Infants, and Children Supplemental Nutrition Program (WIC). Cuts began in 1982 when WIC and children's school breakfast and lunch programs were cut by $1.5 million dollars. That same year, the food stamp program was also cut, by $1.7 billion, which jeopardized the nutritional status of pregnant women. Participation in the WIC program can decrease the rate of low birth rate babies by 75%, yet this program can now serve less than one third of those eligible.[23]

There are 3.4 million women who are just above the poverty level and therefore do not qualify for Medicaid. The poorest one fifth of American families is headed by black women whose disposable income has dropped by 9% over the last 5 years. These women are particularly hard hit by budgetary cuts because so many are in the childbearing years and in need of prenatal care. Inadequate prenatal care, which is defined as no doctor's visits within the first 3 months or fewer than eight visits through term, is associated with premature birth, high infant morbidity and mortality, and low birth weight.[8]

A decline in prenatal visits, according to studies, is associated with an increase of maternal anemia with associated low birth weight and diminished intellectual and physical development in infants.[21] The March of Dimes' statistics indicate that babies weighing less than $5^{1}/_{2}$ pounds are 40 times as likely to die during their first month of life and five times as likely to die before reaching their first birthday. Currently the United States is 17th among nations for infant mortality (see Table 4-2). The National Academy of Science Institute of Medicine estimates that $3.3 billion is spent annually on neonatal intensive care that could have been prevented by adequate prenatal care at one third the cost. The Institute of Medicine in Washington estimates that for every $1 spent on prenatal care, $3.38 can be saved in neonatal intensive care costs.[15] An additional $6 is saved if all costs associated with caring for disabled children is included. Low birth weight infants are highly susceptible to neurological developmental handicaps and have a higher risk of developing illness throughout childhood.[8]

Table 4-2 Infant mortality table

Rank	Country	Rate*
1	Japan	6.0
3	Finland	6.5
5	Denmark	7.7
7	Netherlands	8.3
9	Canada	8.5
11	Hong Kong	9.0
13	Belgium	9.4
15	United Kingdom	9.6
17	German Democratic Republic (East)	10.0
18	United States	10.6

* Rate represents deaths under the age of 1 year per 1000 births.
Source: DHEW, National Center for Health Statistics.

Although infant mortality rates seem to be declining, that perception may be misleading. Infant deaths in the first month of life are down, however there is an increase during the following 11 months. It appears that high-technology and skills of nursing and medicine in neonatal intensive care units save premature and low birth weight neonates, whereas lack of supportive services precludes adequate care in the next critical months. Since nutrition and immunization programs were cut there have been increases in infant anemia, diarrhea, failure to thrive, and communicable diseases.[21] Most of the information related to increased health risks and disease is anecdotal, based on individual studies in various areas of the country. This is in direct relationship to the ever increasing budget cuts, since 1981, at the National Center for Health Statistics and other data collecting agencies throughout the federal government.

Elderly

The older population, defined as those 65 years of age or older, numbered about 30 million in 1988. They represent approximately 12% of the US population. The ratio is 147 women to 100 men. Since 1900 the percentage of 65-year-old persons has tripled. The average life expectancy is 74.7 years and if one lives to 65 there is an average life expectancy of an additional 16.8 years. Further, the older population is itself getting older. The 65 to 74 age group is nearly eight times larger than in 1900, the 75 to 84 age group is 11 times larger and the 85+ age group is 22 times larger. By the year 2030 there will be about 65 million older Americans.[2] This is commonly referred to as the *graying of America.* The bulge in the aging population expected between the years 2010 and 2030 will be caused by a cohort of the population born between 1946 to 1964, commonly called *baby boomers,* that reflect an exceptionally high birth rate for the twenty years after World War II.

The median income in 1988 of older males was $11,854 and $6,734 for older females. Black families headed by persons 65 or over have a median income of $11,937, whereas it is $19,813 for white families. Thirty-five percent of families with an elderly head of household had incomes above $25,000 and 15% had incomes below $10,000. The major source of income for older families is Social Security (35%). Other forms of income are pensions, earnings, and assets. About 3% of the elderly remain in the work force. The median net worth of older persons' households is $60,300. Net worth was below $5000 for 16% of the older population, the majority in households headed by black women. There are about 3.5 million elderly persons living at or below the poverty level, which according to 1985 standards was $6503 for couples and $5156 for individuals (based on data from the US Bureau of the Census). Seventy-five percent of older householders own their own homes, which may be a mixed blessing because their homes are older also and may require increased maintenance that cuts into their spendable income.

For the majority of elderly in America, access to health care is provided, and limited, by Medicare. The majority (70%) of older Americans consider themselves to be in good health with fewer than 30 days per year in which activities were restricted due to illness or accidents. However most older persons have at least one chronic disease and some have multiple health problems. The leading complaints are listed as follows[2]:

1. Arthritis
2. Hypertension
3. Heart disease
4. Orthopedic impairments
5. Cataracts
6. Diabetes
7. Hearing and visual impairments

The elderly account for 31% of the total health care expenditure of the United States. On the other hand, out-of-pocket expenses rose to $1666 per person in 1985, which means that each older person must underwrite about 25% of their yearly health care costs because higher deductibles and a decrease in the amount of reimbursement are now a part of the Medicare program. In 1986, older persons spent almost $12 billion to meet cost-sharing (deductible or coinsurance) requirements.

In the summer of 1988 Medicare was expanded to include catastrophic coverage. After the patient pays $560 for the first day of hospitalization, they may have unlimited days of hospital care. In addition Medicare covered prescription drugs up to 50%, after the patient paid the first $600 per year. Included also was respite care, with the government paying for the costs of 80 hours a year for a nurse or home health aids to come to the home to give the family time off from the duties of caring for the patient. Hospice care was increased to an unlimited number of days for the terminally ill. Skilled nursing care was expanded to cover up to 150 days after an acute illness. There was no change in custodial care, the most potentially devastating financial blow to a family's income; there is still no coverage. These new features were to be financed by Medicare beneficiaries by higher monthly premiums and a special surtax. However, because of the increased expense of the coverage, politically active seniors rallied the older population to protest the coverage. On January 1, 1990, this coverage ended. Relatively well-off persons may purchase Medi-gap insurance to cushion against the huge expenses that Medicare does not cover. Those elderly citizens who live at or below the poverty level can afford no such cushion.

The average hospital stay is $7^1/2$ days; those who suffer longer illnesses will face staggering bills. The hospital charge of $592 must be paid at the beginning of each 90 day benefit period, and there are no benefits for a 60 day period between illnesses. Skilled nursing facility benefits revert to the old rules, which allow entry into the skilled facility only if it is preceded by a minimum 3 day acute hospital stay. Coverage is limited to 100 days for each benefit period, and 60 days must pass after the 100 day benefit is exhausted before readmission from a hospital to the skilled facility is permitted. Furthermore, after the first 20 days, the patient must pay $74 a day out of pocket.

Fortunately, Congress adopted tighter controls over physicians' fees for Medicare patients. The controls were phased-in January 1, 1990, and will be fully implemented over a 5 year period. The overall limit set by the Catastrophic Insurance coverage is gone, however. Premiums for medical coverage will cost $26.60 a month in 1990. In addition, the patient pays the first $75 of the physician bills each year plus 20% of the remaining approved physician charges.

Medicare, which has a multibillion dollar budget, spends about 30% of it on patients who have less than 1 year to live. This is primarily spent in high-technology areas using life-extending techniques on patients who, if given a choice, would probably prefer to be at home as long as comfort and support were available. With the new changes in Medicare coverage, that may soon be a possibility. As health care consumers become more open in their communication with family and physicians, they can guide the level of care they wish to receive.

In a time when the aging population is on a geometric increase they are poorly protected against the costs of chronic illness. Although some of these costs are covered under Medicare, Part B, with the shifts from in-hospital care to out-patient care the overall costs can become impossible to manage on fixed incomes.

In 1983, the exploding cost of health care caused significant changes in Medicare payments within hospitals. Under the Prospective Payment System, hospitals were offered incentives to shorten the length of stay for Medicare recipients. Length of stay was predetermined by a diagnostic-related grouping (DRG) so that an average number of days for a specific disease was determined; hospitals were then reimbursed for the predetermined stay rather than on the actual number of hospitalized days. Therefore if a DRG designated a 5 day stay and the patient was discharged earlier, the hospital could keep the difference. However, if the patient exceeded the allowed period, the hospital had to absorb the difference. This has significant impact on Medicare beneficiaries, decreasing the length of stay (averaging about 6%) and increasing early hospital discharge. Also, because of increased deductibles, many are more ill on admission. Common DRGs with the sharpest decline in length of stay were hip and femur procedures, joint replacements, fractures of the hip or pelvis, and cerebrovascular disorders.

Early discharge has lead to a proliferation of home health care agencies. More patients are discharged to skilled nursing facilities and require more acute care in those facilities. According to *Health Care Financing Review,*[11] patients discharged with large length of stay reductions increased their use of a skilled nursing facility (SNF) care by 83% and increased their use of home health care by 102% between 1982 to 1987. In addition, the increase of day surgery has led to increased demand on home health care. Because Medicare is focused on acute care, home health care is provided as a fol-low-up to an acute episode rather than chronic care. Medicare provides unlimited home health visits under rigorous criteria but it must be related to recovery from an acute ill-ness and must require skilled nursing, speech and/or physical therapy, or a home health aide. Medicare provides limited coverage in skilled nursing facilities, with very rigid requirements. It is available only after a hospitalization, limited to 100 days per benefit, and requires around-the-clock skilled care. Such shifts in coverage expose older people to continuously rising financial liability. To the extent that older Americans must forego health services because they can not afford it, they are denied access to care and deprived of even the basic quality of health they could enjoy.

Access to health is denied to many others as well. Increasing reports regarding migrant workers, the undocumented, and the homeless indicate that they receive little or no care, thereby jeopardizing their health and the population at large.

Poor, Migrant Workers, Homeless

In the United States, poor people are more ill than nonpoor people. Blacks, chicanos, native Americans, and migrant workers, and the homeless are more ill than suburban, white, white collar-employed people. And they get less medical care. At least 35 million people have no insurance to pay for their health care. Some are ignored by the system and some encounter barriers when attempts are made to reach them. Lack of informa-tion, lack of transportation, inability to pay, a complex bureaucratic system, and lan-guage differences are all barriers to the health care delivery system.

The homeless number in the millions across the country. There are numerous reasons for their plight. Rising rents, low paying jobs, and the loss of affordable and federally subsidized housing have contributed to the problem. Some, who might be able to afford the monthly rent, can not afford the 2 months rent in advance required by many apart-ment owners. The homeless constitute the following three distinct groups[16]:
1. Have-nots—working people who are underemployed or have had a temporary setback
2. Can-nots—those disabled by substance abuse, poor health, mental illness, or illit-eracy
3. Will-nots—those so incapacitated from years of mental illness and living on the street that they are willing to accept only limited assistance

Migrant workers tend to belong to large families. Half of the workers are less than 25 years old, with a life expectancy of 49 years. Although illegal, children often work in the fields to supplement the family income. Because work is episodic and the families travel to crops that are ready for harvest, schooling is limited and fewer than 50% complete the ninth grade. Health problems include the following:

1. Tuberculosis
2. Parasitic diseases
3. Pesticide poisoning
4. Multiple pregnancies with little prenatal treatment

Such illnesses contribute to high infant mortality and high morbidity and mortality among the rest of the migrant population.[10]

Most Americans assume that Medicaid pays health care costs for the majority of the poor; actually only about 31% are covered. Five million people annually report that they do not seek medical care because they cannot afford it. Medicaid is a joint federal-state program designed specifically for the poor. Because each state administers its own program, resulting in essentially 50 different programs, eligibility requirements and coverage differ from state to state. At a minimum, those who qualify include the following:

1. People in welfare programs
2. Those enrolled in Social Security Supplemental programs
3. Those enrolled in Aid to Families with Dependent Children (AFDC)

Each state sets its own welfare criteria. Therefore, many underprivileged people slip through the cracks. The following are some of the reasons for lack of aid:

1. No eligibility for welfare
2. No permanent address
3. Fear of deportation
4. Lack of understanding of the complexities of the system

Many public health nurses complain that they find it difficult to access the right agency through the bureaucratic maze and can well understand clients' problems.

Literacy and language problems foil attempts to fill out forms or understand instructions. Health teaching becomes impossible because directions are poorly fathomed. Nurses' own values often conflict with the realities faced each day by the poor and the homeless. Sterile techniques for dressing changes become impossible when one lives on the street with a cardboard box for a shelter. Compliance is perceived as poor when directions are not followed, medications are taken incorrectly, or treatments are not completed as prescribed, when it is lack of language or literacy that may be at fault.

There are severe restrictions in access to health care as a result of cutbacks in funding over the past few years. In 1981 cuts in funding for AFDC resulted in a reduction of aid to 500,000 families. When the food stamp program was reviewed 1 million persons lost eligibility. This may be further reduced as a result of unusual rises in food costs during 1990. By 1983, 600,000 people were deleted from medicaid coverage, which now covers only 31% of all poor Americans and in some states only 20% are covered. Children have been hardest hit by these decreases, as a result of cuts in actual aid, cuts in immunization programs, and reductions in WIC and school lunch programs. The results were almost inevitable: a rise in the incidence of pertussis, measles, and malnutrition. It is because of all the cutback programs that there is increasing discussion about the rationing of health care in America.

Rationing of Health Care

Twenty years ago, making health care available to the poor and the elderly through Medicare and Medicaid appeared to be a first step toward a national health insurance program. Today, public policy has shifted away from expanding access to health toward cost containment. Americans have always been opposed to rationing, except in case of emergency, but more is being written about rationing of health care than ever before. This is certainly not a new concept; it has been practiced with varying degrees of intensity throughout time. The quality and quantity of health services in this country have always been predicated on the person's ability to pay. Those who could afford the best received it. Heart transplants are an example of this; those who have $150,000 have access to the physicians and hospitals performing the procedure.

Rationing was also based on other means. When kidney dialysis was new, access to the limited number of machines was determined by such "objective measures" as quality of life, potential contributions to the community, and age. Triage is another form of rationing wherein those who are most critically ill take precedence over those who are not.

Rationing is an accepted fact in industrialized countries such as Britain and Canada where age limits access to high-technology procedures. In those countries, persons over the age of 55 are excluded from procedures such as by-pass surgery and transplants. The trade-off is that all people have equal access to comprehensive personal health care. Does this make a difference? British life expectancy is slightly longer and infant mortality is lower than in the United States.[12] Canada has a longer life expectancy and a lower infant mortality rate, spending 8.6% of its GNP on health, whereas we expend a staggering 11.4%.[3]

Must rationing be an accepted fact? Many people believe so; people from such diverse fields as ethics and government are beginning to discuss the topic in forums all over the country. One leading proponent is Daniel Callahan of the Hastings Center, who argues that many medical initiatives benefit the elderly at the expense of better care for younger people. He states that eventually there will be an age-based standard for the termination of life-extending treatment. Richard Lamm, former governor of Colorado, created a furor when he stated that people who were terminally ill have a "duty to die." He argued that the money spent on transplants could be better spent on prenatal care. Taking an alternative approach, Edward Schneider believes that using age as a criteria is a step backward from ethics.[29] He contends that savings gained from denying the elderly would not necessarily be reallocated to the young. The savings might go toward defense or farm subsidies. Few health care professionals, particularly nurses, have spoken out on this topic. Yet they are the ones who will ultimately be involved in the outcome.

QUALITY AND ALLOCATION OF HEALTH CARE
Basic Levels of Care: For Whom, By Whom?

In 1971, Elliot Richardson, then Secretary of the US Department of Health, Education and Welfare, testified that:

> In general our critical health problems today do not arise because the health of our people is worsening, or because expenditures on health care have been niggardly, or because we have been negligent as a nation in developing health care resources, or because we have been unconcerned about providing financial protection against ill-health. We must look elsewhere. I should like to suggest that our present concern is a function of two broad problems. The first is the inequality in health status and care, and in access to financing. The other is the pervasive problem of rising medical costs. . . .[25]

Although that statement is almost 20 years old, little has changed and it is still applicable. The government, with the introduction of prospective payments and DRGs, is still spending approximately 10% of its Gross National Product on health care. In 1986, hospitals had a total of $180 billion in revenues, 7% more than in the previous year. The figures are not in for 1990, but it is estimated that hospital profits will continue to grow at a rate of 10% or more per annum.[19] Incomes of the medical and allied health community have not decreased either. What remains is a two-tiered system in which those with the ability to pay have different health care and access to that care than those with limited ability to pay. According to Congressman Ronald Dellums in his introduction to The Health Service Act:

> We have in this country today a health delivery system where the quality of health care received is determined by race, language, national origin, or income level. Health is a commodity to be bought and sold in the marketplace, it is not viewed as a right of the people; a service to be provided by the government. However, financing is not the only problem facing the people when it comes to the delivery of health care. Other, equally important, problems are the maldistribution of health manpower, the unequal access to services, the unreliable quality of care, and the lack of public control over health care. No matter how much we guarantee the payment of services to the people, it is of little comfort to them if there is no one around to provide the service.[6]

Despite highly sophisticated technology available to 85% of Americans with some form of health insurance or private funds, there are 37 million who receive little or no health care and whose access to high-technology is limited. High-technology can detect diseases and provide treatment that was unimaginable 30 years ago. Among the technologies introduced over the past years are computerized automated tomography (CAT) scanners, positive emission tomography (PET) scanners, artificial organs, parenteral nutrition, and organ transplants. These technologies save lives, but at extraordinary costs. A coronary bypass costs around $30,000 and is gaining as much reputation as the hysterectomy in frequency of abuse. Heart transplants cost about $150,000 with multiple organ (heart and lung) following closely. Overall the

United States spent over $2 billion for neonatal care, $2.2 billion in renal dialysis, $1.5 billion for coronary bypass, and nearly $0.25 billion on transplants.*

Each year technology becomes more complex with newer machines and procedures, and increasing costs. Every hospital demands the newest and finest equipment with little thought of sharing the technology. After the equipment is in place, the numbers of patients needing it begins to escalate.

Many people simply can not afford the cost involved. Mammography, CAT and PET scans are out of the question for millions of citizens. Yet the demands increase every day. It is deeply touching to hear the pleas of parents requesting an organ transplant for a sick child. Seeing a once healthy young male on television while his family urgently requests funds for a heart transplant causes many generous people to open their hearts and purses to assist. But what of the thousands of others who have no platform? Do they have an equal right to the care they need? While one state (Illinois) may underwrite the costs of high technology, another (Oregon) refuses to do so. Each has compelling reasons for its decisions and complex problems are the result. Illinois has promised $200,000 to those in need of transplants, while those in need of prenatal care go wanting. Oregon insists that every citizen of Oregon have access to basic care, while children in need of transplants die. Because of regulations that transfer national funds to each state in the form of block grants, each state has the right to make such determinations. Many states have little regulation and attend to each issue in a hit-or-miss fashion, for who would like to decide whether it is better to save 2000 children's lives through pre- and post-natal care or to sacrifice the lives of several transplant patients?

AIDS

Access to adequate health care has also been denied people with AIDS. The debate on financing AIDS services will assuredly include the issue of budgetary constraints and unequal access. As of May 1989, blacks and Hispanics accounted for an estimated 20% of all AIDS cases. Many of these patients rely on publically sponsored health services. Even those fortunate enough to have health insurance ultimately run out of benefits. Yet, in recent years only two fifths of the poor qualify for Medicaid; therefore it can not be viewed as a panacea. The system has not taken the necessary steps to anticipate the needs of people with AIDS. Catastrophic health insurance remains a future dream for people with AIDS, and people who have cancer.

In 1988 there were 64,506 cases of AIDS reported in the United States, with 36,255 known deaths. The year 1989 saw the approach of nearly 100,000 cases. The mortality rate is about 56%. The Public Health Service predicts that 1 to $1^1/2$ million Americans are currently infected with the virus and will manifest the symptoms of AIDS or AIDS-related illnesses. Public Health Service experts project that 365,000 cases of AIDS will have occurred by 1992, with a mortality of 262,000. The population at greatest risk are intravenous drug users, homosexuals, bisexuals, and people with multiple sexual partners.

*Figures are based on 1984 statistics.

A group of increasing importance is children with AIDS. More than 1600 pediatric cases are reported, 618 cases in a year between 1988 and 1989, and the majority of patients become infected as a result of the drug culture. Human Immunodeficiency Virus (HIV) transmission is established as resulting from blood and body secretions. It is not a highly contagious disease if the proper precautions are taken. Former US Surgeon General C. Everett Koop recommended that monogamous relationships, the use of condoms, and avoidance of dirty needles will protect the majority of persons. Health care personnel are cautioned to use standard precautions for blood and body secretions. The Center for Disease Control (CDC) cites universal precautions as the most effective way health professionals can protect themselves from contracting the disease.

Unfortunately, AIDS victims are faced with discrimination at every level throughout this country. Health care personnel discriminate, families discriminate, whole communities discriminate. Potential victims are afraid to come forward for testing, many refuse to disclose their sexual contacts, and some have lost jobs and homes based on a positive HIV test. Until the issue is faced squarely, it will be impossible to solve many of the problems associated with the care and treatment of AIDS patients.

Mental Illness

Although mental illness has limited coverage under some health insurance policies, and no coverage under many, it is a big budget item costing $9.4 billion a year. This cost is an out-of-pocket expense for some or is provided by local and state government. With the deinstitutionalization of the mentally ill, many were seen in county outpatient clinics, some were placed in halfway houses, and some have become the homeless. Incapacitated, unable to work, and unwilling to join the "system," the homeless mentally ill populate parks, street corners, and grates and public buildings of every inner-city in America. This problem poses many ethical questions. Are the mentally ill capable of making their own health care decisions? Should society allow them freedom of choice or, for their own welfare, should the mentally ill be placed in protective environments and given the health care they need? Who should decide? The individual, the family, the government? Should there be some minimal standard of living to which all of us are entitled? For further discussion on this topic, see Chapter 7.

Can the United States afford to care for infants, migrant families, AIDS patients, the homeless, and the mentally ill? Uwe Reinhardt writes that this nation could well afford to spend 11% of the GNP for health care, if only there was agreement on the ethical issue of right to health care for all versus the moral obligation to the poor. Considering past history, Reinhardt surmises that Americans believe that health care is a moral obligation of local communities and not a right. If that premise is correct then he proposes the following hierarchy:

Tourist class care—publicly financed health care with some form of rationing
Business class care—health care financed through employer-paid health insurance
Designer class health care—health care delivered in luxury suites and paid for by
the well-to-do[24]

In previous years, national health insurance plans have been defeated, often through heavy lobbying by health care providers. The decision between high-technology or prevention has yet to be decided. As telethons and televised pleas indicate, Americans are a generous people. Will they be willing to pay, through taxes, what is willingly donated so that everyone has equal access to health care?

Political and Social Systems and Their Impact

Because so much of the funding for health care comes from the government through laws that are enacted, one must be acquainted with the political and social system that shapes the legislation. This country has a two party system, but that says little about the shades of political and social philosophy that molds the thought processes of legislators. Although Republicans are presumed more conservative than Democrats, there are many overlapping beliefs at the center of each party. A review of the voting record on any social issue will indicate the extent to which centrists of either party cross over to join likeminded legislators of the opposition. The latest Medicare expansion was supported by an overwhelming majority of both parties in the House and Senate, but it was no giveaway program because it was designed to be self-supporting. It was therefore acceptable to liberals and conservatives from both parties.

To find actual differences in political beliefs, one must look at the extremes of each party, because they more accurately reflect what the public believes the party stands for. The stereotypical ideology attributed to the Republican Party is that of the conservative, "less government intervention is best government," business oriented, rich man's party; whereas Democrats are supposedly for the working man, government intervention, and legislation to address social ills. Actually, it is the conservative versus the liberal belief that is reflected. Each party has a range from conservative to liberal, and it is necessary for the voter to be well informed of the philosophical stance of each candidate, as well as party affiliation. However, to vote in an election one must declare a party affiliation, be an independent, or decline to state, which eliminates one from primaries. Demographics indicate that the majority of Democrats are working people, minorities, and people living in large cities. Republicans tend to come from Midwest farm land, Deep South, and Mid-Atlantic States, and, increasingly, are younger members of the whitecollar labor force.

The Constitution assigns Congress all legislative powers; therefore the Congress enacts laws. The President executes laws and the Supreme Court interprets the law. The President has the right to veto a law, but Congress may override the veto. Each state in the Union has a similar system to enact, execute, and interpret state laws.

Both state and federal legislators are representatives of the electorate and, to survive elections, they must demonstrate their ability to enact legislation and secure resources that are beneficial to their constituents. The Senate is the smaller body because each state is allowed only two senators, whereas House membership is based on population—the most populous states receive the most representation. A bill must clear both houses before it is sent for Presidential signature.* A bill enacted into law must also

---

*The way a bill becomes a law is beyond the scope of this chapter. For more information, see Mason D and Talbott S: *Political action handbook for nurses,*[20] Menlo Park, Addison-Wesley publishers.

have an appropriations bill, to have funds necessary for putting the program into effect. Traditionally, the House of Representatives has the power to originate tax bills, and it assumes the power to initiate appropriation bills also. The President submits a budget to Congress each January, which contains the programs for the year. The budget reflects the President's political and social philosophy. Decisions related to the federal budget are based on a variety of political, social, and economic issues. Each governmental agency wants a larger part of the budget, yet dividing the limited funds among the competing forces is necessary. Which agency gets the largest cut depends on the President's vision of the country's needs, based on personal philosophy and ability to gain support of the legislators. After Congress reviews and revises the President's budget, it is returned for presidential signature. Under President Reagan, the Department of Defense received the largest share of the budget with sizeable cuts coming out of The Department of Health and Human Services. To meet increasing defense spending, Congress reduced the budget for Medicare and Medicaid by $13 billion.

By assessing the political and social philosophy of the majority of the legislators and the President during the period of 1980-1984, one sees that a conservative budget was appropriated. The Republicans, for the first time since 1954, gained control of the Senate and increased their numbers to 192 in the House. By adding 30 conservative Southern Democrats the Republicans counted on at least 212 votes to the Democratic 243, some of whom joined the conservative coalition. Under the Program for Economic Recovery, the Reagan administration replaced many of the federal health care grant programs with unrestricted block grants to the states. The health planning system that attempted to contain health costs and insure proper distribution of services was dismantled. Funding to the states was cut 25%. The theme of the recovery program was that a safety net was to be provided for the truly needy, but no one defined the terms.

In general, since 1960, major legislation for health and human rights was enacted by a Democratic president and a liberal Democratic Congress. Bills such as the Civil Rights Act, the Food Stamp Act, the Health Manpower and the Nurse Training Act were initiated in the 1960s. Under Republicans in the 1970s funding for these were expanded, the WIC program was funded, as was the Sudden Infant Death Syndrome and Child Abuse prevention program. Curtailment of funds for social policy became noticeable in the early 1980s, when disillusionment with previous policies, an escalating inflation rate, and increased taxation caused a conservative backlash. The magnitude of this is illustrated by the fact that in the 97th Congress of 1981, only 46 Senators and 236 Congressmen had four or more years of experience.[17]

In 1988, voting resulted in the election of a Republican president, George Bush, and a change to a Democratically controlled legislature. The 101st Congress contained 262 Democrats and 173 Republicans in the House and 56 Democrats and 44 Republicans in the Senate. Because the census was taken in 1990, the entire House of Representatives will stand for election in 1991.

President Bush, in campaign promises, stated that he planned no major changes in the governing of the country. Analysts believe that the majority of voters supported

Reagan policies and therefore voted for Bush. The following issues led to this support:
1. Peace
2. National security
3. Economic prosperity
4. Concerns about higher taxes
5. Crime

Although most Americans reported satisfaction with the general state of national affairs, they were not satisfied with the state of the health care system. A national survey indicates that 89% of the American public thought that fundamental changes were needed in the health care system. No major changes appear imminent, although discussion about some form of national health crops up with increasing regularity. Polls by the Gallop and Harris organizations, completed in 1989, indicate that 75% favor the concept of national health insurance. However, the budget remains a largely conservative one with no massive infusion of dollars for social problems.

The Supreme Court may also acquire a conservative or liberal flavor depending on the justices' point of view regarding the construction of the Constitution. Presidential appointment to the court is based on judicial experience, political involvement, and philosophy. Strict constitutional constructionists tend to be conservative and to be appointed by conservative presidents. However, once appointed to the court, most justices appear to migrate 'toward the center' so that few ideologues have been on the recent Courts. Former President Reagan appointed the last justices, notably the first woman to hold that office, Sandra Day O'Connor. The Reagan court was, for the most part, strict constructionist and conservative. Because Justices of the Supreme Court rule on the constitutionality of the law it is vital that their decisions remain constant over time or every contested law would be argued endlessly. One such issue is the one on abortion.

Pro-life vs Pro-choice

In 1973 the Supreme Court, in *Roe v. Wade,* ruled that any state laws that prohibited or restricted a woman's right to abortion during the first 3 months of pregnancy were illegal. This resulted in conflicting ethical and social opinions. One group, the pro-life movement, believes that conception marks the beginning of new life and that any move to terminate that life is analogous to murder. The second group, pro-choice, believes that each woman has the right to determine what she wants to do to, or have happen to, her body and if she chooses to have an abortion, it is her legal right to do so. For some, life must be regarded as sacred and termination of life at any point is a crime. Others believe that although abortion is distasteful, there are circumstances in which it is justifiable, such as incest or rape. Still others believe that early termination of a deformed or defective fetus is acceptable. Another group believes that early termination, during the first trimester, is acceptable but late termination is not.

The pro-life group cites various religious beliefs that do not allow interference of the procreative process and views abortion as tantamount to infanticide. The group works ceaselessly to repeal the Supreme Court decision. Unfortunately, in the last few years some fanatics bomb abortion clinics and, in general, act in ways that detract from the overall ethical stance of the group.

Those who argue in favor of abortion emphasize a woman's control over her own body. They explain that the quality of life is as important as the right to life and suggest that the quality of life for an unwanted baby is minimal. Although many agree, most people do not support abortion as a form of birth control and have negative feeling about abortion after the fifth month for anything but the mother's safety.

In its 1989 decision in *Webster v. Reproductive Health Services,* the Supreme Court narrowed the federal interpretation of the right to abortion. With this decision, the court upheld the constitutionality of a Missouri law that sharply restricted the availability of publically funded abortions, and also required doctors to test for viability of a fetus at 20 weeks. Although this appeared to narrow the focus of *Roe v. Wade* and invite individual states to address the issue of abortion, it did not overturn Roe entirely. The results of this decision are still being explored and there are other states' cases that remain to be heard. In a poll conducted in 1989 by *Newsweek* magazine, the majority of Americans support abortion in some form, whether it be unrestricted or with special circumstances, and this issue crosses party lines. One fact has emerged: both pro-life and pro-choice movements are becoming more vocal and each side threatens to have abortion become a key issue in the coming elections. Florida's governor, Bob Martinez, called a special session of the legislature to consider enacting strong, new abortion-limiting legislation. The lobbying by pro-choice and life advocates was heavy. In the end, not one of the governor's proposals passed. Was this a prediction for the future? So far the answer is still in doubt.

HEALTH PROMOTION AND DISEASE PREVENTION

It is a paradoxical government that pays farmers to grow tobacco, warns citizens of its dangers, and supports medical care for those who choose to use tobacco. It is also a paradox that this nation spends billions of dollars to treat diseases arising from environmental pollution, poor nutrition, stress, and toxic waste, and spends very little on prevention. Streams, lakes, and oceans are giving clear messages that the food chain is being irreparably damaged, yet nothing is done about it. Science has eradicated small pox, prevented polio, diphtheria, and whooping cough, but it can not cure the common cold. Antibiotics can cure bacterial infections but viruses are becoming more deadly. Payment is made to a health delivery system for illnesses incurred, not for maintenance of health. Medicine does not equal health, yet physicians earn considerable salaries, vast prestige, and millions of research dollars, whereas those involved in prevention gather little recognition. In fact, the physician who knows less about the whole patient may have more status and collect larger fees (e.g., the cardiologist versus the family practitioner).

Another paradox is that illness can be defined and measured by morbidity and mortality tables; health is more complex, and often defined as the lack of illness. Although life expectancy rates are increasing, it is not because of better health, but because bacterial infections are not fatal, nor are there wildfire pandemic diseases such as the plague.

Widespread problems arise from lifestyle problems, stress, poor diet, smoking, the use of alcohol and other drugs, lack of exercise, and pollution. The Surgeon General's office estimates that as much as half of the United States mortality is due to unhealthy behavior or lifestyle; 20% to environmental factors. Thus while the population looks to medicine to cure the disease, the true cure lies in behavior changes that are difficult to accomplish. It seems easier to cope with a coronary bypass than it is to eat sensibly, exercise regularly, and abandon smoking. Humans engage in magical thinking, believing that they will know when they are about to become ill so that they can give up the behavior that is causing it. It seems less expensive to tolerate filthy waterways and polluted air than to restore the environment to healthy levels. Again, as with other health issues, this nation does not have a social policy that can shape the manner in which public funds are distributed. At present, public funds are invested largely in illness, with miniscule amounts (less than 1% of the health care budget) distributed to health promotion and disease prevention. Yet, while all other consumer prices increased by 1% in 1987, medical costs escalated to 7.7%. In the long run, prevention may be the best investment, with fewer dollars needed and more people served. This works well with the economist's theory of "more bang for the buck." The Public Health Research Group estimates that $100 billion is spent each year on preventable illnesses, yet today we have an ". . . armamentarium of preventive principles that work and work well. Prevention holds significant promise for problems as diverse as stroke, immune disorders, and a huge range of chronic, debilitating disease from pernicious anemia to osteoporosis.[4]

Nor have the health care professions served society well. Ivan Illich states that by transforming pain, illness, and death from personal challenge into a technical problem, medicine expropriates the potential of people to deal with their condition in an autonomous way.[14] Physicians and nurses have done little to teach the consumer how to stay out of the system, to manage their own wellness, and to live healthier lifestyles. Nursing in particular has health as a primary agenda and should be on the forefront of health promotion, yet the majority of nurses do not assume that responsibility. Even worse, they do not see health as an area of expertise.

School Health

The World Health Organization (WHO) defines health as the state of complete mental, physical, and social wellbeing, not just the absence of disease. Certainly this is an holistic view encompassing all the factors that contribute to the quality of life. With that definition, school systems could design health programs from kindergarten through college. In the primary grades, schools focus on prevention with programs for immunizations and hearing and eye checks, but all too often the programs are underfunded. School nurses are almost always the first to be discharged when budget cuts are made. Health promotion is either ignored or relegated to a small portion of the curriculum borne by the already overburdened primary teacher. With content as complex as substance abuse, HIV infections, and sex education, the primary source of information should be a nurse who has had the educational preparation to impart that information. In addition, the school nurse can spot first signs of alcohol or other drug abuse and intervene at an early stage.

But education should not stop in the primary grades. High school and college students can profit from classes on healthy lifestyles and how to achieve them. Certainly it is important for students to learn how the health care system works. In addition, they need to learn about health insurance, selecting a primary care provider, use of generic drugs, how to get a second opinion, and how to get good care within the hospital.

Sex Education

Parents are often so busy with their own work schedules they are not involved with the school system to any large degree. Teachers complain that there is no one available in the home to assist the student with homework or study. Yet when content regarding sex information is discussed, parents are at PTA meetings and at schoolboard meetings in full force. All too often, parents demand to be the sole provider of sex information to their offspring. This information is frequently inadequate, incorrect, and given too late. Children with little information regarding their sexual health are having children in epidemic proportions. Teenage pregnancies are altering millions of lives and costing the government billions of dollars a year in subsidies. What is lacking is adequate information regarding birth control, whether it be in the form of self-control, the pill, or other forms of contraception. Besides increases in teenage pregnancies, there are increases in sexually transmitted diseases, including HIV infections.

This is another example of a failed social policy. Because our culture is traditionally conservative in sexual matters, sex was once a forbidden topic. Currently we are bombarded with sexual images in commercials and movies. Television is a major purveyor of sex, vividly demonstrating intense love scenes. However, the same medium that extols the thrill of sex can not advertise contraceptives. Children learn the excitement of sexual activity but not the possible sequelae—unwanted pregnancy and disease. Nowhere in our culture is there systematic information regarding human sexuality, disease transmission, pregnancy, and contraception. In this area, the public operates under Puritanical rules, while allowing permissive sexual display. Prevention is always the least expensive form of intervention. This nation needs a policy that encourages sex education beginning in the primary grades and continuing through high school and college. Contraception information should be available so that sexually active teens can learn how to protect themselves. Moral issues should be addressed in homes and places of worship while information is disseminated in the schools.

Stress Reduction

Society is fast-paced and complex, with rapidly changing social and cultural norms. People are placed in competitive arenas where success is the order of the day: sometimes the competition comes from within. Wherever its source, the feeling engendered can be overwhelming. Work, play, and particularly human relations, can disrupt the internal sense of harmony and peace and produce stress. All stressful situations are not harmful; anticipation of a long-awaited kiss can produce the same physiological response as a minor automobile accident. Heartbeats increase, blood pressure elevates, and butterflies invade the stomach, resulting in the stress response. Some stress is necessary in life to motivate people to accomplish tasks, confront challenges, and pursue goals so the individual can grow and change. Some people thrive on stress and others become ill. Certain diseases such as ulcers, colitis, asthma, eczema, psoriasis, and migraine headaches are thought to be stress-induced. The physiologic response to stress activates the nervous and endocrine systems releasing epinephrine, norepinephrine, and other catecholamines.

Scientists propose many theories regarding the causes of stress. Some believe it is the accumulation of life events such as marriage, divorce, becoming widowed, even Christmas, or taking a vacation that can induce feelings of stress.[13] Others suggest that personality characteristics and stress are related. Cardiologists Friedman and Rosenman[7] conducted studies of people they called type A and found that they were constant hurriers, highly competitive, worked on multiple tasks at one time, aggressive, and hated waiting in lines. They often had higher incidents of heart disease than their peers who had a more relaxed approach to life. On the positive side, behavior can be learned to reduce the effects of stress on the physiological system.

Because stress-related illness depends on mental processes, it is possible to exert control over the processes. Change in a disruptive situation such as work or interpersonal relationships may be possible. Seeking counseling may assist in the search for alternatives to high-stress situations. Often relaxation techniques can inhibit the physical response to stress. Biofeedback is one form of relaxation that is proven effective on stress management. Meditation is a centuries-old form of relaxation that is simple, inexpensive, and effective. Meditation requires a comfortable chair, a quiet room, freedom from distraction, and a 20 minute period of time, preferably twice a day. To meditate, one simply becomes comfortable and clears one's mind of extraneous thoughts. A mantra, or single syllable word, helps keep focus. *Oom* or *won* are often used but any word will do. By eliminating stressors in the environment or by controlling reactions to the stressors, one may achieve a healthier lifestyle. Even more potent is the fact that health care is the responsibility of the individual, and decision-making is under individual control.

Stress reduction techniques are easily taught and certainly within the nurse's realm, yet nurses rarely initiate such teaching. If nurses believe in health promotion and primary prevention, they will address the issue of stress control by learning and teaching techniques that will assist clients.

Women's Health and Men's Health

Women were considered the heartier of the sexes because they lived longer and had fewer incidents of heart disease, ulcers, and lung cancer. But this has changed. In past decades, women had limited choices and most became wives and mothers, but with the women's movement came wider choices and increased stresses. Today women contend with the same problems that men face in the workforce—desire to advance, income to support the family, and status gained from work. In addition women often work 8 hours at one job and then work another few hours at home. Some women must decide whether to forego children for work; others worry about child care. With the increase in smoking, stress in the work setting, and a polluted environment, women are rapidly approaching men in stress-related illnesses.

Prevention of illness is the best defense against the health care industry. Getting a second or third opinion is the second best line of defense. Patients, at one time, were loath to ask their physicians for referral for another opinion. Now almost every insurance company requires it. Even so, many procedures are performed for little reason. In a Rand study completed in 1988, only 56% of the coronary bypass surgeries performed were appropriate. Hysterectomies fare little better when 33% of the operations performed per year are unnecessary. Prostates are performed 29% of the time without good reason. One research group estimates that more than $10 billion is spent each year on surgical procedures that are not necessary.[5] In America, mastectomies are performed more often than lumpectomies, even though research in Europe, over a 10 year period, indicates that survival rates are as good with the less intrusive procedure.

Prevention of illness includes the following:

1. Sensible diet to maintain weight
2. Exercise
3. Stress reduction
4. Elimination of smoking
5. Limiting alcohol consumption
6. Balancing work and recreation

Although prevention for men and women is essentially the same, there are a few differences. Women need monthly breast examinations, yearly Pap smears, and, if over forty, regularly scheduled mammograms. Men need prostate check-ups on a regular basis. In addition a baseline electrocardiogram is probably a good idea for anyone over forty years old. The greatest barrier to routine check-ups is the lack of coverage for preventive examinations, which leads to out-of-pocket expenses of several hundred dollars.

Substance Abuse

Although death from infectious diseases declined as a result of antibiotics, there is a new group of health problems—respiratory diseases such as emphysema, chronic bronchitis, and lung cancer. Social problems such as alcoholism and drug addiction are front page news as movie stars and sports figures join the ranks of street people in "doing drugs." Cocaine was considered a recreational drug until the first 21-year-old athlete died of a massive heart attack after cocaine use. According to Joseph Califano, former Secretary of Health, Education, and Welfare, addiction is one of America's greatest health problems. He estimates that there are 50 million Americans addicted to cigarettes, 13 million abuse alcohol, and uncounted millions are addicted to heroin, marijuana, cocaine, barbiturates, and other forms of drugs.[5]

Yearly, smoking contributes to 130,000 deaths due to lung cancer, 170,000 deaths due to cardiovascular diseases, and 60,000 deaths due to respiratory diseases other than cancer. In 1984, Surgeon General C. Everett Koop stated that pollution from secondhand smoke in homes and the workplace can contain more contaminants than is permitted by most occupational and environmental regulations. Yet this same government that warns about the dangers of smoking provides subsidies to farmers who grow tobacco. The tobacco industry was forced to place warnings about the dangers of smoking on each package of cigarettes, yet they spend $2.5 billion advertising their product. In the past few years, nonsmokers have become more aggressive in securing rights to a smoke-free environment. Many localities have ordinances prohibiting smoking in public buildings and providing smoke-free areas in restaurants and in the workplace. In 1988 smoking was banned on airline flights of 1 hour or within the borders of some states. In 1989, the push was for a smoking ban within the borders of the United States. The decade of the 90s may see in-flight smoking banned internationally.

Another lifestyle problem, alcohol, contributes to the untimely death of citizens through cirrhosis of the liver, esophageal hemorrhage, cancer, and suicide. Include the numbers of deaths and maiming resulting from automobile accidents caused by drivers under the influence of alcohol and the statistics are staggering. There were over 28,000 highway fatalities in 1986. Alcohol and other substance abuse added $40 billion to the health budget. The incidents of family violence, and work and school absenteeism is escalating. There is no evidence that drinking alcoholic beverages in moderation is harmful to health but there is overwhelming evidence that abuse of it can cause significant physiological damage to the brain, the liver, and the gastrointestinal tract. Advertisements lead people to believe drinking is sophisticated, that chic and up-and-coming executives use it to become successful, or that it is wonderfully relaxing to have a drink after work. For some that may prove correct. For others it is deadly. The ads never show the deadly aspects of drinking. Social policy needs to be developed that bans advertisements glamorizing cigarettes and alcohol. Laws regarding smoke-free environments and the legal ages for purchasing or use of cigarettes and alcohol should be strictly enforced. Mandatory jail sentences for drunk drivers should be enacted and enforced in every state. Physicians and nurses need to have substance abuse content added to their curricula so they can diagnose and counsel at the early phase of a problem. Education regarding hazards of substance abuse must become part of every schoolchild's learning. Nurses must begin to shape social policy so that policy focuses on health promotion and prevention issues, rather than on restoration. Here is a void that nurses can fill with their knowledge and expertise and thus contribute to the health of the nation.

COMPETING SOCIAL ISSUES

Despite the fact that government has interceded in many areas of life, it normally is considered inappropriate for it to encroach too far into family life. Because the family represents personal freedom, the government has established very few laws regarding marriage, divorce, or childrearing. In general, there are laws for the protection of women and children, particularly in the area of family dysfunction. The government sees the family as the traditional two-parent family, with the father working and the mother managing the home. All other family structures are seen as deviant. Much has changed over the past decades and there are now multiple forms of family structures, without much policy to assist in their support.

Single-parent Families

There was a time when divorce was a social stigma and women with children had few skills to enable them to consider divorce an option. Now divorce no longer stigmatizes the family and the majority of married women with children are already in the workforce. But somehow the image of the perfect family is retained—two kids, mom in the kitchen, and dad in the office. Yet, the increases in divorce rates and numbers of single-parent families causes growing concern over family breakdown. Single-parent households account for 15% of American families. By age 18, nearly half of the children will have lived a period of time with a single parent.[30] Single parenthood is seen as a transitional state but all too often, especially past age 30, remarriage is not occurring. A recent study indicates that fewer than one fifth of unmarried head-of-household women remarried within the 5 year study period. Single parents are classified in one of the following ways:

1. Widowed
2. Divorced
3. Separated
4. Unmarried

However they are classified single-parents, and their families suffer from the public image of the perfect family.

In the perfect family, men bring home the money needed to support the family. The latest study by the Joint Select Task Force on Changing Families (1989) indicates that only 15% of families live in this traditional mode. Today most mothers, 62% nationally, work outside the home, and even though society knows the perfect family image is not reality and that even two-parent families need the mother's salary to live at middleclass levels, the myth that women work for pin money remains. Thus, often doing the same work, women earn less than men—about 60 cents to every dollar men earn. This also applies to women who are heads of the household. The result of this form of discrimination is that three out of five poor children come from single-parent families.

Working mothers have problems other than money. Job structure is usually inflexible and long, leaving little time or energy for homemaking and mothering. Just getting the children to the dentist or doctor is a major problem because the hours conflict with the wage earner's hours. Childcare is expensive and in short supply. Many single mothers have informal arrangements with grandparents, other relatives, or neighbors. School-age children may become part of the "latch-key kid" solution to childcare because they are unattended, from the time school lets out until the parent comes home. Single parents, because of job- and home-related time constraints, have little time for social interaction and may feel socially isolated.

Although lip service is paid to "equal pay for equal work," the overwhelming evidence is that it is not happening. This has increased the numbers of the working poor. Low paying jobs often do not offer health care insurance but pay enough to prevent the family from qualifying for Medicaid. Childhood diseases may become a nightmare from which no budget can recover. There is no one to care for the sick child, and the parent is forced to stay home to provide care while sacrificing the much needed paycheck. Sadly, many childhood diseases are preventable with proper immunizations, which are not universally available in this country.

What is needed is public policy that affords children access to free or affordable health care, resulting in primary prevention rather than tertiary intervention. Most industrialized nations have health coverage for all children; the United States does not. Also needed are enforceable laws that do not tolerate fathers avoiding child support.

Childcare is another social policy issue that has been overlooked. One option that government can take is to award tax breaks to companies that have in-house childcare facilities. School districts could combine after school activities at schools with a low fee, which would afford children the protection of supervised play. Stricter enforcement of childcare regulations would preclude molestation scandals, which are becoming more prevalent at childcare facilities. Childcare is on the agenda for the legislative year of 1990. It will be interesting to see what form it takes.

Alternative Family Styles

Divorce rates are rising continuously in the United States. Divorce affects each member of the family because children are deprived of the constant interaction of one parent and their divorced parents are concerned about finances, social relationships, and diminished time to meet family needs. When the single parent remarries, children from a previous marriage are often added to the family unit. There is little to guide blended families to resolve the complex problems remarriage brings. Even language is not supportive, because *stepmother* and *stepchild* are viewed as pejorative terms. What does a child call a parent's new spouse? Is is permissible for a stepparent to discipline the children: whose, his, hers, theirs? Step roles must be achieved rather than ascribed. Stepparents must earn love and respect; it is not automatic because they are mother or father. After remarriage, the incidents of failure to provide child support increases and the law is lax in enforcing the natural father's obligations. Sexual abuse of children is increasing. Children complain that other children are being treated better. Such problems are widespread, and each family has its own myriad of smaller or larger ones. An additional problem is that there are no social norms to assist the family to achieve the new roles required in the blended family. This problem is verified by the statistic that the divorce rate in remarriage is higher than the divorce rate in first marriages.

Living Together

During the 1980s, cohabitation increased rapidly as society began to accept it as an alternative to marriage. In a national sample, the majority of couples questioned believed that living together was a prelude to marriage. For many, it was an attractive alternative to marrying again. During the last census, the government developed an acronym for this phenomenon, *posslq,* which stands for people of the opposite sex sharing living quarters. In that census, 1.8 million couples were living together, more than double the number obtained in the previous census. Traditionally, couples who chose to live together come from the very poor; now however, another class has joined them—well-educated urban professionals and the somewhat less-educated previously married. The legal system has not resolved the legal ramifications involved in long-term cohabiting relationships. There are serious economic and social complexities stemming from this arrangement that have just begun to be addressed. The case of *Marvin v. Marvin,* involving property rights distribution between Lee Marvin and Michelle Triola-Marvin, his long time live in partner, indicates that the law is beginning to address what has become a societal norm. Seventeen states now recognize *de facto* marriages as having nearly the same rights as *de jure* marriages.

Homosexual Families

The alternative family lifestyle that has accrued the most stigma is the homosexual family. Homosexuals are "coming out of the closet" in ever increasing numbers. Their problems are much more societal than legal. Numerous laws have been passed assuring their civil rights, but society retains a largely negative prejudice against this group, making it more difficult to achieve their rights. Homosexual parents have difficulties obtaining custody of their children. They are not considered fit adoptive parents. Society is outraged when long-standing homosexual relationships seek the sanctity of marriage. With the advent of HIV infections, homophobia may well increase, rather than homosexuality becoming an acceptable alternative family style.

The Sandwich Generation

Aging parents live with their adult children for the following reasons:
1. Death of a spouse
2. Limited resources
3. Chronic illness
4. Emotional dependence

The burden of caring for aging parents often falls on women, traditionally the eldest daughter. However, approximately 60% of these women work outside the home. Increasingly the middle-aged generation is sandwiched between aging parents and young adult children. They are faced with the problems of their own careers and marriage and the problems encountered by their children and by their parents. Emotional and financial resources may be strained by the needs of both ends of the generational lifespan, resulting in conflict and guilt when the needs of one intersects the needs of the other. On a more positive note, the generational differences are not as great as the generations age. The three generations are usually in close touch with one another, giving aid and exerting influence.[28] Most adult children develop warm and loving relationships with their aging parents. The aging parent becomes a model for successful aging. However, when parents become frail and need supervision, problems arise.

Adult Day Care

An area of social concern is care of the elderly. Most elderly people live full and meaningful lives. Some become debilitated by disease and must reside in long-term care facilities. Others are primarily independent and need only supplementary home care. In addition, there are increasing numbers of frail elderly being cared for by their aging children. Often the caregivers are gainfully employed, not ready for retirement, and must face the problem of how to care for the parent who can not be left home unattended for long periods of time.

Daycare centers may help the older adult remain independent. They offer activities such as arts and crafts, exercise, health education, continuing education, and reality orientation and remotivation. Nutritionally balanced meals are served for a nominal cost. Daycare can fill a void in the older person's day. It can also provide a secure and nurturing environment while the caregiver continues to work. Some centers are allied with agencies such as the following:

1. United Way
2. Red Cross
3. Nursing homes
4. Acute hospitals

Some centers are associated with nursing homes or acute hospitals but are separate entities and are self-supporting. Some daycare centers are particularly innovative. They combine childcare with adult daycare, giving both generations the opportunity to spend time together. Surrogate grandparents have the warm love of the children and the children have a "family" during daycare hours.

Problems arise from costs and transportation. Most centers try to keep costs at a minimum, because almost everyone has a limited budget. If the caregiving family covers the cost, there is no tax incentive, no write-off, no tax shelter. Elderly parents who live with a child and who receive Social Security afford no tax advantage to the caregiver. The costs of food and shelter, as well as daycare, must be underwritten by the family.

Long-term Care

Nursing homes provide a vital function in the overall health care system. Although thought of as permanent homes for the elderly, they also serve many short-term functions such as rehabilitation. The following three levels of care are offered by nursing homes:

1. Skilled nursing—for the person who needs intensive 24-hour supervision and treatment by a registered nurse or other skilled rehabilitation service and paid for by Medicare or private funds
2. Intermediate care—for persons who do not require intensive care or treatment, but who, because of their mental or physical status, require care above the level of room and board
3. Custodial care—for persons who can no longer attend to their personal needs and need supervision with activities of daily living such as eating and hygiene

Intermediate and custodial care are paid by Medicaid or private funds, whereas Medicare covers the cost of acute and skilled care only.

Nursing homes charge a daily rate, depending on the level of care, that can cost between $2000 to $3000 a month. Long-term care is covered by Medicare for a period of

100 days for each benefit period, if it follows an acute illness. Furthermore, there must be a 60 day hiatus after the 100 days is exhausted before readmission from a hospital to a nursing care facility is permitted. There are some private insurance companies that provide long-term care insurance and some that provide Medigap insurance, but these vary in amount and kind of service. Medicaid insurance is available for low-income people and for persons who have exhausted their resources paying for long-term care. Because Medicaid payments are much lower than private pay or Medicare, many long-term care facilities limit the number of admissions or do not accept Medicaid patients at all. Some states use a policy called *deeming*. A couple living together has funds that are considered (deemed) available to pay each other's medical bills. Therefore the Medicaid applicant must deplete the spouse's assets before receiving coverage. Even if the spouse's name appears on a pension or Social Security check, it is not a joint income, but must be used to pay for the Medicaid care. This may cause the well spouse to become impoverished to maintain long-term care for the Medicaid patient. Now some states split income and assets in half when determining a spouse's eligibility.

In 1987, Medicare covered less than 2% of the $35 billion dollars spent on nursing homes. Families finance aid for more than half, $18 billion dollars, with Medicaid picking up the rest of the bill. Contrary to popular belief, only 5% of the elderly population are in long-term care facilities at any given time. Much of skilled nursing care goes toward rehabilitation costs. Although the stereotypical picture of long-term care is of very old and senile people, in reality, skilled nursing care is given to those recuperating from accidents, strokes, and complicated surgeries. Except for the family, medicaid is the only source of funds for custodial care, and the numbers of custodial care admissions are increasing. High-technology, while giving and maintaining life, has not improved the quality of life. Therefore, victims of irreversible head trauma, degenerative muscle and nerve diseases, Huntington's chorea, and Alzheimer's disease, after depleting all other resources, including those of the family, find themselves in long-term care. At any given time, one may see a mix of chronic debilitating physical diseases, vegetative states, or psychopathological diseases. There are very few rewards for caregivers in this arena.

Long-term care is fraught with problems that stem from a lack of coordinated policies, goals, and methods. There are no well-defined standards of care that provide minimum protection for the patients. There is a serious shortage in the numbers of nursing homes, so that even those who qualify find it difficult to find a vacancy.

Further the use of qualified, licensed personnel is severely limited. Often the staff consists of aides who have a few months of limited training and are paid minimal wages. Supervision is either lax or lacking. Because there are repeated accounts of patient abuse and neglect, cruelty, and violations of whatever health and safety rules exist, most states have commissions investigating complaints. A further problem is that physicians have generally avoided the responsibility of the care and treatment of nursing home patients. Nursing home care is considered a low status job for registered nurses, who tend to choose intensive care and acute hospitals. In the past, those with the best education were least available. This void facilitated the type of neglect previously mentioned.

Nursing home administrators list problems within the system: overwhelming red tape, confusing rules, insufficient funds, and skyrocketing costs.[26] Medicaid pays less than $25 per day for care of its beneficiaries and that must cover the total care required by the patient.

Because long-term care facilities are in short supply and also to control escalating costs, alternatives to institutionalization had to be found and financed. There are many programs that can assist the client to stay within the community, such as home health care, day care, respite care, and homemaker and nutrition services.

Home Health Care

Home health care is considered a provision of skilled nursing services provided by a licensed nurse; rehabilitation services such as physical, occupational, or speech therapy; and personal care such as bathing, eating, and ambulation. Home health care agencies pioneered the pricing of nursing services, because nursing care was always considered a revenue-producing center, as opposed to hospitals, which included nursing services in room and board charges.

Home care is made available based on need as assessed by a health professional or by a multidisciplinary team. There are four agencies generally involved in the delivery of home care: public agencies, Visiting Nurses, agencies operated by hospitals, and proprietary agencies. Because agencies are growing rapidly and there are a variety of providers, the quality of services vary.

Cost savings resulting from the provision of home care services provide incentives to use those services (see Table 4-3). Congressman Claude Pepper estimated that the average cost of 1 hospital day is $400, whereas the cost of 1 home care day ranges between $25 and $75 dollars. In another study, Visiting Nurses Service of New York demonstrated that AIDS patients could be cared-for at home for $800 a day, whereas the costs of hospitalization would be $3000 a day.

Instituting the DRG system led to shorter hospital stays as a result of fixed hospital reimbursement from government and third party payers (insurance companies). Patients are discharged "sicker and quicker." The flood of still acutely ill discharged patients encouraged the growth of the home health industry. In 1988 estimates indicated a revenue of $12.2 billion dollars. The major identified problem with home health is quality

Table 4-3 Typical costs of care: home versus hospital

	Hospital ($)	Home ($)
After surgery	300-500 / day	25-75 / day
Chronically ill elderly	(LTC) 75-150 /day	50-75 / day
Ventilator dependent	60,900 / month	20,200 / month
Cancer chemotherapy	10,500 / month	3,500 / month
Kidney dialysis	2,000 / month	1,200 / month
Quadraplegic care	23,888 / month	13,900 / month

Source: U.S. News and World Report 1/25/88.

control. Quality assurance tools that measure patient outcomes, an adequate surveillance system, and a monitoring mechanism that surveys patient benefits from treatment are not standardized. Providers of care, accreditation agencies, and legislators must work together to insure the adequacy of care.

Barhydt-Wezenaar[3] propose that the new focus of the home as a setting of choice will enhance the quality of life of those who receive care. However, home care is increasingly complex as a result of early discharge under the DRG system and it is no longer unusual to deliver care to a respirator-dependent client at home. Nurses are delivering home care to patients on chemotherapy, intravenous hydration, intravenous antibiotic therapy, and parenteral and enteral nutrition. Clients are taught self-care of parenteral feedings, kidney dialysis, and Hickman catheters. Furthermore, self-care at home decreases iatrogenic infections and allows the client a greater degree of freedom. Unfortunately, there is often little time in the hospital for the necessary teaching to provide the client with the requisite skills for the task. However, with home health, a licensed nurse can follow up on the level of knowledge and skill that a client and family has. To receive home health coverage under Medicare, the beneficiary must meet the following criteria:

1. Be homebound
2. Require skilled nursing or therapy
3. Have physician certification
4. Be cared for by an authorized agency
5. Be re-evaluated every 2 months

If the plan of treatment is approved by a physician, a home health aide and medical supplies can be included. Fortunately, home health nurses are knowledgeable in the intricacies of Medicare's prescribed care planning and charting, and can assist the client and the physician in gaining the best compensation for the treatment needed. Even with the best documentation, benefits are often denied as part of governmental cost cutting.

Under Medicaid there are fewer restrictions. There is a wider range of health and personal services, if they are ordered by a physician. These can include personal care services such as assistance with dressing, hygiene, and meal or housekeeping tasks. These are subject to review every 60 days.

Homemaker and housekeeper services are provided under Title XX directly through a county department of social services or provider agencies. Because of the cost saving factors, many private insurers are providing home health protection with their policies.

Hospice

The modern hospital with all the marvelous technological advances is the best of worlds and the worst of worlds. Many lives are saved by the latest medical breakthrough. However, many lives are prolonged needlessly by the very same method. Often the higher the level of technology the more dehumanizing the treatment may seem to the patient and the family. For persons with terminal illnesses, the emotional cost of hospitalization is exceeded only by the enormous financial burden. Society is beginning to understand and accept that death is a normal process and therefore does not require the sterile efficient machinery offered in an acute care setting. Because many people do not want their dying postponed by machines, and because of the government's interest in cost saving, alternatives to hospital care for the dying have become more acceptable. One alternative is hospice, which has the following as its philosophy:

Dying is a natural process whether or not resulting from disease. Hospice exists neither to hasten nor to postpone death. Rather, hospice exists to affirm life—by providing support and care for those in the last phases of incurable disease so they can live as fully and comfortably as possible.[22]

Hospice is specifically for clients and their families who have decided to forego treatment that focuses on curing a terminal disease. Instead, they chose to receive pain relief, palliative care, and emotional support at home. Hospice care provides or arranges for the following:

1. Nursing and physician services
2. Social work
3. Pastoral counseling
4. Psychological services
5. Therapies ranging from physical to pharmaceutical
6. Home health aides
7. Homemakers
8. Equipment and supplies

To be truly effective, hospice must be the key part of an interdisciplinary service. Hospice must be available 24 hours a day, 7 days a week. The goal of hospice is to provide comfort and peace in the familiar setting of the client's own home.

Hospice addresses physical, psychological, spiritual, and social needs of the client and the family. Pain relief is a primary task, whether it be physical or psychological. Removing the client's fear of pain through proper management is essential. Working with the nurse and the physician, the client can be taught to anticipate and administer the appropriate treatment to alleviate physical pain. The client and the family need assistance in acceptance of the dying process and in dealing with the stress that the knowledge of dying engenders. The nurse is the patient's advocate in providing care that leads to a comfortable, pain-free atmosphere. The nurse facilitates interaction between patient and family so that adequate physical and psychological caring is shared.

Although the hospice movement is usually associated with cancer, people with other terminal diseases such as amyotrophic lateral sclerosis, HIV infections, and end stage renal or cardiac disease are also using the service. Hospice is paid by Medicare, if the patient is eligible; through private insurance; and in some states, by Medicaid. Because both government and private insurers view hospice as a valuable and cost cutting service, it has moved into the mainstream of health care delivery.

• • •

Although the government has no Bureau of Family and few laws regarding family life, its authority is felt in subtle ways. Because of its size and influence, the federal government has great impact on family life. Tax policies regarding home mortgage deductions, credits for child care, and deductions for dependent children directly influence family life. Legislation regarding aid to dependent children, Medicaid, Medicare, and school lunch programs influences the lives of low-income families. Tax breaks afforded the affluent influence the monetary gifts given to offspring. Although one may argue that government policy is too little in many areas, unfair in some, and too much in others, the general consensus is that a successful family perspective is one that affords the greatest freedom, yet protects individual environments so that children and the less fortunate are protected.

Futurists predict that health care will consume an even larger portion of the nation's income, possibly up to 15% by 1995. Payers will attempt to hold down health care spending, through cost sharing or through rationing. Americans fret over the spiraling costs of health care but seem unwilling to support any increase in taxes to provide the level of care they desire.[9] If current needs are not met, demands for future needs will be even greater. One solution may be to closely examine the biomedical model, which has been ineffective in the areas of stress, substance abuse, infant mortality, the aging population, chronic diseases, and the wise use of technology. Public policy will need to include nurses as primary caregivers and recipients of third party payments. Nursing has demonstrated the cost effectiveness of home care, primary care, and the value of prevention over restoration to health. It is time for nursing to become involved in policy formation to provide care for the least advantaged, as well as for those who are fortunate to have adequate health coverage.

Certainly there is public policy that has never been successfully resolved. The issue of national health insurance is a problem that continues. Bioethical concerns regarding life and death genetic engineering, fetal transplants, and rationing of health care will continue well into the 1990s. The American people are becoming involved in these issues through a rapidly growing grass roots movement. Community health decision projects are indirect agents of change. Through public forums, people come together to think about and discuss their own health beliefs and values in an attempt to influence public policy. There are community health decision groups in Oregon, California, Iowa, Illinois, Maine, and Washington. Each is successful in influencing public policy on health care issues related to distribution of block grant funds, access to health, and health

---

SOCIAL CONCERNS OF AMERICANS

Drug abuse	Plight of farmers
Cost of medical care	AIDS
Federal budget deficit	Poverty
Unemployment	Smoking
Crime	Pornography
Loss of manufacturing jobs	Threat of nuclear war
Alcoholism	

insurance. Possibly, these projects are the wave of the future, and "we, the people" may indeed resolve the remaining difficult health care decisions, rather than await governmental action. The primary social aspects that concern Americans today are listed in the box.

STUDY QUESTIONS

1. What factors are in favor or against national health insurance? What is the reader's position?
2. What are major obstacles to accessibility to health care in the United States?
3. How can nurses affect policy and programs to improve people's accessibility to health care?

REFERENCES

1. American Association of Retired Persons: Aging in America, Washington, DC, 1988, American Association of Retired Persons.
2. American Association of Retired persons: A profile of older Americans, Washington, DC, 1988, American Association of Retired Persons.
3. Barhydt-Wezenaar N: Home health and hospice In S Jonas, ed: Health care delivery in the United States, ed 3, New York, 1986, Springer Publishing Co.
4. Berger S: What your doctor didn't learn in medical school, New York, 1988, William Morrow & Company, Inc.
5. Califano J: America's health care revolution, New York, 1986, Random House.
6. Dellum R: The Health Service Act. H.R. 2969. Washington, DC, Congressional Record, 125(33), 1979.
7. Friedman M and Rosenman R: Type A behavior and your heart, New York, 1971, Alfred A Knopf.
8. Harrington C and Lempert L: Medicaid: a public program in distress, Nurs Outlook 36(1):6-8, 1988.
9. Harrison I et al: 1989 National healthcare poll #1, Boston, 1989, John Hancock Financial Services.
10. Hawkins J and Higgens L: Nursing and the American health care delivery system, ed 2, New York, 1985, The Tiresias Press, Inc.
11. Health Care Financing Association: Health Care Financ Rev 9(3):68-76, 1988.
12. Hiatt H: Medical Lifeboat, New York, 1987, Perennial Library, Harper and Row, Publishers.
13. Holmes T and Rahe R: The social readjustment rating scale, J Psychosomat Res 11:213-218, 1961.
14. Illich I: Medical nemesis. In P Lee, N Brown, and I Red, eds: The nation's health, San Francisco, 1980, Boyd and Fraser Publishing Co.
15. Institute of Medicine: Preventing low birth weight, Washington, DC, 1985, National Academy of Science.
16. Johnston M: Homeless are more than homeless, Los Angeles Times, part II, June 22, 1988.
17. Kalish B and Kalish P: Politics and nursing, Philadelphia, 1982, JB Lippincott Co.
18. Kaufman R: Abortion. In M Hiller, ed: Medical ethics and the law, Cambridge, 1981, Ballinger Publishing Co.
19. Kimball M: Hospital Medicare profits collapsing, Health Week 2(3):1, 36, February 1, 1988.
20. Mason D and Talbott S: Political action handbook for nurses, Menlo Park, 1985, Addison-Wesley Publishers.
21. Mundinger M: Health services funding cuts and the declining health of the poor, New Eng J Med 313(1):44-47, 1985.
22. National Hospice Organization: hospice principles and standards, Washington, DC, 1979, National Hospice Organization.
23. Popp R: Health care for the poor, J Nurs Admin 18(1):8-12, 1988.
24. Reinhardt E: Rationing the health care surplus: an American tragedy, Nurs Econ 4(3):101-108, 1986.
25. Richardson E: Health care crisis in America, 1971. Testimony before the Subcommittee on Health of the Committee on Labor and Public Welfare, US Senate, Washington, DC, Feb 22, 1971, US Senate.
26. Rowland D: Meeting the long term care needs of an aging population. In CJ Schramm, ed: Health care and its costs, New York, 1987, WW Norton & Co.
27. St. Joseph Hospital: Guidelines for "no-code" orders, Orange, 1980, St. Joseph Hospital.

28. Schaie KW and Willis S: Adult development and aging, ed 2, Boston, 1986, Little, Brown & Co.
29. Schneider E: A debate: should health care be rationed on the basis of age? The aging connection, 1X(2), 9, 1988.
30. Shorr A and Moen P: The single parent and public policy. In Skolnick A and Skolnick J, eds: Family in Transition, ed 4, Boston, 1983, Little, Brown & Company.
31. Spector M: Searching for the best medical care money can't buy, The Washington Post National Weekly Edition, December 25-31, 1989.
32. US Bureau of Census: Statistical abstract of the United States (105th ed), Washington, DC, 1984, US Bureau of Census.

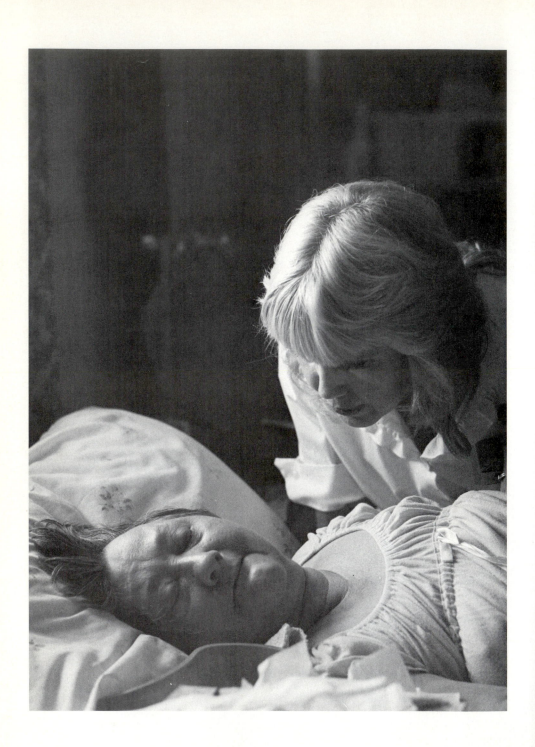

CHAPTER 5

CULTURAL INFLUENCES ON NURSING

Sharon Minton Kirkpatrick
Grace L. Deloughery

OBJECTIVES

After completing this chapter the reader should be able to:

- Define culture and how it manifests itself

- Describe the changes in American society since the melting pot theory was predominant

- List some physiological and physical characteristics that nurses must assess accurately when caring for various ethnic people

- Identify some ways in which cultural beliefs and values of an individual may alter a nurse's plan of care for that individual

- Give several examples of how a nurse can achieve a desired goal for a patient or client while staying within the context of that person's cultural patterns, beliefs, and values

- Make a general overall cultural assessment of an individual, family, and group

- Describe the reader's own cultural beliefs, values, and behaviors that can affect nursing care if not recognized and accounted for when caring for a patient or client of another culture

This chapter is divided into the following three major content areas:
1. Philosophy of transcultural nursing
2. History of transcultural nursing in the United States
3. Practical tools to provide nursing care to persons of other cultures

Having achieved an increased awareness for the need to incorporate cultural concepts in nursing practice, the reader will be asked to evaluate his/her own cultural background. Awareness of one's thinking and behavior patterns can help accommodation of these patterns to situations in which communication differences arise as a result of cultural factors.

Self-satisfaction is gained when the nurse skillfully crosses cultural lines and provides excellent nursing care to patients and clients. This results in increased awareness and respect of people from other cultures. Hopefully students today will find the need for this knowledge as basic as that of basic skills taught in schools of nursing during earlier decades.

Because of limited space in the text, the reader is encouraged to follow up with additional readings other than those suggested here.

PHILOSOPHY OF TRANSCULTURAL NURSING

The world becomes smaller daily as the activities of those who live on the opposite side of the ocean are brought directly into living rooms thousands of miles away. The advent of satellite technology makes communications faster and more readily available as news is transmitted around the world as quickly as it was once relayed across the backyard fence. Modern transportation makes access to remote corners of the earth an every day occurrence: jet travel takes hours, whereas more primitive modes of travel used to take weeks and even months to accomplish. Not only are people around the world more aware of each other, they are also intermingling to a greater extent as immigrations and migrations make the world a giant mobile society. The ultimate outcome of these changes is an increased merging of the global population, which brings with it demands for new cultural understandings.

Nursing is one of the frontline professions that keenly feels the impact of this diverse population shift. It is no longer sufficient to practice an ethnocentric nursing protocol and expect it to meet needs universally. Each culture has a set of values and beliefs that are inextricably intertwined with health care behaviors. Lessons from the past have taught that the ability of nurses to help others is not always accompanied by a sound cultural knowledge base that would promote understanding of health care practices in transcultural situations.

MEANING OF CULTURE

Culture is an accepted set of values, beliefs, and behaviors shared within a social group.[26] Culture influences the ways in which people express themselves, as well as the foods they eat, and establishes the rules—spoken and unspoken—within which people operate.[17]

Many variations exist within, and between, cultures. Each person may belong to more than one subculture within a major culture. For instance, there are over 226 million people in the United States[25] who form the American culture, and within this culture there are numerous subcultures that share common characteristics within the group but not necessarily the American culture as a whole. Although born in the same country, teenagers living on farms in rural Iowa may find it difficult to relate to teenagers raised on the streets of Los Angeles; they may speak the same language but have so many diverse experiences and perspectives that they cannot relate to each other.

Culture is like a template used as a pattern to make duplicate copies. Members of a society attempt to preserve the status quo for the next generation by replicating their values, beliefs, and behaviors, much like a template would be used to make copies. Imagine, however, a template made of soft cardboard. After multiple tracings the edges begin wearing and the new copies differ somewhat from the previous ones. After awhile, the original template is discarded and the copies, each of which has taken on its own unique variations, are used as new templates. Imagine also that periodically someone introduces a variation of the template, which is thought superior to the old one, resulting in a new line of copies that develop their own changes over time. For many reasons, the templates of culture develop mutations and variations that result in changes from one generation to the next, as well as in a multiplicity of subcultures.

CULTURAL DIVERSITY

The United States has been described as a melting pot, in which diverse groups from all over the world gather and are encouraged to forsake many of their native traditions and become homogenized into Americans. In the past, those who attempted to retain native beliefs, customs, and language were often scorned and ridiculed, and otherwise made to feel like misfits.

Fortunately, the melting pot theory is slowly changing to appreciation and acceptance of other cultures, described as the *stewpot theory*.[11] Like stew, each ingredient is enhanced and becomes more flavorful from exposure to the distinctive flavors of the others; so does a society in which people of various cultures are exposed to each other.

The mingling of cultures can be likened to the stewpot. When each individual culture is allowed to exist, and more importantly is appreciated and valued for its unique contribution to society, the cultural stewpot will become more "flavorful." One's perspective on the world in general and one's own culture in particular will be broadened and enlightened when an appreciation is gained for cultures different from one's own.

EXAMPLE: A friend relates an experience that occurred repeatedly in his childhood. When he and his mother were going somewhere in the car she would often choose a new route, even though their destination was one to which they went frequently. On one of these routing trips, they found a bridge closed and detour signs posted. The detour was creating general havoc for the majority of travelers, who knew only one route. For this child and his mother, however, it was only a momentary delay. They had learned multiple routes and therefore had more than one option; they were not solely dependent on the route across the bridge.

Learning about other cultures also increases one's options by providing a wider perspective out of which decisions can be made. Choices and decisions made by people of various cultural backgrounds will surprise the nurse who does not know, or does not try to learn, what the choices are that patients (clients with that background) are *apt* to make.

Timely and appropriate nursing care is not always instituted, because of a basic lack of knowledge about other cultures. Frequently, health care workers learn only one route to a destination. According to Branch and Paxton,[9] ethnic people of color are not receiving safe nursing care because of this lack. Recognizing cyanosis in a patient with dark skin can be a challenge for nurses who have only worked with patients who have light skin. Nurses should be taught assessment skills for noting signs and symptoms such as cyanosis and jaundice in people of all skin colors. Health and illness are defined in various ways. Culture influences the values, beliefs, and behavior of individuals, families, and communities regarding health and illness.

Nurses must be aware that certain disease conditions are prevalent in certain population groups and relatively nonprevalent (or even absent) in others. For example, phenylketonuria is a chronic condition that is especially prevalent in infants of European descent. It occurs rarely among blacks. On the other hand, sickle cell anemia is found only among blacks.

Cultural factors that affect an individual's illness and is a concern of nursing services include the following:

1. Patient's role and status in the family
2. Social, material, and professional support
3. The way a patient with a chronic illness is treated by families and groups
4. Ways in which symptoms of illness are identified and interpreted
5. Ways in which pain and discomfort are dealt with

For example, young Amish men are taught to be stoic in the face of excruciating pain, whereas Philippine women have what appears to be a very low tolerance for pain.

Cultural factors also influence the ways in which people interact with health care professionals. Cultural and ethnic differences influence differences in delivery of health and social service. However, while considering group differences within the larger cultural (ethnic) group, one must be aware of individual differences within the groups.

CULTURAL BELIEFS

Cultural beliefs that may appear strange and unfounded to persons from other cultures can be deeply rooted and greatly influence behavior. Some beliefs produce positive effects, and others produce negative ones. Certain beliefs of the Masai women of Kenya, Africa, are good examples of those that produce beneficial effects.

EXAMPLE: Because the Masai are primarily nomadic herdsmen, they acquire very few material possessions. Their simple grass thatched dwellings are furnished with little more than the skins stretched and preserved from their herds. The only beds available are animal skins laid on the bare ground. The women believe that laying a newborn baby on this hard surface is detrimental because a baby's head is still soft and forming. To prevent this problem from occurring, the women in the tribe take turns, night and day, holding newborn babies throughout their first week of life.[19]

Health care workers know that one of the primary causes of neonatal deaths in Third World countries is hypothermia,[18] of which the Masai women are unaware. They may hold newborns to protect their heads from hard surfaces, but it is probably the 98.6 degree human incubator effect that is the beneficial factor. Regardless of the rationale behind the belief, the fact remains that the end result is a positive one.

On the other hand, some of the Masai beliefs can be quite detrimental. They believe, for instance, that if a woman eats very little when she is pregnant, she will have a small infant, which will assure an easy delivery. Pregnant women are, therefore, encouraged to eat nothing but a porridge made of maize. The end result may indeed be a small infant, but one who has not had the advantage of good prenatal nutrition. An additional effect of this nutritional deprivation is the physical depletion of the mother, which results in an inability to sustain successful breastfeeding.[18] It is obvious that this belief has a negative effect.

In other cases, beliefs have neither obvious positive nor negative effects; they are simply used to explain the unexplainable.

EXAMPLE: A common belief among Haitian mothers living in the bateys or sugar cane fields of the Dominican Republic is that of *mal de ojo* or the evil eye. One of the mothers relates an event in which her two-month-old daughter was taken to the small store on the batey by an older sister. A Haitian woman, who was also shopping at the store said, "Be careful, don't let the baby fall down. Give her to me. I will hold her while you shop." When the woman took the baby, she exclaimed, "What a beautiful baby. She's such a beautiful child!" The mother relating the story went on to explain that this interaction, the verbal admiration or *mal de ojo*, caused the infant to become seriously ill. When the baby arrived home, the mother immediately discovered it had a high fever, a cold, and diarrhea. She contended the baby was very healthy before going to the store. She also said she believed the only reason the baby survived the spell was because the curandera, or local healer, was consulted and invoked a " friendly" spirit to deal with the evil spirit cast by the *mal de ojo*.

During one of the first trips to the bateys, the author observed that many of the babies had red rags or red strings tied around their wrists. When asked about the reason for this, the mothers stated it was to protect the child from *mal de ojo*. When the author noted a young mother hurriedly tying a red string around her infant's wrist as she approached, the author suddenly realized that she was suspected of having the power of *mal de ojo*. When the interpreter was asked if that was a possibility, he said, "Of course, because you are a stranger and she doesn't know you." It was later learned that in addition to persons with supernatural powers, it is commonly believed that ordinary people, male or female, can be born with the power to give *mal de ojo*. It is believed they are not necessarily evil people; they are simply victims themselves, because they cannot rid themselves of the power.

A nurse in this culture discovers that it is extremely important to be aware of this belief. Verbal admiration of a child, which is highly valued in some cultures, could be viewed in other cultures as a threat to the child and render the nurse powerless because of the mother's fears. In that case, a nurse who maintains a sincere, but strictly professional interest, in a child will more likely earn the trust of a mother more quickly than one who tried to create a more personal relationship by admiring a child.

CULTURAL VALUES

Values are beliefs about which one feels strongly and will go to great lengths to preserve. Values vary significantly from culture to culture and are sometimes diametrically opposed. The wide diversity of some commonly held values is illustrated in the box. If persons from a variety of cultures were given this questionnaire, some would strongly agree with the beliefs listed on the left, whereas others would strongly agree with the opposite viewpoint listed on the right (see box).

Those who view their own culture as superior and reject all other cultures as being underdeveloped, inferior, or second-class hold a belief called *ethnocentrism*. The problem that evolves from ethnocentrism is not necessarily the belief that one's culture is best. As a matter of fact, this belief would usually suggest one has adapted well to a specific culture.[28] The problem occurs when the health care professional attempts to impose personal values on others, believing not only that they are the best way but the only way. Ethnocentrism can be extremely limiting in the health care field because the nurse who holds this belief may assess, plan, intervene, and evaluate the client based on personal perceptions and values without taking into account those of the client. Health care managed in this way often fails from the beginning, because of the lack of communication and understanding between the health care worker and the client.

One of the areas in which cultures tend to develop strong values is sexuality. Because strong sexual values are brought from the nurse's own cultural background, a state of tension sometimes develops between the nurse and a client with a different sexual orientation. Each culture assigns a socially approved sexual role to each sex, as well as a given set of approved behaviors.[10] These roles and behaviors may vary dramatically from culture to culture. For instance, in the United States coitus between consenting adults who are married is socially valued, whereas adultery and prostitution are discouraged. The stance or at least tolerance toward adultery, premarital sex, and having children out of wedlock, however, has changed dramatically in the last few years. In previous generations unmarried pregnant women were secretly sent away to homes for unwed mothers to await the arrival of a baby that would then be placed for adoption. Today the number of unwed teenage mothers has grown tremendously and the trend is for them to keep their babies.

On the other hand, even though prostitution continues to be negatively sanctioned, it also continues to be "judged" with a double standard. The prostitute is sanctioned for selling sex, but the customer who pays for the sex is not. A case in point is the American custom of regularly incarcerating prostitutes while allowing the customer to go free.

CULTURAL VALUES

Directions

| Circle 1 if you strongly agree with the statement on the left | Circle 3 if you agree with the statement on the right |
| Circle 2 if you agree with the statement on the left | Circle 4 if you strongly agree with the statement on the right |

1. Preparing for and influencing the future are important parts of being a responsible adult — 1 2 3 4 — Life follows a preordained course; the individual should follow that course

2. Vague and tentative answers are dishonest and confusing — 1 2 3 4 — Vague answers are sometimes preferred because they avoid embarrassment and confrontation

3. Punctuality and efficient use of time are reflections of intelligence and concern — 1 2 3 4 — Punctuality is rarely important and should be subordinate to such concerns as maintaining a relaxed atmosphere, enjoying the moment, and being with family and friends

4. When in severe pain, it is better and more appropriate to remain stoic — 1 2 3 4 — When in severe pain, it is better to vent the discomfort vocally and physically

5. It is presumptuous and unwise to accept a gift from someone you do not know well — 1 2 3 4 — It is an insult to refuse a gift when it is offered

6. Addressing someone by their first name shows friendliness — 1 2 3 4 — Addressing someone by their first name is disrespectful

7. Direct questions are usually the best way to gain information — 1 2 3 4 — Direct questioning is intrusive, rude, and potentially embarrassing

8. Direct eye contact shows interest — 1 2 3 4 — Direct eye contact is intrusive

9. Ultimately, the independence of the individual must come before the needs of the family — 1 2 3 4 — The needs of the individual are always subordinate to the needs of the family

---

Adapted from Renwick GW and Rhinesmith SH: An exercise in cultural analysis for managers, Chicago, Intercultural Press.

In Thiederman S: Ethnocentrism: a barrier to effective health care, Nurse Practition 11(8):54, 1986. Used by permission.

Incest between parent and child is almost universally negatively sanctioned. Brink[10] reports, however, that there are subcultures, such as those of some alcoholic families, in which the father and daughter believe it is the father's duty to "deflower" his daughter before marriage. Other societies have socially sanctioned incest in ways quite different from those espoused in the United States. In ancient Egypt, for instance, a royal marriage between siblings was not only expected but required.

Traditions for choosing a mate vary widely from culture to culture. The American culture values the freedom of an individual to choose one's own mate. Other cultures believe this should be the responsibility of parents. One Japanese man stated, "I wouldn't dream of choosing my own bride. That is one of the most important steps I will ever take and deserves the wisdom, insight, and objective love that only a parent can provide."

Cultural values sometimes change significantly and then come back full circle to previously held values. Breastfeeding is an example of this change in the United States. In pioneer days, women breastfed because it was the only practical option they had. With the advent of bottles and readily available formulas, however, bottle feeding grew in popularity and breastfeeding fell into disfavor. However, as the benefits of breastfeeding, for both mother and baby, become more widely publicized, breastfeeding is once again highly valued in the United States.

CULTURAL BEHAVIORS

Cultural behaviors grow out of beliefs and values held by a group within a society. Frequently the behavior is more obvious than the belief which precipitated the behavior.

EXAMPLE: The first time I took students to Grand Cayman for an elective transcultural nursing experience, I was frustrated by the seeming indifference of the Caymanian nurses to efficiency and time schedules. The students were told by the Caymanian nurses to report for work each morning at 8:00 am. When they arrived, however, they frequently found nurses visiting with one another and the morning's work not even considered for over an hour. As everyone became better acquainted it was learned that this was not a disregard for schedules but a very important part of the day. Showing interest and concern for coworkers' personal lives was highly valued by Caymanians and was reflected in their social behavior. This same pattern was noted in telephone conversations, which often began with a rather lengthy period of social amenities before proceeding to the business at hand. To ignore this tradition would have offended coworkers and made a less effective member of the team.

CROSS-CULTURAL COMMUNICATIONS

The establishment of effective communication between a nurse of one culture and a patient of another is facilitated by the nurse's identification of areas of commonality between self and patient.[24]

EXAMPLE: While conducting research by interviewing mothers in Haiti and the Dominican Republic, I found the establishment of trust and rapport key elements in the research process. Each interview began with an introduction of self as a nurse and a mother. When the title of *nurse* was mentioned the mother being interviewed usually acknowledged my statement by nodding respectfully. When the term *mother* was mentioned however, there was almost always a visible change in the mother's body language as she made eye contact, leaned slightly closer, and smiled.

It was the mother role that the nurse and patient had in common and therefore the one logically pursued in establishing rapport. By the nurse's briefly sharing some hopes, dreams, and concerns as a mother, the mother being interviewed felt freer to share in return.

In addition to establishing areas of commonality to encourage good communications, it is also important to be aware of misunderstandings because of language barriers. Orque[24] relates a case in which an English-speaking nurse gave a nonEnglish-speaking patient preoperative instructions. The nurse explained the way in which povidone-iodine (Bethadine) should be used to prepare the area preoperatively; the patient nodded and smiled, indicating she understood. Unfortunately the patient had not understood and drank the bottle of solution, rather than use it topically. Fortunately the error was discovered immediately and appropriate measures saved the patient's life. Demonstrations followed by return demonstrations are usually a more appropriate way of validating understanding across language barriers than relying solely on spoken language. Ideally, of course, both nurse and patient speak the same language.

CULTURAL ASSESSMENT

A specific means of communicating cultural beliefs, values, and behaviors that are important in health care is through a formal cultural assessment. Cultural assessment places the nurse in a better position to meet the patient's needs by enabling the nurse to understand cultural factors that influence people's health behaviors. If culturally specific care is not achieved, clients become unhappy, uncooperative, and ultimately withdraw from the relationship. Remember that maintaining the dignity of the persons involved requires treating each as an equal, who brings important and relevant cultural beliefs to the relationship.

•   •   •

Culture is defined as a system of values, beliefs, and customs that an individual learns while growing up in the environment; it is an unconscious learning process.

People of different cultures define health in different ways. They describe disease causation in different ways. They may describe a disease as having natural causes or as having supernatural causes, such as spirits or other phenomena. The Navajo Indian, for example, theorizes that illness has natural causes, whereas another tribal group explains the illness of a child as being caused by envy of an adult who admires the child (a result of what they label the *evil eye*). It is necessary that nurses are cognizant of the way in which the patient or client is enculturated to view his/her condition of illness.

Compliance with nursing and medical protocol also depends on the acceptance or way in which people deal with chronic illness and/or defects. A congenitally malformed child who is considered a shame and hidden from public view is likely not to keep appointments when parents feel the lack of acceptance and support from their social group or health care professionals. Nurses must learn to identify cultural variables and be able to alter nursing care interventions so that they are congruent to the patient's cultural pattern beliefs.

History and Evolution of Transcultural Nursing

Long before nurses routinely performed cultural assessments, they were aware of the needs created by cultural differences, and began to formally describe this specialty area of nursing. A variety of terms and definitions have been used over the past several years and are continuing to evolve at present.

Early terms to describe a cultural focus in nursing include the following:
1. Transcultural nursing
2. Ethnonursing
3. Cross-cultural nursing

Transcultural nursing is the branch of nursing that focuses on comparative study and analysis of cultures with respect to nursing and culturally determined health-illness practices, beliefs, and values. The goal is to develop a scientific and humanistic body of knowledge to provide caring, culturally based, nursing care.

Roots of Transcultural Nursing

Unfortunately, Florence Nightingale did not leave nursing a legacy of works entitled "Transcultural Nursing Notes." She did, however, leave a philosophy that helps nurses prepare for this subspecialty. Dr. Alfred Worcester, who visited Miss Nightingale in 1895 in her home in London, was later to report: Miss Nightingale "recognized that if ever she were to have opportunity of doing good work in nursing she must first learn her business."[30] Learning about other cultures was part of her life-long business. She was fluent in Greek and Latin, as well as French, German, and Italian; she traveled extensively; and also lived abroad for long periods of time.[30]

Nightingale's concerns for the people of India are further indications of her transcultural interests. When she was asked by the Sanitary Commission of Bengal to suggest a plan for organizing nursing services in India, she quickly noted the contributions only people familiar with the Indian culture could make. Native-born Indians, as well as non-native-born people who lived in the country, could join the nursing services and "be very useful from their knowledge of the native language and of local circumstances of which persons arriving from England would necessarily be ignorant."[23]

Nightingale strongly advocated that nursing could meet the needs of unfamiliar social groups by studying their habits and knowing their desires. In an address to women workers, which focused on the needs of the rural poor, Nightingale asserted, "*You* could not get through the daily work of the cottage mother—the washing, cooking, cleaning, mending, making. So ask what plan *she* would *recommend* to carry out your suggestions rather than what she *does*."[23] She went on to say, "without knowing the wants, the difficulties, temptations, fatigues, of their daily lives—without a serious study of their world—we cannot help them."[23]

FORMALIZATION OF TRANSCULTURAL NURSING

Increasingly in the past several years, nurses are aware of a lack of professional training to prepare them for cross-cultural experiences. Some learn by doing, as they travel to new environments and live with people in cultures different from their own. Some have frustrating experiences in other cultures, as a result of a lack of understanding; out of this frustration, however, emerges a movement to become better informed about cultural beliefs through formal nursing education and interactions.

One of the pioneers in this new area of transcultural nursing is Madeleine Leininger. In 1955 she founded the field of transcultural nursing as a formal area of study and practice. Working as a psychiatric clinical nurse specialist in a guidance home for disturbed children in Ohio, Leininger observed the children's different reactions to nursing activities. Because they came from diverse cultural background, such as Afro-American, Spanish-American, Jewish-American, and Appalachian, she began looking at the association between their backgrounds and their actions.

Leininger was one of the first nurses to seek additional academic preparation through graduate study in anthropology at the University of Washington in 1959. She conducted fieldwork in New Guinea to become the first professional nurse to complete a doctoral program in cultural anthropology. In 1968 she organized The Committee on Nursing and Anthropology of the American Anthropological Association. The primary goal of this committee was to "help nurses and anthropologists work together to incorporate anthropological knowledge into nursing curricula."[15]

Leininger saw the critical need to prepare nurses in anthropology to develop the new field of transcultural nursing. Under her leadership, educational programs in transcultural nursing began to develop. In the late 1960s and early 1970s, she encouraged a core of nurse educators and practitioners to prepare in anthropology to assist in the development of the new discipline of transcultural nursing. She was instrumental in establishing the first transcultural nursing courses at the University of Colorado and, since then, has provided leadership in establishing graduate programs in transcultural nursing in several other universities.

As health care workers became involved in cultural settings different from their own, the following problems were identified:

1. Lack of knowledge about diversities in cultural beliefs and practices
2. Health care personnel difficulties in identifying relationships between social structures and health systems
3. Cultural shock, or feelings of helplessness and disorientation felt by the health giver, leading to ineffectiveness
4. Cultural imposition, or the imposition of the health worker's beliefs on another cultural group, resulting in distrust and, many times, failure of proposed health interventions

These cultural problems were graphically illustrated in nursing education in the early 1970s. Two private schools of nursing sent their baccalaureate nursing students to Alaska, South America, and Africa for a ten-week course in nursing, without providing knowledge or even an orientation about the culture in which they would work. Several other schools of nursing sent culturally unprepared students to foreign countries because they believed they would obtain better clinical experiences. Experiences such as these resulted in culture shock for the students and a reliance on cultural imposition as the method of procedure. As more schools offer courses in transcultural nursing, preparation for such experiences will enhance the quality and success of the endeavors.

Transcultural Nursing and Curricula

During the early 1970s, several nurse-anthropologists encouraged the Western Commission on Higher Education in Nursing to help faculty members in schools of nursing to develop cultural concepts in nursing curricula. By 1975, the word *culture* was appearing in nursing philosophies, objectives, and course descriptions of various schools. Several articles have since been published that give guidelines for including transcultural content in curricula.[8,15,20] In 1972, the University of Washington initiated a master's degree program in transcultural nursing, and Pennsylvania State started a similar program in 1974. A more recent program is the Nursing School at Wayne State University. The University of Utah approved a master's degree program in transcultural nursing in 1977, and later that same year initiated the first Ph.D. program in the field. By 1984, there were four masters and five doctoral programs that focused on transcultural nursing, whereas over 20% of the baccalaureate and associate degree programs included courses or material on transcultural nursing.[16] More schools have added cultural concepts to their curriculum since that time.

The University of Miami School of Nursing, which emphasizes transcultural nursing, emerges as one of the leaders in providing educational opportunities for nurses interested in cultures other than their own. Their undergraduate and graduate nursing programs incorporate a transcultural nursing curriculum. A $1,000,000 endowment establishes funding of the William R. Ryan Distinguished Chair in Transcultural Nursing, as well as a Transcultural Nursing Research Institute.

The impetus for providing multicultural content in nursing continues to increase. The American Nurses Association (ANA), in 1976, adopted the following statement as part of its Code for Nurses: "Consideration of individual value systems and lifestyles should be included in the planning and health care for each client."[1] The ANA's Standards of Nursing Practice further indicate that health status data should include cultural background.[7] The National League for Nursing supplied guidance for those responsible for providing nursing curriculum, by affirming in 1977 that: "the curriculum is based on the philosophy, purposes, and objectives of the program and recognizes the contribution of nursing and other disciplines toward meeting the health needs of a diverse and multicultural society."[22]

In addition to transcultural nursing, some nurses also pursue degrees in related fields. Between 1965 and 1972, 28 nurses obtained a graduate degree in anthropology. By the late 1970s, there were an estimated 55 nurses in the United States who held masters' degrees, and 45 who had doctoral preparation in anthropology.[15] Appreciating cultural diversity, nurses recognize the need to shape nursing to meet the population's cultural needs, rather than expect the entire population to conform to one's ethnocentric model.

A third social factor that affects the multicultural emphasis in nursing is the civil rights movement. Although this movement lost momentum in the 1970s, it resulted in other rights movements, one of which was affirmative action programs. These federally backed programs opened doors for minorities in employment opportunities. Around 1970, nurses, who at first represented only their own group, later pursued equal rights for the following four minority groups:

1. Afro-Americans
2. Chicanos
3. Asian-Americans
4. Some North American Indian groups

Their contributions helped promote cultural awareness of the needs of these specific ethnic groups. The main thrust, however, was on recruitment and retention of minority students.

Even though nurses displayed a long-time interest in transcultural nursing, the events of the 1960s and 1970s added impetus for formal organization. Nurses' interest in transcultural nursing certainly was not generated in a vacuum; rather, it emerged simultaneously with concerns in society at large. Interest in transcultural nursing and its relevance to care and health increased. Care behavior in transcultural nursing was later reflected in the organization of the Annual National Caring Conference, first held in 1978.

Transcultural Nursing Organizations

In 1974 a national transcultural conference on communications and culture was held at the University of Hawaii School of Nursing. That same year, under the leadership of Leininger, plans for a series of transcultural nursing conferences were initiated, with the objectives of bringing together nurses, anthropologists, and other social scientists who had expressed an interest in shaping the field of transcultural nursing.

The first National Transcultural Nursing Conference was held in 1974 at the College of Nursing at the University of Utah. Subsequent conferences were held annually through 1978, with Leininger serving as conference chairperson. The first three conferences were organized around the life cycle, and the presentations focused on specific age categories. The fourth conference departed from the life cycle framework and focused on cultural change and ethics related to nursing care.

Subsequent conferences resulted in a desire to organize ongoing activities and inter-actions; this was formalized in the founding of the Transcultural Nursing Society in 1975. Originally initiated at the University of Utah, the Transcultural Nursing Society became independently and legally incorporated in 1981 and presently has a membership of over 1000.

Soon after the Transcultural Nursing Society was organized, a group of nurses began to express concern for the ethnic composition of the nursing profession itself. In 1977, the Division of Nursing of the US Department of Health and Human Services conducted a survey with the ANA to determine racial and ethnic composition of the registered nurse population. The study indicated 6.2% of all registered nurses with active licenses were of an ethnic minority background.[6] Soon after the release of this report, the 1980 ANA House of Delegates reaffirmed the Association's commitment to increasing ethnic minorities in the nursing profession by adopting resolution number 52, which addressed the "recruitment, retention and graduation of minority persons in baccalaureate and higher degree programs in nursing."[6]

About the same time, the ANA Commission on Human Rights sent a questionnaire to all ANA members who had identified themselves on their membership applications as members of an ethnic-minority group.[3] Responses to the questionnaire indicate these members wanted to become more involved in their professional organization, but felt it did not allow them to do so. The Human Rights Commission members proposed the for-mation of a council to provide direction in the development of programs of human rights concerns, and to increase the responsiveness of nurses to cultural and ethnic variances among patients.[4] To obtain an indication of level of interest in their proposal, the Commission surveyed its members at the 1978 and 1979 conferences. Approximately 130 members expressed an interest in joining a council that would focus on cultural and ethnic concerns.[3]

Nurses' interests in intercultural affairs were officially recognized by the ANA in 1980 with the establishment of the Council on Intercultural Nursing. Approximately 30 ANA members applied for membership on the council at that time and plans were made for election of an executive committee later that year. This council, initially under the chairmanship of Mildred Cox, was directly accountable to the ANA's Commission on Human Rights. Short-term goals adopted by the newly elected Council Executive Committee focused on involvement in national legislative issues concerning human rights and the dissemination of information regarding human rights issues to the mem-bership at large.[2] In the first *Council of Intercultural Nursing Newsletter,* which was pub-lished in February/March, 1981, Chairperson Cox noted:

While we have needed such a council over the past year—it is most apparent at this time that the number of ethnic minorities comprising our patient population is ever increasing. Nurses by necessity will be in the forefront of promoting safe and effective health care. Efforts of the council will be to focus on developing a mechanism to bring this about—to share with constituent nurses.[6]

In 1984, the ANA moved the Council from the Human Rights Commission to the Cabinet on Nursing Practice and changed the name from the Council on Intercultural Nursing to the Council on Cultural Diversity in Nursing Practice. The purpose of the move was to focus the attention of the council on the improvement of nursing practice through incorporation of cultural awareness. In addition, the council accepted as its 1984 goal, the commitment "to promote the development of nursing curriculum models to provide culturally specific nursing care."[5]

The 1981 membership roster for the Council on Intercultural Nursing revealed a wide variety of culturally diverse surnames.[12] Membership of ethnic minorities on the council was undoubtedly encouraged by the original inquiry of interest that was targeted at nurses of ethnic and cultural minority backgrounds. This was further encouraged by ANA activities in the early 1980s that focused as much attention on the ethnic nurse as the ethnic patient. With council purposes increasingly concerned with nursing practice, it is possible that educators and nurse clinicians, who confront ethnic and cultural issues for their patients, rather than for themselves, will be more inclined to support the council on cultural diversity.

Transcultural Research

Research and the acquisition of a sound knowledge base are crucial to the development of transcultural nursing. The primary goal for health personnel working in transcultural settings is to determine the dominant culture values, priorities, and characteristics of the cultural group, and then ascertain how best to provide for the needs of people.

As early as 1960, nurses began to use the ethnoscientific method to address a lack of knowledge in nursing. Encouraged by Leininger, nurses began a rigorous system to collect carefully documented statements of the idigenous people's views about *their* health care system."[14] According to Leininger,[13] advantages of the ethnoscience approach include the following:

1. A more accurate picture of a cultural group
2. An emphasis on importance of viewing health care from the patient's viewpoint
3. Data for a sound basis for prediction studies and generalizations
4. Generation of nursing theories
5. Reduction of intuitive nursing

Nightingale once suggested, "in beginning new things we commence with the easier, and having mastered that, proceed to the more difficult."[23] Leininger also believed ethnoscientific methods should be implemented first on a small scale by studying one or two cultures in depth and then by following up with field studies. The knowledge base gradually expands as more in-depth studies are conducted and a variety of cultures is compared and contrasted. Tripp-Reimer[29] suggests that one of the reasons for lack of progression in this area is because cross-cultural research is conducted in a horizontal manner, i.e., one culture described, then another culture, and then another. Instead, she says, knowledge should be linked vertically, i.e., studies replicated or hypotheses retested so that the knowledge base can become more substantive.

Ultimately this classification and testing of transcultural knowledge "should generate new theories, different practices, and clues for the prevention of illness . . . "[14] Variables to investigate should include biophysiological, genetic, environmental, social, and general cultural ways.[15]

In some of her later writings, Leininger recommended, in addition to the ethnoscience approach, the following methods[15]:

1. Participant-observation
2. Descriptive-survey
3. Experimental and control laboratory
4. Hypothesis-testing
5. Paradigm and model

While nurses were organizing professional interest groups and defining the domains of the new subspecialty, culture, society was not stagnate. Governmental decisions, grass-roots pressures, and shifting populations were all changing and ultimately added impetus to the transcultural nursing movement.

Societal Factors Affecting Development of Transcultural Nursing

Social programs of the 1960s brought health care attention to a previously neglected group: the poor.[27] Health insurance, as a fringe benefit of employment, brought health care to the working class in the 1940s and 1950s. Social programs, specifically Medicare and Medicaid, helped fill this need for the poor in the 1960s. In 1964, the nonpoor saw physicians about 20% more frequently than the poor; by 1975, however, this ratio reversed and the poor visited physicians 18% more often than the nonpoor.[27]

The social programs of the 1960s made a significant impact on nursing. Nurses began to see more poor patients, because the physicians who were seeing these patients were also admitting more of them to hospitals for nursing care and making referrals for follow-up nursing care in the community. The numbers of these patients seen by nurses increased.

Minority groups traditionally have been among the poorer segments of the population. Poorer people receive more health care as a result of increased social welfare funding. The ethnic-minority groups are often recipients as well. Increased ethnic-minority groups in the health care system brought a new awareness of their needs to the nursing profession, which in turn added impetus to finding ways for better understanding of their unique needs.

A second social factor that brought pressure on nursing to address multicultural needs was the rapid influx of immigrants. During the 1970s, an average of half a million immigrants entered the United States legally each year. Two minorities in particular added considerable numbers to the American population: 15 million Spanish-speaking and 3½ million Asian Americans. Previously, blacks were the only minority of significant number.[21]

Three major minorities now exist in the United States. The largest minority is blacks, with 26 million, or about ¹/₁₀ of the US population. No longer are Americans either black or white. The world is no longer structured to encourage uniformity, but rather diversity. When blacks were the only recognized ethnic group, they encountered racial and ethnic prejudice; whites, who were themselves ethnically diverse, tried to emulate (subconsciously perhaps) the WASP ideal.

In the past, new immigrants experienced a process of *enculturation* until they were homogenized with the American people. In the process they retained little of their former heritage. However, there is now more of an appreciation of cultural diversity and the melting pot ideal has faded.

•   •   •

Over the past 25 years, transcultural nursing emerged as a formal area of study and an explicit practice in nursing with a definite set of goals and purposes. A variety of societal factors, including the advent of Medicare and Medicaid, the rapid influx of immigrants, and the civil rights movement influenced the direction of nursing toward multicultural interests.

As the need for a better understanding of ethnic-minority cultural values became evident, educators addressed the problem by incorporating transcultural content into nursing curricula on the undergraduate and graduate levels. Nurses, who shared a common interest in advancing the field of transcultural nursing, joined forces and organized national conferences, societies, and councils.

Technical advances continue to bring peoples of the world closer, creating a greater demand for nurses who understand other cultures. Nurses made marked progress in the past 2 decades toward seeking a better understanding of other cultures. In view of the size and complexity of the world, however, the challenge still lies before nurses, who haven't finished the task but have only just begun.

MAKING CULTURAL ASSESSMENTS*

Rather than impose personal cultural care values on others, the professional nurse is an active listener and analyst who develops appropriate care plans based on the insights, knowledge, and beliefs of other cultures. The problem in implementing this philosophy is the inclination of nurses to use their professional and culturally-determined personal values and beliefs to give care to others.

Beliefs, customs, and values are variables at three levels: the patient or client, the nurse, and the health care facility, or agency (see box). When one is incongruent with any other, the incongruencies must be resolved. The format in the box can be used to measure the degree of congruency or incongruency. Following this format, the nurse may begin to plan nursing action and interventions.

Perhaps one of the greatest mistakes nurses make in working with culturally different

---

*Parts of this section are contributed by Tony Tripp-Reimer.

ASSESSMENT OF CULTURAL VARIABLES AT THREE LEVELS

	Beliefs	Customs	Values
Patient or client			
Nurse			
Health care facility or agency			

people is transferring expectations based on their own cultural background. This is easy to do and makes one feel secure, but the outcome may be a failure to obtain desired behavioral results.

A second mistake is that of making generalizations about culturally different groups. Groups have subgroups, whose core beliefs may be shared, but language, customs, beliefs, and values may differ significantly. Subgroup ideas about the cause and cure of illness and health may or may not be shared.

When language barriers are present it is difficult to assure that patients or clients are given care within the standards of the Patient Bill of Rights. For example, informed consent is not possible when the health care team and patient speak different languages. The patient may have a different set of beliefs regarding the meaning of a procedure based on values. An interpreter may be the only means of communicating. Because of fear and difference in values, it may be necessary to keep the number of procedures to a minimum for culturally different patients.

A culture is composed of a group of persons with a common set of beliefs, customs, and values, which dictate behavior that is overall to the group. For a cultural assessment a systematic study must include these factors.

A number of cultural assessment tools have been developed for use by health care professionals. Some are short and specific, whereas others are lengthy and comprehensive. Whether nurses choose to integrate cultural assessment in the nursing process or

---

PARTS OF A CULTURAL ASSESSMENT

Values	Beliefs	Customs	Social group factors
Health	Health	Communication	Family structure
Nature of man	Health maintenance	Verbal	Religion
Man, nature	Illness	Language	Politics
Time	Cause	Speed of Talking	Education
Activity	Diagnosis	Style	Economy
Relationship	Treatments	Nonverbal	Health systems
	Religious	Touch	Formal
	Other	Space, interpersonal	Informal
		Silence	Alternative
		Eye contact	practitioners and
		Decision-making	facilities
		Religion	Ethnic identification
		Food	History
		Family roles/	Art
		behavior	Physical environment
		Death, dying	Other
		Other	

---

conduct a very specific and separate assessment should depend on the health problem and clinical setting. Regardless of how it is accomplished, cultural assessment should be including in the nursing process cultural assessment. Guidelines are listed in the box.

The importance of accurate assessment of individual families and groups in planning nursing and overall health care cannot be overemphasized. The planning of residential communities often does not accommodate cultural preferences, and consequently nursing and health care is affected. People of certain European nationality and enculturation, e.g., Czechs, Hungarians, Romanians, may prefer to live in their own homes, but when that is not possible they are likely to accept long-term care facilities much more readily than people of Amish or Greek origin. When working with patients or clients of a given background, it is necessary as well to understand how families of these patients or clients feel. If not congruent, then there are additional factors that must be worked out.

One example is that of nursing home planning. Adjustments can be made within the environment to simulate the preferred living situation of persons for whom the facility is the least desirable care option. Amish patients may prefer an area of the building where noise and clutter of radios and TV are less. The nurse, caring for a person from that culture, should make, as part of the nursing care plan, a goal of providing an environment in which mechanical technology and its noise output are kept to a minimum. As patient advocates, nurses must be creative about making such adaptations, and also in suggesting actions can make life more satisfying and humanistic, e.g., the Amish nursing home resident can benefit from leave for short visits to a family farm to check on a horse. Restrictions from all that is meaningful can cause a patient to become belligerent.

Psychiatric nurses who work with depressed patients need to look for insights into the cause of the depression by obtaining data specific to the cultural background of the patient. It may be that the depression has its basis in conflict between cultural expectations of the group or community and reality of what is possible.

EXAMPLE: A young Greek man is depressed, because he thinks he has betrayed the family's status of honor by moving his father to a nursing home.

Cultural data makes the nurse alert to social factors that may be the basis for depression and other conditions. This is useful in making an assessment and planning nursing interventions.

Nurses must include a cultural assessment in nursing care plans and while caring for individuals, either well or ill. Factors to consider are individual, but also influenced by cultural factors. Some factors to identify are whether the individual is a part of a cultural group that is predominantly made up of nuclear families, isolated individuals, or extended families. Also consider whether the society is male-dominated, female-dominated, or equalitarian. One must be aware of the difference between being strong and being dominant. For example, black women demonstrate strength to preserve family life, but they are not necessarily dominant. Further, the nurse must recognize the overall characteristic, in this case male/female dominance, but remember that individual variations occur within the predominate pattern.

Basic cultural data include the following ethnic deviations or affiliations:

1. Religious preference
2. Pattern of family makeup (eating patterns, food preferences)
3. Patterns of caring for health

This knowledge can provide all the information that the nurse needs in many situations. When the patient or client is inexplicably noncompliant with a recommended plan of care, knowing how to explore cultural data in greater depth is necessary to explain the patient/client's behavior.

Cultural assessment tools have been devised by numerous nurses. However, the goal here is to assist the student-reader to gain awareness of cultural patterns and differences and, as a professional nurse, apply them to the assessment of patients or clients. Assessment models have been developed by Orque, Brownlee, Black, Tripp-Reimer, Admodt, Leininger, and Branch. Included here is a basic assessment format (see box).

After the nurse identifies the patient/client's ethnicity, degree of identification with ethnic roots, religion, and decision making process the next step is to obtain more specific data. To do so, pertinent questions must be answered. Appropriate questions for obtaining cultural information about specific health problems are provided in the following six sample questions:

1. What do you think caused your problem?
2. Why did it start?

_____ PROCESS OF CULTURAL ASSESSMENT _____

	Beliefs	Customs	Values

DATA COLLECTION
General content
  Ethnicity
  Degree of affiliation
Problem content
  Diabetic diet
  Pregnancy
Intervention			

DATA ORGANIZATION General content Problem content Intervention			
DATA INTERPRETATON General content Problem content Intervention			

---

2. Why did it start?
3. How bad/serious is your illness?
4. How does your sickness work?
5. What treatment do you think will make you well?
6. What frightens you about your sickness?

Before planning nursing actions or interventions, the nurse needs further information that is designed to obtain cultural data. The following six sample questions can be useful:

1. Is your situation good or bad?
2. Have you had this problem before and what do (did) you do for it?
3. What should a person do if they have this problem?
4. What are you planning to do with your situation?
5. How should a person in your situation (with your sickness) be treated by your family?
6. How should people in the community treat you?

Values have been categorized into the following four aspects:

1. **Time** is past, present, and future; cultural groups vary in the emphasis placed on one versus the other
2. **Personal activity** orientation of a culture has emphasis on either doing or being;

larly for accomplishments. A culture that is being-oriented values a person simply for existence, e.g., being a link between generations
3. **Relationship orientation** can be broken down into several categories: in societies such as Russia and Israel, a collateral pattern of rational behavior predominates because individuals are concerned with others on a lateral plan as members of their own group; other societies stress the importance of lineage, and kinship is emphasized in terms of maintaining lineality, usually stressing that the male carry the major responsibility for lineage
4. **Orientation of the individual to nature** described how the culture views man and nature, and which has major emphasis, e.g., nature over man, man over nature

An aspect of nursing care is concern for nutritional status. Cultural differences within the mainstream of American society affect nutritional status. Persons born in the United States have profound differences in food habits, depending on ethnic origin, beliefs, or religious background. These habits can serve as risks to good health. People of Scandinavian origin prefer cheese and fish; Mexicans tend to eat cornmeal and highly spiced foods; and Asians like fish and vegetables. To determine nutritional balance in a person's diet, have patients/clients keep a 7-day dietary record of all foods eaten; at the end of that period review the record for congruency with the requirements of a well-balanced diet.

Religious affiliation also influences food intake and nutritional status. Orthodox Jews eat only foods of a certain kind that are prepared according to Jewish law. Some conservative Christian denominations sponsor frequent church suppers or potluck meals, which are heavily concentrated with high calorie desserts, salads, and macaroni dishes that have little meat.

The nurse receives verbal or nonverbal messages from patients/clients to indicate whether an accurate assessment is made and nursing care given that is congruent with that patient/client's expectations, i.e., the nurse and/or health care facility has appropriately crossed cultural lines; now the patient, nurse, and facility are on the same wavelength.

Some behavior that may be observed when providing care to culturally different people is passive obedience. This may be explained in various ways, but could be due to a belief by the patient that the nurse or other health care worker is an authority figure or an expert. The Southeast Asian person is apt to cope with uncertainty and authority in the same way, i.e., to be passively obedient. Instead of asking questions when uncertain, such a person may conceal lack of knowledge by being obedient or compliant.

Sometimes when patients/clients are labeled as noncompliant, it is because of an inaccurate cultural assessment by the nurse or other health workers. The patient may not understand or may be unable to accomplish expectations. Noncompliance among persons of different cultures may have bases associated with cultural perceptions of the patient/client. Reasons for lack of compliance with planned care, in the case of a Vietnamese refugee, may be disappearance of the symptoms, inconvenience, and lack of precedent for continuing the regimen. This lack of compliance is reinforced when there is a relative lack of other supports such as family and social encouragement, absence of knowledge about treatment of asymptomatic conditions, and the precedent of traditional self-care and self-medication.

Refugees, in general, tend to seek care from health care providers because they feel alone, are alienated socially, and other sources of institutional support (school, church) are not available to them as a result of language and various barriers. They form a bond with people who demonstrate a caring attitude.

• • •

Nurses accept individuals as they are, regardless of the setting or circumstances. In present American society, few nurses are limited to caring for people exclusively from backgrounds that parallel their own. In the past, native Americans, blacks, Mexicans, and people from Northern European cultures composed the major groups with which nurses interacted in daily practice. With the recent great influx of Southeast Asians, South Africans, people from the Mideast, and now people from the Eastern Block, nurses are challenged to learn how to cross cultural lines and break down communication barriers.

One mistake a nurse can make is to generalize. For example, nursing care to the Native American cannot be planned and provided universally to all Native Americans without consideration of subgroup differences created by tribal differences.

The nurse should remember that cultural assessments and judgments are relative, based on one's experience, and experience is interpreted by people based on their own enculturation. One stereotypes people unconsciously on the basis of one's own value systems. Therefore, when performing a cultural assessment it is important not to stereotype, because there may be persons in a cultural group who are more acculturated to the dominant society rather than to their group of origin.

Significant changes in US demographics require nurses to attune to the philosophy that serves as a foundation of transcultural nursing. Nurses must be able to cross cultural lines with ease. Theories from anthropology and other fields are important, but each nurse must establish a foundation that has a nursing perspective.

Transcultural nursing is developing through research and experience with ethnic and cultural groups. Regretfully, not all who have contributed to the body of knowledge as *transcultural* have been acknowledged.

The second section of this chapter deals with the practical aspects of making a cultural assessment. Because this is not a textbook and space is limited the discussion is not in great detail but gives the nurse a format, some examples, and a basis for thinking of patients/clients from a cultural viewpoint. For further detail the reader is referred to books, articles, and research reports on transcultural nursing and health care.

STUDY ACTIVITIES

1. Describe your own background in cultural terms using the three major categories of data (beliefs, values, customs).
2. Describe a situation you have encountered in which you feel you could have given better nursing care had you known the patient/client's cultural background better.
3. Review briefly the history of transcultural nursing in the United States.

REFERENCES

1. American Nurses' Association: code for nurses with interpretive statements, Kansas City, 1976, American Nurses' Association.
2. American Nurses' Association: commission on human rights, Council on International Nursing, Executive Committee meeting minutes, December 5-7, 1980, American Nurses' Association.
3. American Nurses' Association Commission on Human Rights: historical background (unpublished).
4. American Nurses' Association Commission on Human Rights: guidelines for Council on Intercultural Nursing (unpublished).
5. American Nurses' Association: Council on Cultural Diversity in Nursing Practice Operating Guidelines, (unpublished), 1984, The American Nurses' Association.
6. American Nurses' Association: Council on Intercultural Nursing Newsletter, 1(1), Feb-March, 1981, American Nurses' Association.
7. American Nurses' Association: standards of nursing practice, Kansas City, 1973, American Nurses' Association.
8. Branch M: Models for introducing cultural diversity in nursing curricula, J Nurs Educ 15, March 1976.
9. Branch M and Paxton P: Providing safe nursing care for ethnic people of color, New York, 1976, Appleton-Century-Crofts.
10. Brink P: Cultural aspects of sexuality, Holistic Nursing Practice 1(4):12-19, 1987.
11. Donders JG: African Institute lecture, Notre Dame University, 1987.
12. Johnson C: Data on ethnic nurses, Council in Intercultural Nursing Newsletter, 1(1), February/March 1981.
13. Leininger M: Ethnoscience: a new and promising research approach for the health sciences, Image 3(1):22-28, 1969.
14. Leininger M: Transcultural health care issues and conditions, Philadelphia, 1976, FA Davis Co.
15. Leininger M: Transcultural nursing: concepts, theories, and practices, New York, 1978, John Wiley & Sons.
16. Leininger M: A decade of growth, discovery, and recognition. Paper presented at the Tenth National Transcultural Nursing Society Conference, Boston, October 1984.
17. Major ML: Developing cultural sensitivity, Calif Nurse 83(2):5, 1987.
18. Morley D: Personal interview, July 6, 1988, London, England.
19. Munyere A: Personal interview, July 18, 1988, Kenya, East Africa.
20. Murillo-Rohde I: Cultural diversity in curriculum development. Paper presented at "Chautauqua '76" sponsored by the Colorado Nurses' Association, Vail, Colorado, July 1976. In Leininger M: Transcultural nursing: concepts, theories, and practices, New York, 1978, John Wiley and Sons.
21. Naisbitt J: Megatrends: ten new directions transforming our lives, New York, 1982, Warner Books, Inc.
22. National League for Nursing, Council of Baccalaureate and Higher Degree Programs: criteria for the evaluation of baccalaureate and higher degree programs in nursing, Pub. No. 15-1251 (ed 5), New York, 1983, National League for Nursing.
23. Nightingale F (1865): Suggestions on a system of nursing for hospitals in India. In Seymer L (compiler): Selected writings of Florence Nightingale, New York, 1954, MacMillan.
24. Orque M (1983): Orque's ethnic/cultural system: a framework for ethnic nursing care. In Orque M, Block B, and Monrroy L: Ethnic nursing care: a multicultural approach, St. Louis, 1983, The CV Mosby Co.
25. Rand McNally Road Atlas, 1986, Library of Congress No. 79-62950.
26. Spradley B: Community health nursing: concepts and practice, ed 2, Boston, 1985, Little Brown.
27. Starr P: The social transformation of American medicine, New York, 1982, Basic Books, Inc.
28. Thiederman S: Ethnocentrism: a barrier to effective health care, Nurs Pract 11(8):56-59, 1986.
29. Tripp-Reimer T: Research in cultural diversity: directions for future research, West Nurs 6(2):253-255, 1984.
30. Worcester A: Nurses and nursing, Cambridge, 1927, Harvard University Press.

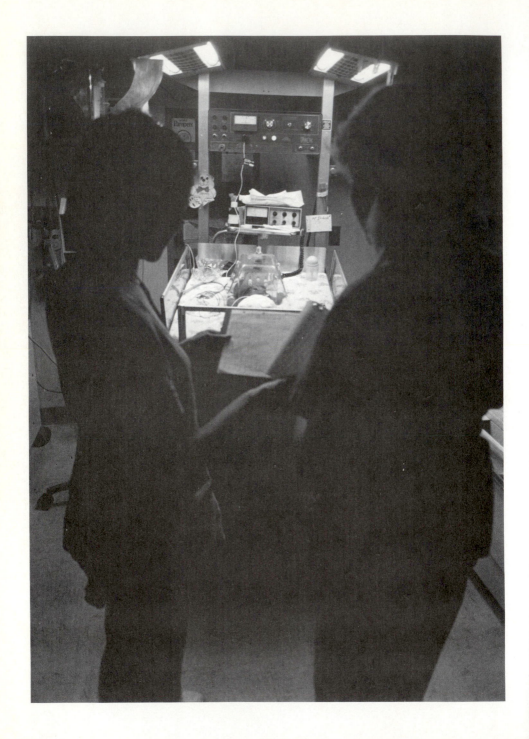

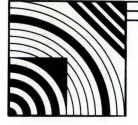

CHAPTER 6

LEGAL ASPECTS OF NURSING

Cheryl Hall Harris

OBJECTIVES

After completing this chapter the reader should be able to:

- Identify three major sources that provide laws

- Differentiate between statutory law, common law, and administrative law

- Distinguish between criminal law and civil law. Give examples of how these may be breached by the nurse

- Identify at least three areas within the category of civil law and provide explanation of each

- Define the difference between negligence and malpractice

- Explain how a complaint case moves through the court system

- Define liability

- Identify and describe three types of professional liability insurance nurses may carry

- Discuss some areas out of which lawsuits often originate such as informed consent, do not resuscitate (DNR), physician orders, and documentation

In a civilized society, a system of laws promotes order, protects the rights of citizens, and provides the framework for a wide variety of relationships. Laws help establish order within a society for the common good of all. In today's complex world, with advancing technologies and an array of societal problems, legal issues are an important aspect of life. For nurses in practice within the current health care system, knowledge of basic legal concepts is vital.

Nurses have been legally accountable for their actions for many years, and current trends regarding the legal ramifications of nursing practice compel nurses to learn the legal aspects of their field. Many contemporary nurses are functioning in more autonomous roles, in which legal exposure increases in proportion to their level of independence.

In addition to the altruistic motivation of providing the highest quality of care to their patients, nurses need to understand the parameters of nursing practice within their state and country, as governed by nurse practice acts and standards of care established by organizations and the employing institution. As nurses adopt the role of patient advocate, they should promote concepts of patient rights. Finally, nurses must be aware of legal implications of nursing practice because present day society is litigious, and an increasing number of nurses have been named as defendants in malpractice lawsuits.

How LAWS ARE ESTABLISHED

The following three major sources provide laws for society:
1. **Statutory laws**—generated by various legislative bodies such as state legislatures or the Congress of the United States
2. **Common law**—evolves through the court system as judicial decisions are made in various cases; through the concept of setting precedents, the decision made in one case may affect the decision made in a later and similar case; each state develops a body of common law through previous rulings
3. **Administrative law**—provided by a legislative body, which gives authority to some other agency to regulate procedures; e.g., a state board of nursing is often authorized to publish and promote certain regulations regarding nursing practice[17]

LEGAL CATEGORIES

The legal system may be divided into two categories: criminal law and civil law. Criminal law relates to a violation of law. In criminal cases, an individual commits a crime and faces trial in the criminal court system, and, if convicted, expects some form of punishment. The purpose of the punishment is to discourage others from committing the same crime, as well as to punish the person who violates the law.

Civil law deals with disputes over legal rights and duties of individuals in relation to one another. In a civil action, compensation or damages may be awarded to the injured person from the other person(s) who caused the harm. It is possible for nurses to be in a situation that involves both civil and criminal laws. This may result because civil and criminal components are included in both statutory and common law.[7]

EXAMPLE: Horsley[13] describes a case in which a home health nurse overstepped nursing boundaries. A Visiting Nurses' Association (VNA) nurse, Mary was assigned to visit a patient under emergency circumstances, when a physician believed the patient might have suffered a cardiovascular accident (CVA). In her initial assessment, Mary reported the symptoms to the physician, who diagnosed a transient ischemic attack (TIA) and prescribed medication to decrease the patient's blood pressure. Mary continued to provide care.

A month later, Mary received an emergency call from the family. She neither notified the VNA nor the physician, but rushed to the patient's home to examine him. She assessed his condition as another TIA, and then made a severe error: she instructed the patient to take the remaining portion of the medication, even though she still had not contacted the physician. This constitutes the practice of medicine, which is illegal, because Mary was not licensed to do so. Unfortunately the patient suffered a massive CVA that night, and suffered from weakness and aphasia nearly 2 weeks later when he was released from the hospital. This patient charged Mary with professional malpractice. Horsley reminds nurses that no matter how autonomous the environment in which they practice, they must never diagnose, prescribe, or direct treatment.

Criminal Law as it Relates to Nursing

There are instances in which a nurse breaks a law and is tried in the criminal court system. An example of criminal activity involves a nurse who misappropriates controlled substances, either for her own personal use or to sell to others. This circumstance usually includes falsification of records to "cover" the misdeed.

In *State of New Jersey v. Winter,* a conviction of manslaughter was judged against a nurse who had transfused incompatible blood into a patient, concealed her conduct, and falsified the records. The patient died of a transfusion reaction.[17] Northrop and Kelly further note that, "In some jurisdictions, alterations of a medical record or creation of a false medical record is a misdemeanor in itself."[17]

The expanded role of the nurse, including anesthetists, midwives, practitioners, and clinical specialists has led to development of new statutes and regulations, as well as increased legal exposure. One of the important areas of clarification involves legal distinctions in the definition of nursing practice, as opposed to medical practice.

In most instances, additional education and/or certification in a specialty are required for a nurse to practice in this extended capacity. "Some states have specific advanced practice laws authorizing nurse practitioner practice...Many state laws require that nurse practitioners be certified by the applicable professional association."[17] Practice laws carefully define the scope of nursing practice within these specialized fields.

Besides specified expanded roles of nursing, there are specialty areas of practice, such as the recovery room after surgery.

EXAMPLE: In *Laidlaw v. Lions Gate Hospital,* a patient was taken to the recovery room still unconscious from an uneventful cystectomy. The charge nurse was alone because her staff nurse had left the unit for a work break. At the time Ms Laidlaw was taken to the recovery room, there were three other patients under the charge nurse's care. When the charge nurse rendered care to another patient, and accepted a phone call, she left Ms Laidlaw unattended. The patient stopped breathing, and after resuscitation, suffered permanent brain damage that required lifelong care.[6]

In the court decision, the hospital was found not liable because the unit had an appropriate number of staff, although they were not present at the time. The anesthesiologist was not liable because there was no evidence that the physician knew that there was only one nurse in this eight bed unit. Both nurses were found negligent: the charge nurse because she allowed the staff nurse to leave, and the staff nurse because she did not consider the patient load with anticipated arrivals of other patients.

In the decision, the legal opinion held that a recovery room is a highly specialized area requiring the nurse to provide "…frequent and careful observation of patients who are under the influence of anesthesia." and "…close scrutiny and ever present watchfulness are required in this room and the patient is entitled to expect the same."

Cases such as this one delineate the scope of nursing practice.[6] Similar cases will further define the role of nurses in specialty areas.

Civil Law

Several areas of civil law that affect nurses are tort law, contract law, antitrust law, and other civil laws such as employment discrimination and labor laws. Only tort law will be discussed in this chapter, although the other areas are important as well.

Tort Law. "A tort is a legal or civil wrong committed by one person against the person or property of another."[7] There are *intentional torts* (e.g., false imprisonment, or assault and/or battery) in which the injured party may seek damages for personal injury and punitive judgment against the person who injured them. In an intentional tort, the injured person must prove that there was actual intent to harm. In an *unintentional tort,* (e.g., professional negligence) there is no intent to cause harm. In a negligence case, no punitive damages are sought.

Cushing[5] defines the difference between *negligence* and *malpractice.* Negligence pertains to a person's failing to do something that a reasonable and prudent person would do, or doing something that a reasonable prudent person would not do. Malpractice involves professional wrongdoing or remarkable lack of skill in performing expected professional duties.

A civil case is heard before a judge, and a jury, unless the plaintiff waives that right. A procedural pattern ensues after a civil case is initiated (see box).

In the initial stages of a negligence suit, the complaint must contain the following four distinct elements:

1. A statement that the defendant has a duty to perform in a certain manner

---

PROCEDURE PATTERN FOR A CIVIL CASE

1. A person *(plaintiff)* files a complaint against another person *(defendant)*.
2. The complaint includes allegations of wrongdoing, which the plaintiff must prove.
3. After the complaint is "served" to the defendant, litigation procedures begin.
4. Pretrial exploration of the facts are completed by both sides. This may include witnesses to support the allegations or defense.
5. The trial begins with selection of a jury. Then the plaintiff and the defendant state their positions, often with attendant corroborating evidence.
6. After all the information is revealed, the jury deliberates and makes a decision.
7. If one of the parties believes the decision is in error, they may elect to appeal the decision by taking it to a higher court.

---

2. An allegation that there was a breach of that duty
3. A statement of proximate cause (that the error caused a problem)
4. A demand for compensation to cover damages

Common cases of negligence include foreign objects (such as sponges) left inside a patient, burns caused by equipment or solutions, falls that cause injury to a patient, serious inaccuracies in administration of medications, and failure to exercise reasonable judgment.[4]

IMPORTANT LEGAL CONCEPTS FOR NURSES

Many key legal concepts are important for nurses to understand. As nursing practice evolves, these fluid concepts are refined and change. For example, many standards of care are well defined and long-standing, but as the practice of nursing develops with new areas of specialization, new standards are formulated to address these changes. These legal concepts apply to all areas of nursing practice and are not restricted to any specific segment.

Standards of Care

Standards of care are provided by statute, by professional organizations, and by the nurse's employing institution. The nurse is expected to know all of these standards as they apply to nursing practice. For example, all states have Nursing Practice Acts to govern the parameters of nursing practice within their jurisdiction. The ANA has specific standards of practice in general and in several clinical areas.[21] Finally, the employing institution should have a carefully defined system of policies and procedures that prescribe specific nursing tasks and duties.

In the event of a claim of malpractice, one important issue will include whether or not the nurse followed the expected standards as defined by these sources. It is possible that all of the standards of care applicable to the situation may be introduced as evidence to determine whether or not the nurse met the criteria. Therefore, it is important for nurses to determine the standards that apply to their specific area of practice.

Reasonably Prudent Nurse

The practice of nursing not only requires a high degree of education and knowledge, but also involves the use of common sense. If a nurse's performance is in question, those functions will be measured against the norm of how another comparably educated nurse, within a equivalent setting, using good judgment, would have acted in the same situation. Naturally, nurses within specialized areas of practice who have received additional education will be required to perform a higher level of care than a nurse who has not received additional training.

Kelly describes that in many cases, physicians testify as expert witnesses as to whether or not a nurse functioned according to standards of care.[17] Kelly asserts that professional nurses should serve as expert witnesses regarding standards of care in any nursing malpractice case. This is the position adopted by The American Association of Nurse Attorneys and represents an emerging trend.[17] In addition, Rabinow[20] believes that, as the nurse's role in assessment of patient conditions becomes more recognized, nursing assessment may become a focal point for lawsuits in the future.

Informed Consent

Many procedures performed within the health care setting, such as surgery, require consent from the patient. Each person has the right to authorize or to refuse medical treatment. Although the physician is legally responsible for obtaining a patient's consent, nurses are often involved. Rabinow[20] asserts that as physicians assign increased responsibility for patient teaching to nurses, the nurse will experience increased obligations for obtaining informed consent.

There are several key elements to ensure that the patient actually gives informed consent (see box).[17]

Ellis and Hartley[7] suggest that nurses must obtain consent for nursing measures. For example, if a nurse enters a patient's room to administer an intramuscular medication, the nurse should inform the patient of the intended procedure. If the patient turns over to receive the injection in the buttocks, that constitutes implied consent.

Consent to Experimental Treatment

Protocols for studies that use human subjects for experimental purposes must pass a stringent review process by an institutional review board before they are approved. When experimental drugs and some techniques are employed, the Federal Food and Drug Administration is also involved in the review process. If a patient enters such a study, a highly detailed consent form is presented for signature, and the patient has the right to withdraw from the study at any time.

KEY ELEMENTS FOR INFORMED CONSENT

1. The consent must be given voluntarily by a mentally competent adult. The patient should not be coerced into giving consent.
2. Patients must understand exactly what they are consenting to. If a patient speaks a foreign language or is deaf, an interpreter must explain the consent.
3. The consent should include risks to the procedure, alternative treatments available, and prognosis if the treatment is refused.
4. The consent is usually written, to provide a record of the transaction.
5. Consent to treatment for a minor is usually given by the parent or legal guardian; but, increasingly, children who are at least 7 years old are included in the decision-making process.

Refusal of Treatment

If recommended treatment is refused, a patient must be notified of the consequences of rejection of the intended procedure, and refusal must be noted in the health care record.

EXAMPLE: In a recent Texas case, parents who were members of the Jehovah's Witnesses faith refused a blood transfusion that would save the life of their child. The child was made a ward of the court for the purposes of receiving the lifesaving transfusion. A judge ruled that although parents are adults and may choose to become martyrs, they are not allowed to make martyrs of their children.[4]

Remanding such cases to a court for decision is relatively commonplace.

Right to Privacy and Confidentiality

Patients who enter the health care system have a right to privacy of their personal lives. As society relies more heavily on computerized information and health care institutions enter the computer age with patient records, patients become more apprehensive about possible invasion of privacy. In particular, patients who are infected with human immunodeficiency virus (HIV) are concerned that their privacy be maintained, because of possible repercussions if that information becomes available to outside sources.

Only people directly involved with a patient should have access to patient records. If information is given without patient or legal guardian consent, a nurse can be held liable. Many health care institutions have rigorous policies about issues of confidentiality and the right to privacy. Nurses must be aware of these policies to avoid a breach of confidentiality.

As health care agencies begin to use computers to keep records, they must develop policies and procedures to ensure the confidentiality of all computerized information. A system of identification and authorization codes will help maintain the integrity of computer data.[2]

Documentation

Health care records for each patient provide a complete and accurate representation of all care delivered to the patient, including diagnostic tests and their results, physical examination, procedures, assessments of condition, and any therapy ordered and received. Nurses are involved in this extremely important aspect of patient care. If there is a malpractice lawsuit, written documentation of a patient's care may literally determine the outcome of the case.[2]

Important elements of appropriate nursing documentation[2] include the following:
1. Accuracy—a patient's record must never be falsified; entries should be dated, timed, and written in sequence as events occur
2. If an error is written, it is marked through with a single line, the word "error" written and initialed; do not erase or obliterate the error
3. Completeness—it is important to record all nursing and health care interventions and their outcome
4. Nursing charting should be objective with factual data
5. Documentation must be legible and permanent

Quality Assurance

Quality Assurance is a program adopted by an institution that is designed to promote the best possible care. These systems include ongoing education of staff, evaluation of staff performance on a routine schedule, and an audit of selected activities on a regular basis. If a problem surfaces, efforts will be made to correct it.[17]

EXAMPLE: A nursing service department develops the expectation that every patient will have an individualized nursing care plan within a certain period of time after admission. Using a system of routine monitors, they determine whether or not the expectation is being met. If patients do not have nursing care plans, the department works to correct that problem.

Risk Management

Risk Management is usually related to quality assurance and may overlap functions; however, it is designed to identify problems, and to evaluate and correct problems to decrease the possibility of financial loss to the institution or individual. Typically, risk identification involves a specific patient care problem such as an unusual incident. A medication error, a patient who falls, or an IV that infiltrates and leads to further complications are examples of unusual incidents.

In a system of risk management, an incident report is filed describing the error. After the report is completed, it is analyzed by a risk manager who looks for possible trends within a nursing unit, or the entire institution. If a trend is noted, corrective actions are initiated to decrease occurrence of the problem, and then an evaluation of effectiveness of these activities is completed. Bowyer predicts an increase in risk management in the future because it not only decreases liability, but also benefits health care.[17]

Diagnostic Related Groups

DRGs are a classification system based on diagnosis of illness, with typical length of stay and hospitalization costs attached to the diagnoses. Currently, payment for Medicare patients is based on the DRG system. However, Kelly suggests that, "insurance companies are considering adopting the DRG-based prospective payment system."[17] Kelly describes studies that demonstrate some patients suffer complications as a result of discharge from an intensive care unit (ICU) before their condition warrants this action. She further submits: "To the extent that the decision to admit or discharge a patient from the ICU depends on a nursing assessment, the nurse may be implicated in liability for early discharge (abandonment) or failure to admit."

Floating to Another Unit

In many health care institutions, nurses are required to work in settings other than their normal area of practice. The practice of "floating" nurses from one unit to another usually results from inadequate numbers of staff. As the current staffing crisis in nursing increases, this problem may intensify. If a nurse is floated to an area in which she does not feel qualified, she may present the supervising nurse with a written protest to the assignment. In fact, Kelly describes a document, known as an *assignment despite objection,* developed by The California Nurse's Association, for this express purpose.

There are other options for nurses who experience this situation. They may request a restricted set of duties within the role required of them. For example, if floated to an intensive care setting, a nurse might assess vital signs and give medications—tasks with which the nurse is familiar—but another nurse might closely supervise and perform tasks that the floating nurse is not comfortable in doing—tasks such as caring for a central line.

Nurses who perform outside of their accustomed area of practice may do harm to a patient. Creighton[4] describes a case in which an obstetrical nurse, floated to an emergency room, administered a markedly increased dose of lidocaine to a patient. The patient suffered cardiac arrest and subsequent irreversible severe brain damage. The hospital and the nurse were named as defendants in the lawsuit, which the plaintiff won.

Short Staffing

Staffing ratio guidelines, based on the level of acuity of the patients, have been established by the Joint Commission on Accreditation of Hospitals. If required to accept an assignment to provide care for more clients than is reasonable, a nurse should write a protest to the supervising nurse. Although this protest would not relieve the nurse from responsibility if a problem ensues, it would demonstrate that the nurse was attempting to act in good faith. Nurses should not refuse assignment in such a situation and leave the area, because this could lead to a charge of abandonment by the patients.[12]

Decreasing Risk of Malpractice Lawsuits

Although the societal climate is favorable towards initiation of lawsuits, nurses can take some actions to decrease the risk.[7] Generally, patients want to be considered as individuals and not as just another number. Therefore, any nursing activity that helps to personalize care will set a positive nurse-patient relationship. Formulating individualized nursing care plans is a way to accomplish this goal.

If the patient believes the nurse is trying to render the best possible care, the patient is less likely to sue, even if unforeseen circumstances arise and some problem develops. Nurses must be sensitive to patient needs and try to respond in a timely fashion. As Rabinow[20] affirms, "A patient-centered attitude will go a long way toward minimizing your liability."

Naturally, following accepted standards of care and attempting to give the best possible care is the best means of decreasing risk. Nurses must continually update their education and maintain competency in their area of practice, as well as maintain good rapport with their patients.

Liability Insurance

If named as a defendant in a malpractice lawsuit, the costs incurred in a nurse's defense may be prohibitive. In the current legal climate of our society, the number of lawsuits initiated has risen dramatically, the size of monetary awards has increased, and some attorneys generate large fee charges. Therefore, nurses are encouraged to carry individual malpractice insurance to help defray the costs of defense. Some state legislatures address these problems by drafting laws to permit awards that cover only actual losses and cost of care, but which limit awards for intangible factors such as claims for pain and suffering.[7]

The following are three types of professional liability insurance[17]:

1. **Individual professional liability**—insures the individual nurse for any professional actions performed at any time, or any place; the nurse should look for several elements such as coverage period, limits on coverage, and the authority to select an attorney
2. **Institutional Liability**—provides coverage for nurses if they are acting within their scope of employment in their institution
3. **Commercial Liability**—covers partnerships, corporations, or business ventures

Baldwin-Mech[2] suggest that nurses should be sufficiently protected by individual policies, or institutional policies, before they practice nursing. Frequently, individual policies are available from professional organizations such as the ANA. Ford[9] describes a lack of professional liability insurance as the "Ultimate Malpractice Pitfall." He relates, "...if you're ever sued and found liable for damages, your insurance may be all that stands between you and serious financial hardship."

Physician Orders

Physicians are responsible for directing medical treatment, and nurses are obligated to follow physician's orders unless they believe the orders to be in error and that they would cause harm to the patient. If a nurse performs an order in question, both the nurse and the physician could be liable. "The courts increasingly have begun to recognize that the scientific knowledge base on which nursing relies increases the duty nurses owe to the health care consumer."[5] In the event a nurse questions an order, the physician continues to confirm that order, and the nurse still believes it is inappropriate, the supervising nurse should be notified. The supervising nurse should help to resolve the questionable order.[11]

Physician orders should be written; oral orders are not recommended because of increased possibility of error. The legal editor of *Nursing '89* wrote a review letter in which a nurse accepted a verbal order from a resident. When the attending physician questioned the order, the resident denied having given it. Therefore the nurse appeared to have acted without authority. The legal editor suggests that a nurse accepting a verbal order should have another nurse listen, and then cosign the order as verification.[14] If an oral order is necessary during an emergency situation, it should be written and signed within 24 hours if possible.

Do Not Resuscitate Orders

Historically, when a heart stops beating, a patient is declared dead. However, in modern health care institutions, resuscitation for cardiac and pulmonary arrest is commonplace. When a *Code* to prevent death is required, an entire system of emergency and extraordinary care is initiated to return a patient to a viable state. Our technological advances have led to dramatic and emotional decisionmaking situations.[16]

In many intensive care settings, Do Not Resuscitate (DNR) orders are common, and most hospitals have policies to address this important issue. Physicians are responsible for writing a DNR order, although the decision to receive life-sustaining measures rests with the patient.[17] Kelly presents key elements, proposed by a number of professional organizations, that should be included in a DNR order (see box).[17] The issue of resuscitation provides some clear cut and specific actions to be withheld. Recent cases describe patients or family members who wish to stop other means of supportive treatment such as long-term ventilatory support, or tube feedings. The legal dilemmas presented in these cases are often decided in the court system. The ethical

---

KEY PRINCIPLES FOR A DNR ORDER

1. Statement of policy of the institution that resuscitation will be initiated unless there is a specific order to withhold resuscitative measures
2. Statement from the patient regarding specific desires
3. Description of the patient's medical condition to justify a DNR order
4. Statement about the role of family members or significant others
5. Definition of the scope of the DNR order
6. Statement about the initiation of the DNR order
7. Delineation of the role of various care givers

Adapted from Northrop CE and Kelly ME: Legal issues in nursing, 1987, The CV Mosby Co.

component to deciding these and other cases are frequently reviewed by hospital bioethics committees.

Hospital DNRs on individual patients may require updating, for example, every 72 hours. Rigid protocols delineate how a DNR is assigned and who participates. Nurses are often involved in the dilemma of an expiring DNR, or caring for patients whom they feel should have such status. Currently, some humanistic-thinking professionals, and the public in various states, are taking radical steps to assure individuals a graceful end to life, when it is the individual's willful desire. Ethical, social, economic, and other factors mandate our society to face the overwhelming task of maintaining persons on life support machinery.

Advanced Directives

Karen Ann Quinlan was attached to a respirator for many months before her parents requested it be turned off. The physician and hospital refused, believing they would be responsible for her death. Her parents sued for the right to do so and in a landmark decision by the New Jersey Supreme Court, their request was granted. The Quinlan case jolted other state legislatures into looking at a method for individuals to inform their loved ones and physicians of their desires regarding health care, if they are unable to do so themselves.

In the Fall of 1989, the Supreme Court made medico-legal history when it heard the case of Nancy Cruzan, the first case involving the right of an adult patient to forgo life-sustaining treatment. Nancy Cruzan at 31 years of age, has been in a persistent vegetative state since 1983 as the result of a car accident. She is kept alive by fluids and nutrients administered through a gastronomy tube. In 1987, her parents requested that the treatment be stopped, stating that Nancy would not want to continue to live under such circumstances. The hospital refused to comply with the parents' request. Although lower courts agreed to the withholding of food and fluid, the Missouri attorney general appealed the case to the state supreme court, which ruled, in a four to three decision, that the artificial feeding must continue. The case was appealed to the federal supreme court, which must ultimately decide whether to stop the artificial feeding. Generally, the right-to-die revolves around the following key issues:

1. Do an individual's constitutional and common law rights outweigh the state interest in life?
2. Do incompetent patients retain the same right to forgo life-sustaining treatment that competent patients possess?
3. Who should make decisions on behalf of the incompetent patient?

Many states have enacted laws that direct a physician in the course of care when a person becomes terminally ill or comatose. The right-to-die laws have differing forms, but they are all advanced directives. Living wills are a written statement that asks that no heroic measures be taken when expectation of recovery from extreme physical or mental disability is unlikely. Directives to physicians permit requests for no extraordinary treatment when terminally ill and treatment would only prolong the dying process. Another form of directive is called the *Durable Power of Attorney for Health Care* (DPAHC), which allows a statement of desire regarding heroic treatment and extraordinary treatment. However, unlike the others, the DPAHC permits an adult patient to designate a surrogate who can direct care when the patient is unable to do so. The DPAHC limits the attorney-in-fact to health care decisions and then only in the limited time when signatories can not make decisions for themselves, such as when comatose or mentally incapacitated. In the state of California, and 35 other states, the DPAHC is a legal document, valid for 7 years and revokable at any time, that affords control over health care when the patient is most vulnerable. It is also a protection to physicians when individual members of the family can not agree on a course of action.

Emanuel and Emanuel[8] proposed the Medical Directive, which contains the following five distinct portions:

1. An introduction that explains the purpose of advance care documents
2. A portion with four scenarios of illness, in which patients can give preferences for medical treatment if such situations apply to them
3. A segment in which patients may name a proxy decision maker
4. A section for patients to give permission to donate their organs
5. Space for the patient to compose a personal statement about values, the limits of life, and goals of treatment

Emanuel and Emanuel further suggest that if medical directives were available in physicians' offices, they would probably improve physician-patient communication in these important issues.

Because each state's statutes are different, it is imperative that health care professionals learn what is operative in their area. There is agreement that the patient is the true "Captain of the Ship" and has the legal right to determine the course of care. Because of that, nurses can no longer be satisfied with only following physicians' orders, and must teach clients about their rights, advocate for their wishes, and be active on committees that serve to meet the client's needs. Life and death decisions are complex, and therefore need educated and caring professionals willing to grapple with the complexities to serve the client well.

PERINATAL NURSING

In perinatal nursing, nurses see effects of their care on both mothers and their infants. Technological advances altered this field immeasurably over the past 2 decades, and new techniques are being developed continuously. Advances in genetics, prenatal diagnosis, fetal surgery, and techniques of newborn intensive care have increased chances for infant survival. However, societal problems such as drug use, spread of sexually transmitted disease, and low rate of prenatal care and immunization among the poor keep infant mortality rates at a high level in the United States.

Maternal Drug Use

One of the most alarming trends to affect perinatal nurses is the rise in drug use among pregnant women. Alcohol, tobacco, and various sedatives have been used for many years, but the increase in numbers of pregnant women who use cocaine and other illegal drugs complicates treatment and nursing care of these women and their infants. The negative effects of maternal drug use for children may produce problems for a prolonged period, perhaps a lifetime.

Experts agree that most drug users are actually *polydrug* users, that is, they use more than one substance at a time. Frequently a drug such as "crack" cocaine will be extended with other drugs such as PCP. Also, sometimes several drugs such as alcohol and cocaine, are used together to enhance the effect. Another alarming aspect of today's societal drug use is that "Thousands of women from middle and upper socioeconomic groups are addicted to this drug (cocaine) of the 1980s."[3]

In some health care facilities, nurses assist addicted patients to enter drug treatment centers. If a mother refuses to do so, then her baby may be removed from her care and placed in protective services or foster care.

Sexually Transmitted Diseases in Pregnancy

Of the more than 20 sexually transmissible diseases, two present serious ramifications because they are incurable and because they cause irreversible congenital effects: herpes and AIDS. Public health officials indicate that the number of infected women continues to rise.[22] The effects of these diseases may prove life-threatening to the newborn.

Many sexually transmitted diseases must be reported to local health departments. The CDC issued guidelines for reporting that stress the importance of preserving privacy for the patient, while promoting public good by disclosing information about the infection. Incidence statistics are compiled using this reported data. Because reporting of this information is mandated, the nurse is immune from a claim of breach of confidentiality if she reports the information. Other than the official reporting of these diseases, confidentiality still applies.[17]

Contact tracing is a difficult issue that arises in caring for patients with AIDS. This program requires the cooperation of the patient identified as a carrier: the patient is asked to reveal names and addresses of any sexual or drug-sharing partners. In such instances the carrier, or index case, is asked to incriminate close associates. Current laws do not compel the infected person to provide such personal information, which represents a significant invasion of privacy.[10] This topic will be discussed later.

Nurse Midwives

Certified nurse midwives function in an expanded role of nursing and currently face a critical problem: the burden imposed by the rising costs of their professional liability insurance. Patch and Holaday[18] report that malpractice insurance rates for these nurses rose from $35 per year in 1983 to $3500 in 1987. These increases do not reflect a higher rate of malpractice litigation because "Nurse-midwives have experienced only a 6% malpractice suit rate over the past 10 years.[18] We conclude that the financial hardships for certified nurse midwives, caused by this trend in insurance, may ultimately limit patient access to quality care.

Abortion

Rarely has a topic led to as much public debate and level of sentiment as the issue of abortion. Two diametrically opposed camps exist: those who believe that the mother has a right to privacy in matters concerning reproduction, and those who believe that once conception has occurred, the baby has a right to be born. The monumental US Supreme Court decision, *Roe v. Wade* in 1973, with several other decisions dealing with abortion during that year, established the rights of women to have an abortion, and to be free from governmental intrusion.[5] Since that time, the debate has raged unabated.

Impaired Newborns

In newborn intensive care units (NICUs), technological advances have led to legal dilemmas for nurses. In the early 1980s, "Baby Doe cases," involving lack of treatment for some handicapped infants, resulted in regulations requiring the reporting of such situations to a hotline number as abuse and neglect. This established an important trend.

In 1984, the US Congress enacted legislation that mandates treatment unless (1) the infant is irreversibly comatose, (2) providing treatment only prolongs inevitable dying, and (3) the treatment would only prove futile regarding survival of the infant and was considered inhumane in itself.[15] The American Academy of Pediatrics Bioethics Committee[1] recommends that decisions be made on each individual case, and that bioethics committees should be established to assist in the decision-making process.

Before these discussions, health care workers in NICUs struggled with the ethical and moral issues involved in these decisions. Current trends suggest that they also need to be concerned with the legal implications.

Home Health Care Nursing

Home health care is a rapidly expanding field of practice for nurses. Not only are patients discharged from the hospital with more complex short-term high-technology care needs, but many more patients with chronic health problems are treated as outpatients. For example, patients on peritoneal dialysis or extended chemotherapy with IVs may be treated at home with sporadic nursing assessments. Infants are sent home who require continuous ventilatory support or central line total parenteral alimentation, and an increasing number of care needs are now relegated to home care. This trend is likely to continue.

Home care nurses must be sure their practice remains within the scope of nursing, effectively document all levels of care, and receive authorization from a physician for all medications and treatments. If home care nurses question a physician's order, they should notify their agency supervisor and follow appropriate channels to clarify the proper course of action.[13]

Hospice Nursing

As federal legislation regulates home health care, so hospice nursing is also regulated. Hospice nursing addresses issues for patients who have no reasonable prospect for a cure for their disease and who are expected to die within 6 months.[17]

Basic legal concerns surround such issues as pronouncement of death. New Jersey passed a law allowing professional registered nurses to determine patient death, make a legal pronouncement of death, and sign a death certificate. The procedure includes notification of a physician, who also signs the death certificate, but the nurse is permitted to specify events surrounding last sickness and the details of death.[17]

MEDICAL SURGICAL NURSING

A number of legal issues affect nurses who practice in the area of medical-surgical nursing. Many malpractice lawsuits are initiated as a result of incorrect administration of medication, patient falls, and other errors. However, within the scope of this chapter, only two trends will be discussed.

Critical Care Nursing

As the incidence of malpractice litigation increases, nurses involved in critical care nursing will also probably experience a higher rate of malpractice claims brought against their highly specialized area of practice. Nurses who pursue this field must receive additional training and maintain competency in their skills. The American Association of Critical Care Nurses (AACN) has standards of care that guide nursing practice in this area.

In this technologically advanced field, reliance on medical equipment is very important. Nurses are responsible for the proper function of equipment. If equipment malfunctions, it must be checked and repaired if necessary. Although critical care nurses are expected to possess a mechanical aptitude, most hospitals have biomedical equipment departments to routinely check equipment and respond if a problem arises.

AIDS

Acquired immune deficiency syndrome was first described in 1981. Since that time, the incidence has increased at an alarming rate, with an anticipated 485,000 cases by 1991. Given the severity of the disease and the current lack of treatment to cure, many legal issues surround this devastating disease.

Screening. There are three groups of people for whom testing for the human immunodeficiency virus antibody (HIVAb) are mandatory: military recruits, blood donors, and immigrants. The AMA recommends mandatory testing for all prison inmates in state and federal prisons. As of 1988, inmates in all federal and 14 state prisons are tested. Prison inmates are a high-risk population because many are IV drug users, and the possibility of homosexual contact exists.

Based on their study completed in 1988, Andrus and his colleagues recommend voluntary, rather than mandatory, testing of prison inmates. The primary reason for a voluntary test system is to inform inmates to whom it applies that they are not infected. Then using a program of education, the desired outcome is to reduce high-risk behavior and thereby the infection rate. Andrus and his colleagues believe this educational emphasis ultimately benefits the prisoners and the society to which they return.

Perhaps this model could be applied to screening of other high-risk populations. The acceptance of an educational paradigm is a long-standing public health technique. Injecting fear of quarantine or other repercussions may only cause possible infected carriers to conceal their condition, thus contributing to the spread of the disease.

Partner Identification. The issue of partner notification presents a dilemma for health care workers. When a person is diagnosed as HIV positive, there is a potential that others may be infected, through sharing of needles during illegal drug use or sexual contact. One of the basic public health infection control measures is to notify partners who may have contracted the disease through contact with the infected person.[19] Historically this technique was used to help control outbreaks of small pox, scarlet fever, and gonorrhea or other sexually transmitted diseases. Currently parents are notified if their school-age child is exposed to chickenpox or other contagious diseases.

Potterat and his colleagues describe that partner notification in relation to HIV positive status or AIDS has produced several objections, including the following:

1. Too expensive
2. Because there is no known cure, there is no reason to notify
3. It may lead to discrimination or stigmatization of infected individuals

We argue that none of these objections is valid. Estimated cost of notification is approximately $2 million dollars at an annual case rate of 100,000. Although this is expensive, it is not prohibitive, and benefits from the expected decrease in infection rate would justify the cost. Also, even though there is no cure to date, there are "life-prolonging compounds," and any method of relaying information about the disease should decrease the incidence of HIV transmission. Finally, current laws regarding confidentiality would help decrease discrimination, and the US public health departments have a "long and distinguished track record for protecting patient confidentiality."[19]

• • •

Legal issues are a major component in contemporary nursing in all areas of practice. Nurses must be informed about the legal implications of their actions and continue to update their information as situations change. Throughout contemporary society, the evolution of societal thought, and the legal ramifications of that thought, continues to affect the practice of nursing.

STUDY ACTIVITIES

1. What are common legal issues that affect nurses practicing in medical-surgical nursing?
2. What are common legal issues that affect nurses practicing as midwives? In home health?
3. What are common legal issues that affect nurses in critical care?
4. Discuss your thinking about who can and should serve as expert witnesses when a case is tried involving a nurse's practice.
5. How can you prepare to serve as an expert witness in a case when a nurse's practice is in question?

REFERENCES

1. American Academy of Pediatrics Committee on Bioethics: treatment of critically ill newborns, Pediatrics 74:306-310, 1984.
2. Baldwin-Mech A: Quality assurance and documentation. In Northrop CE and Kelly ME, eds: Legal issues in nursing, St. Louis, 1987, The CV Mosby Co.
3. Chasnoff IJ: Perinatal effects of cocaine, Contemp Ob/Gyn 26(5), May 1987.
4. Creighton H: Law every nurse should know, ed 4, Philadelphia, 1981, WB Saunders Co.
5. Cushing M: Nursing jurisprudence, Philadelphia, 1988, Appleton & Lange.
6. Cushing M: When the courts define nursing: what it is, what it does, Am J Nurs 87(6):773-774, June 1987.
7. Ellis JR and Hartley CL: Nursing in today's world: challenges, issues and trends, ed 3, Philadelphia, 1988, JB Lippincott Co.
8. Emanuel LL and Emanuel EJ: The medical directive: a new comprehensive advance care document, JAMA 261(22):3288-3293, June 1989.
9. Ford RD and Haston L: Nurse's legal handbook, Springhouse, PA, 1985, Springhouse Corp.
10. Gostin L and Curran WJ: Legal control measures for AIDS: reporting requirements, surveillance, quarantine, and regulation of public meeting places, Am J Public Health 77(2), Feb 1987.
11. Hemelt MD and Mackert ME: Dynamics of law in nursing and health care, ed 2, 1982, Reston Publishing Co, Reston, Va.
12. Horsley JE: Short staffing means increased liability for you, RN 44(73), 1981.
13. Horsley JE: The new risks of home care, RN, 52(1), 1989.
14. Legal Column Editor: Nursing '89, 19(5), May 1989.
15. Moreno J: Ethical and legal issues in the care of the impaired newborn, Clinics Perinatol 14:345-360, 1987.
16. Nolan K: In death's shadow: the meanings of withholding resuscitation, Hastings Center Report 17(5), Oct/Nov 1987.
17. Northrop CE and Kelly ME: Legal issues in nursing, St. Louis, 1987, The CV Mosby Co.
18. Patch FB and Holaday SD: Effects of changes in professional liability insurance on certified nurse-midwives, J Nurs Midwife 34(3), May/June 1989.
19. Potterat JJ, Spencer NE, et al.: Partner notification in the control of human immunodeficiency virus infection, Am J Public Health 79(7), July 1989.
20. Rabinow J: Where you stand in the eyes of the law, Nursing '89, 19(2), Feb 1989.
21. Rocerto L and Maleski C: The legal dimensions of nursing practice, New York, 1982, Springer Publishing Co, Inc.
22. Wilson D: An overview of sexually transmissible diseases in the perinatal period, J Nurs Midwife 33(3):115-128, May/June 1988.

SUGGESTED READINGS

Fiesta J: The law and liability: a guide for nurses, ed 2, New York, 1988, John Wiley and Sons.
Handbook of living will laws: ed 1987, New York, 1987, Society for the Right to Die.

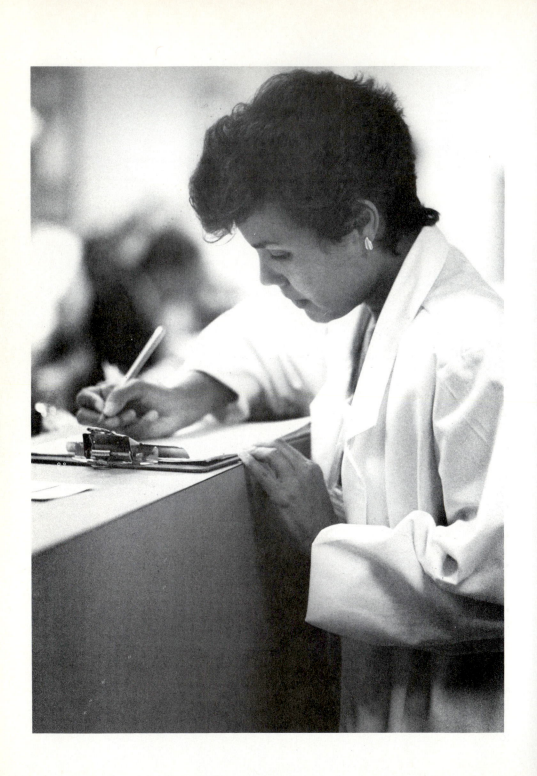

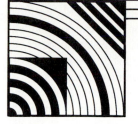

C H A P T E R **7**

ETHICAL INFLUENCES ON NURSING

Fred Hendrickson
Grace L. Deloughery

OBJECTIVES

After completing this chapter the reader should be able to:

- Describe what ethics is and differentiate it from other areas such as law and etiquette

- List at least six major philosophical schools of thought from which ethics is derived

- Name some basic rights of patients/clients as presented in the Patient Bill of Rights

- Identify the professional document/code that guides the nurse in practice

- List a number of current bioethical issues that nurses must understand and deal with in practice

- Identify the most significant role of the nurse in the area of ethical dilemmas with patients and families

Many nurses begin practice without a personal framework from the field of ethics and are therefore unable to make professional judgments based on their own reasoning. Ethics is a more important part of nursing practice than ever before.

This chapter discusses basic approaches to ethics and the major schools of thought, followed by a discussion of the Patient's Bill of Rights and the ANA Code for Nurses.

Practical situations that nurses can identify in everyday experience are incorporated. These vignettes are referenced to the ANA Code for Nurses.

Special categories are examined regarding patients' rights and the nurse's ethical responsibilities to them, to assist the nurse to determine a personal ethical position and professional responsibility. Ethics committees are presented as a recent approach to resolving ethical questions for patients who are unable to decide for themselves. This is followed by discussion of nurses in organizational settings and common dynamics.

The chapter concludes with a summary and questions that are intended to help the reader examine personal ethical thinking and develop an ethical framework from which responsible professional nursing practice can begin.

Foundation of Nursing Ethics

Ethics is the branch of philosophy that deals with the dynamics of decision-making concerning what is right or wrong. Moral decision-making specific to nursing practice, policy making, and research are all elements of nursing ethics. Nursing ethics evolved from philosophical schools of thinking and is specialized to meet the needs of the nursing profession. The need for more understanding and background in nursing ethics is the result of nurses increasing involvement in health care crises. The need is growing as nurses' level of sophistication in the role of client advocate continues to evolve.

Nursing historically has taught its practitioners to promote the wellbeing of clients, families, and the public. However, this conduct was not consistently practiced. For many years, nurses accepted physicians' orders unquestionably and were told to ignore inappropriate or unnecessary procedure that might prove harmful to the patient. If nurses spoke up, they or the institution could be subject to reprimand. Thankfully nursing is now evolving out of this mind-set, and nursing ethics is one of the formidable leaders assisting with the process.

Ethical principles remind nurses that their mission is not an ordinary one. Without advocacy of protection of rights there are no rights. The lives and wellbeing of others depend not only on nurses' technical skills and general knowledge base but also on their professional integrity. To encourage nurses to act according to such principles an ethical framework was developed.

Nurses must have knowledge of ethical principles because the problems they face are often ethical, rather than technical in nature. Knowing *how* to resuscitate a patient involves technical expertise; deciding *whether* to resuscitate may be an ethical judgment.

The following discusses some preliminary observations about common misconceptions regarding ethics.

What Ethics is Not

First, ethics is not *etiquette*. Open-mouth gum chewing, the use of vulgar language, "unprofessional" dress, or the failure to exhibit a cheerful attitude may violate professional etiquette but would not be unethical. However, reporting a physician or nurse for violating a patient's rights may be an ethical obligation, as spelled out in the Patient's Bill of Rights.

Second, ethics is not *law.* Law is the regulations necessary to preserve public order. Often, law and ethics are in basic agreement, as, for example, when the law requires the nurse to furnish the patient with adequate information for making a decision regarding proposed treatment. (Although the minimum legal requirements might fall far short of the ethical requirements of informed consent.) At other times, the judgments of law and ethics are dichotomous. Law, for example, might make a distinction between taking someone off a respirator and not putting the patient on it in the first place; a distinction that many ethicists would not make.

Another area of confusion about the nature of ethics is more widespread than either of the two previously mentioned. This is a tendency to equate ethics with *values clarification.* Values clarification is a process that helps people to:

1. Sort through, analyze, and set priorities of their own values
2. Behave in a way that is consistent with those values
3. Understand personal beliefs and feelings, so that decisions will be based on a conscious awareness of a value system

Although this is a valuable process, it is not ethics, but more accurately belongs in the area of psychology. It helps people identify what they *do* value but not what *should* be valued or how to decide when values come in conflict.

A similar assessment could be made that is often called *descriptive ethics.* The term is self-explanatory. It simply describes the ethical values of a particular culture, or group—what the group considers right or wrong. This, too, can be valuable information, but more accurately belongs in the area of sociology or anthropology; it is not ethics as the term is used in this chapter.

Nursing ethics is not medical ethics and medical ethics texts are not adequate to meet nursing needs. Nursing is a profession with all the rights, privileges, and responsibilities that a profession entails. Thus ethical frameworks must be specific to problems and dilemmas in nursing situations. This leads to the concept of dialectical tension. A dialectical pertains to a way of understanding reality by consciously keeping seemingly opposite values in mind. Nursing is a unique profession; yet it is grounded in the mandates of society. Questions of nursing ethics may be nursing-specific; but the input of a larger social framework is important.

Definitions of Ethics

Barry defines ethics as "the study of what constitutes good and bad human conduct, including related actions and values."[7] Ethics, therefore, is *normative.* It attempts to establish norms or principles by which conduct can be judged. It is not so concerned with what people value or consider right or wrong, but rather with what people *ought* to value and what behavior ought to be considered right and wrong. Ethics is also concerned with *why.* Why is informed consent important? Is there an ethical difference between allowing a terminally ill patient to die and actively terminating his life?

Many authors distinguish between the terms ethical and moral, using the latter to refer to the *actions* or behavior of a person and the former to refer to the *study* of the morality of conduct.[7] In this chapter, however, the terms will be used interchangeably.

Even before Hippocrates, the health care professions were concerned with ethical behavior. Several relatively recent developments in our society have dramatically increased ethical awareness. Among these are:

1. Advances in medical technology. Transplants and artificial organs, amniocentesis, respirators, dialysis machines, etc. have opened the doors to new possibilities for extending or prolonging life, but they are also prompting the ethical question, "It *can* be done, but *should* it be done?"

2. Greater recognition of patient rights. Our society has become more rights conscious, beginning with the civil rights movement and extending to women's rights, rights of children, the elderly, the handicapped, and AIDS victims. Today patients and health practitioners are acutely aware of patient rights and health care professionals' obligation to respect these rights.

3. Malpractice cases and court-ordered treatment. Civil law and the courts intervene more frequently in medical situations to insure that patients' legal rights are protected. This legal intervention emphasizes the existence of ethical issues, but has not always been beneficial in solving ethical dilemmas. Fear of a malpractice suit can produce additional ethical problems, by providing pressure to practice to avoid lawsuits rather than in the best interest of the patient.

4. Scarcity of Resources. Technological advances have created shortages: of machines and qualified personnel, frequently of organs for transplantation, but more frequently, of money. As previously discussed, the issue of the availability and financing of health services is recognized as one of the more important and difficult ethical problems facing the health care field and society itself.

Factors such as these require nurses to make decisions that are not only technically correct, but also morally right or good. There is a need therefore for an understanding of ethics and ethical decision-making. Before discussing the different schools of thought, two approaches to the origination of ethics will be discussed. These two approaches are subjectivism and objectivism.

Subjectivism and Objectivism

If ethics is the study of what constitutes morally good or bad, right or wrong conduct, a fundamental question of ethics is "What makes an act good or bad?" The basic disagreement in this area is between subjectivism and objectivism.[5,26]

Subjectivists maintain that human judgments create morality (see box). An act is right because the individual or the group judges it to be right. The only requirement for acting ethically is to follow your conscience, or "be true to yourself." "If one thinks it's right, that makes it right" summarizes the subjectivist code of morality.

The objectivist, however, insists that human judgment discovers, rather than creates, morality. Right or wrong is independent of what people think and it is the function of human judgment to discover the right or wrong inherent in a particular course of action.

Without an in-depth analysis of these positions, it is evident that any *study* of ethics presumes some sort of objectivist approach. Only if morality is in some way objective can there be any meaningful discussion of principles or codes of ethical conduct.

_____ BASIC APPROACHES TO ETHICS _____

Objectivism: human judgment discovers morality
    Consequentialism: morality is determined by the consequences of a particular act
    Nonconsequentialism: morality is determined by intrinsic characteristics of a particular act
Subjectivism: human judgment creates morality

Consequentialism versus Nonconsequentialism

Objectivists agree that something other than human judgment causes behavior to be ethically right or wrong. They disagree radically, however, on what this something is. The two major theories of objective morality are consequentialism (teleology) and non-consequentialism (deontology).

Consequentialism (teleology). Consequentialists argue that the morality of an act is determined solely by its consequences. Nothing is ethically good or bad in itself; only the results matter. (Consequentialism is sometimes expressed in common language as "the end justifies the means.") An act is considered ethical if it produces, or is intended to produce, the best long-term consequences when compared with all other available alternatives. But, the best consequences for whom? The answer to this leads to the following three distinct classifications of consequentialists.

1. For oneself (egoism). Egoists say that one should always act to produce the greatest ratio of happiness over unhappiness (or good over evil) for the one acting.
2. For everyone (utilitarianism). Utilitarians argue that one should always act to produce the greatest ratio of long-term happiness over unhappiness for everyone (the greatest good for the greatest number of people). Utilitarianism, developed by Jeremy Betham (1748-1832) and further refined by John Stuart Mill (1806-1873), is a widely known form of consequentialism.* Utilitarianism may be divided into two classes—_act_ and _rule_.

   Act utilitarianism maintains that only the consequences of a specific act need be considered (Figure 7-1). For example, in deciding if it is ethical to withhold information about a terminally ill patient's condition, the act utilitarian is concerned solely with the consequences of the act of telling or not telling.

   Rule utilitarianism, on the other hand, maintains that one should consider not just the consequences of a particular act, but rather the _kind_ of act. One should follow a rule about telling or not telling terminally ill patients their condition based on the consequences that generally follow.
3. For some (limited consequentialism). Not all consequentialists judge the morality of an act by consequences for oneself or for everyone. For many, the conse-

---

*For a summary and critique of utilitarianism, see Building a Moral System by Robert B. Ashmore, Englewood Cliffs, New Jersey, Prentice-Hall, 1997.

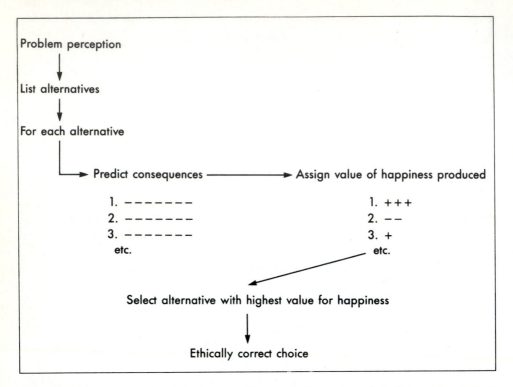

Fig. 7-1 Act-Utilitarian ethical decision-making model (consequential). This method fails if one is unable to (1) predict consequences accurately, or (2) estimate accurate happiness values. *(From Brody H: Ethical decisions in medicine, ed 2, Boston, 1981, Little, Brown, and Company.)*

quences for a specific individual (other than the agent) or number of individuals are the deciding factor in determining the morality of an act. This is especially true in the history of health care in which the consequences to the patient (patient consequentialism) have been the only significant consideration.[26]

Nonconsequentialism (deontology, formalism). Nonconsequentialists reject the consequentialist position that only results determine an action's morality. They maintain that certain things are right or wrong in themselves and not because of the good or evil results they produce. Figure 7-2 illustrates the decision-making process using the deontologic method.

Some nonconsequentialists argue that consequences should not be considered at all. The most influential proponent of this position is Immanuel Kant (1724-1804).[29] According to Kant, nothing is good in itself except good will. "Good will" is the capacity to act according to principle. The basic principle governing behavior is *duty*. When we act from duty, our actions are considered ethical. Kant divides duties into two groups: perfect and imperfect. Perfect duties are those that we are *always* obligated to observe.

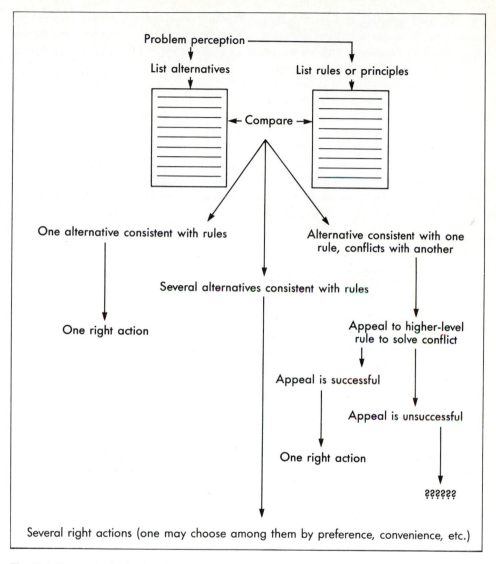

Fig. 7-2 Deontological ethical decision-making method (nonconsequential). *(From Brody H: Ethical decisions in medicine, ed 2, Boston, 1981, Little, Brown, and Company.)*

These are usually negative (e.g., not to harm others). Imperfect duties (usually positive) are those that have obligation to observe (e.g., to render aid).

The basic principle underlying and determining duties may be summarized in a universal law that Kant calls the *categorical imperative*. Kant gives several different versions of this command. The best known formulation is "act only according to that maxim by which you can at the same time will that it should become a universal law."[21]

The way of expressing this command, and one that is probably more meaningful for health care, is "so act as to treat humanity, whether in thine own person or in that of any other, in every case as an end withal, never as means only."[21] Ethically, human beings can never be treated as means to an end.

Kant's ethical formalism is perceived by many as being excessively rigid, and the ignoring of consequences in assessing morality as ignoring a vital element of good decision making. For these people, the ethical act is one that upholds the highest principles (do your duty, do not harm, do not treat a person as a means to an end) while also attempting to obtain the best results.

This ethical position (seeking to combine the best elements and avoid the worst pitfalls), of both a consequentialist and a nonconsequentialist approach, is known as pluralism (Figure 7-3). There are many pluralist theories, all insisting that certain things are

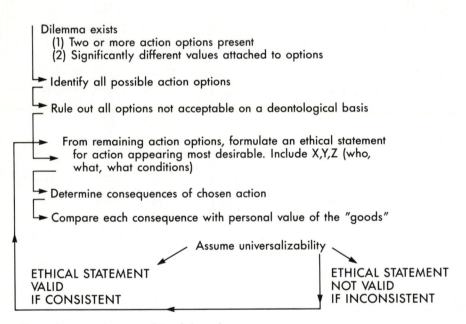

Dilemma exists
   (1) Two or more action options present
   (2) Significantly different values attached to options

Identify all possible action options

Rule out all options not acceptable on a deontological basis

From remaining action options, formulate an ethical statement for action appearing most desirable. Include X,Y,Z (who, what, what conditions)

Determine consequences of chosen action

Compare each consequence with personal value of the "goods"

Assume universalizability

ETHICAL STATEMENT VALID IF CONSISTENT

ETHICAL STATEMENT NOT VALID IF INCONSISTENT

On cycle return in case of invalid result:
   (1) Ethical statement may be reformulated modifying the conditions
   (2) Alternate action option (still available after rule in) may be expected going through all remaining steps

Remember: the decision to take no action is in itself action

Fig. 7-3 Pluralistic ethical decision-making model. An original synthesis of the deontological (nonconsequential) and teleological (consequential) decision-making models. *(From Payton RJ: Pluralistic ethical decision making: clinical and scientific sessions, Kansas City, 1979, American Nurses' Association, 1979.)*

right or wrong in themselves, and not just because of the results they produce, while affirming the importance of producing the best consequences ethical behavior will permit. One position is *Natural Law.* The natural law theory is important, because of its central position in the history of philosophy and because of its influence in health care ethics. This will be discussed in the section on ethical schools of thought.

Ethical theories are difficult. Moral problems are often intertwined. Because it is unlikely that a completely satisfactory solution to any problem will be reached, the majority of ethical questions continue to raise the same problems repeatedly. The choice of approach for resolving a problem is not as important as the fact that the first step in the ethical journey within the nursing career has been taken. Although no solid evidence exists that nurses must choose one ethical theory over another, they should not slip into pragmatism/relativism in an irresponsible manner. Situations are various and often complex. One solution to indecision is dialectical tension. Determining for oneself what should be valued is to establish principles and develop a conscience, which is one's personal guide for applying ethics.

The multiplicity of ethical theories presented here is focused on the inclusion of major ethical schools of thought (see Table 7-1) rather than emphasis based on the author's own value judgments.

ETHICAL SCHOOLS OF THOUGHT
Naturalism

The oldest known philosophy in the Western World is naturalism, which can be traced back to Aristotle in the fourth Century, BC, and was formulated by Thomas Aquinas (1225-1274). The influence of Aquinas resulted in natural law becoming the philosophical basis for much of Roman Catholic moral principles, and influenced the moral principles of other Christian denominations, as well.

Natural law is based on two presuppositions: (1) an action is good if it is in accord with human nature; bad if it is contrary to that nature and (2) the nature of things can be discovered by reason.

Naturalists maintain that there is a dependable and consistent order in nature. They insist that reality and nature are identical and that there is no reality beyond nature. Because of its general simplicity, naturalism has a universal appeal.

To fully appreciate naturalism, one must look at the two schools that have evolved from its overall tenets. *Native* naturalism attempts to designate any one substance as the entire essence of nature explaining all things in terms of material or energy-producing substances. *Critical* naturalism opposes the view that all things are explained in terms of material or energy-producing substances. This school examines the relationship between the constituent parts or events, rather than the parts or events themselves. Because of the process of interaction between constituent parts, laws and relationships continually and persistently run throughout nature. The highest good within the naturalistic school is pleasure. The naturalistic philosopher seeks freedom from internal struggle and pain. This is achieved through as many pleasurable experiences as

Table 7-1 Ethical Schools of Thought

	Spiritual reference (God, afterlife, etc.)	Basis for ethical decisionmaking	Place of mankind	Idea of good
Naturalism (objectivist)	None	Natural elements or forces; scientific laws	Agent within framework of nature, and nature is source of ethics	Harmony
Idealism (subjectivist)	Not determined	Self; universals are subjective	End in itself; Every person has equal importance; man is source of ethics	Harmonious coexistence; nothing is totally right or wrong
Realism (objectivist)	Important as source of universals	Universals are objective; no *a priori* knowledge	Man discovers ethics as objective universals	The good of society is more important than that of the individual; permanent good over transitory good
Utilitarianism (subjectivist)	None	Good results at all costs	Emphasis on the majority; man is source of ethics	Right conduct is determined by useful consequences
Rationalism (objectivist)	Possible source of *a priori* knowledge and truth	*A priori* knowledge; reason alone determines true knowledge	Ideas exist outside of human thought; man discovers ethics as objective universals	Not determined
Existentialism (Subjectivist)	None; the world is uncertain and purposeless	The individual's own conscience and principles	Emphasis on the individual, who is entirely free and must accept full responsibility for individual actions; man is source of ethics	Not determined
Theory of Justice (subjectivist or objectivist)	Not determined	Equal human rights	Man determines or discovers for self certain rights that apply to all equally; man may be source of ethics	Everyone has a right to happiness
Pragmatism	None; here and now orientation	Scientific method; no general rule is appropriate for every situation	Individual act is based on current mores	Resolution of conflict

possible. Although this statement makes naturalism appear hedonistic, many philosophers of this school argue that the highest moral good is that which is to be sought the most.[29]

Two principles of natural law ethics have special importance for health care. These are (1) the principle of double effect and (2) the principle of totality. The principle of double effect has a wider acceptance than the principle of totality, which is considered valid primarily by Roman Catholic moralists.

The Principle of Double Effect. Health care professionals may become involved in situations that result in evil consequences regardless of what course of action is taken. The decision to administer a drug to relieve a cancer patient's pain, for example, may result in a risk of shortening that patient's life; or removal of a pregnant woman's cancerous uterus will result in the death of the fetus. One must consider the morality of such acts. The principle of double effect requires that the following four conditions be met before such an act can be justified[7]:

1. The act itself must be morally good or at least indifferent
2. The good effect must not be achieved by means of the bad effect
3. Only the good effect must be intended (although the evil effect is obviously foreseen)
4. The good intended must be equal to or greater than the evil

This means that one may never ethically intend a major evil, even as a means to achieving a good end. "Major evil" is the violation of a natural right, or the destruction of a good necessary to attain a goal. One may ethically risk or permit a major evil if one has a proportionate reason. A proportionate reason is determined by considering the following criteria:

1. Balancing the effects. Is the good intended equal to or greater than the evil foreseen?
2. Availability of alternatives. Is any other method available for achieving the good that does not involve evil? If so, one is ethically obliged to use it.
3. Likelihood of the evil occurring. When evil is risked rather than permitted, the evil is more likely to result; thus the good must be greater to justify it (e.g., in administering drugs to relieve pain).

This principle of double effect establishes natural law as a pluralist ethical system. While denying that a good end can justify an evil means (thus disagreeing with consequentialism) it still insists that consequences are important. Indeed, they are the deciding factor when evil is risked or permitted (thus rejecting a strict Kantian nonconsequentialism).

The Principle of Totality. According to the Roman Catholic version of natural law, individuals can ethically dispose of their organs or interfere with those organs' ability to function only to the extent that the well-being of the whole body requires it. This principle is the philosophical basis for Catholic opposition to hysterectomies, vasectomies, etc. for the purpose of preventing conception, although the surgeries are permitted to remedy a pathological condition.

Strengths and Weaknesses. The strength of naturalism is its simplicity. It offers individual freedom from presumption and decreases the influence of confusion in our society today. It offers a wholesome simplification reflecting the elementary aspects of nature that have not been corrupted by human artificiality. Further, because man considers nature when exploring the moon, planting crops, constructing buildings, or sailing ships, he has been successful.

The primary weakness of naturalism, again, is its simplification. Life and existence is so simplified that deep insights and adequate explanations cannot be formed. Nature is not completely harmonious in its progression or form, i.e., when it snows in June, when a drought halts the growth of crops. Within the realm of metaphysics, naturalism has not developed sufficiently to be clearly explanatory. The knowledge base cannot be assessed because there is no formal theory base from which to draw.

Idealism

Idealism, not widely held today, is associated with George Berkeley, an 18th century Irish philosopher. Other idealist philosophers include David Hume and Emmanual Kant. The idealist states that nothing exists outside of ideas. The self is the primary reality of any individual's experience. It is the culmination of the body, soul, and the interactions with society. The ultimate reality is the self, which can be an individual, community, or a universe. Mental realities of what exists are personal. Observations are perceptions, thoughts, emotions, and volitions as they pertain to one's self.[18]

Idealism has many variations, including the idea that the self is the primary reality and the experience of a person.[11] Kant[21] believed that these were universal moral laws. He expressed principles common among the idealist school. An individual can morally engage in some act if it is seen that an act cannot be universally practiced by all. For example, an individual murder such as euthanasia might be justified, but if it were applied to everyone, there would be the obliteration of the race. This concept is known as *categorical imperative*. Man has an obligation to act in conjunction with these moral laws. This results not alone from experience but is based on reason and logic. According to Kant, man should be free to act out of desire or intention to do good. Nothing is totally right or wrong. This has a vast impact on nursing practice.

The universe is an all-inclusive self. Each part is an equal member in the universe. Thus no shred of reality, however minute, can be outside of the whole. Critical idealists such as Kant avoid the theory of reality, but believe that every experience that one encounters contributes to reality. Evil is a fact. Men are not completely positive in attempting to achieve their moral goals. They commonly respond not as their brother's keeper, but as a means to an end to satisfy whatever desires they choose.[6] Evil occurs only when people do not assess values and apply them appropriately.

Idealism contends that the qualities we perceive in the world are rooted in their actual existence. Because nothing can exist without relationship to another, reality is a logically connected unified total system. The values of human life exist because there are individuals to possess and enjoy them. The idealist ethic is likely some form of perfectionism. Relations between individuals must be harmonious, because persons are seen as ends rather than means. One individual is just as important as another. In every man there is an innate need to do good. There are said to be at least four other values that are innate to humans: (1) obedience to universal moral laws, (2) the good will of man, (3) the society of ends, and (4) immortality.

Obedience to universal moral laws are ethical values that are essential in relationships because individuals are persons, and as persons they can act only in ways they feel to be the ultimate practice for all men, e.g., dishonesty, murder.

Good will is to do right because one knows that it is right and necessary. Individuals in a society control their actions to result in respect and consideration of all others involved. This is an idealistic society. The corollary is that individual immortality is a value. Because of this, the fulfillment of moral law exists.

All of this is best summarized by Kant's statement, "Act so that in your own person as well as in the person of every other, you are treating mankind also as an end, never merely as a means."[22]

Strengths and Weaknesses. The strength of idealism is that it has a central reality around which it evolves, namely that of the self. This relates directly to existence as a person. The idea of the self is central in obtaining and organizing knowledge. This is especially necessary because idealists see the world as subjective rather than objective. Idealism stresses the human elements in life, education, and work. Although idealists can live with the increased sophistication of science, they insist that the human and personal is more important than scientific advancement. It is a comprehensive theory and deals with metaphysics and epistemology. It is consistent.

One difficulty is the need to sort through and understand. Yet, there is an intuitive understanding of what is good, what is right, and what is best for everybody.

Realism

Realists believe that nature is the primary self-evident reality that is the starting point of all philosophy; the objectivity of things, apart from the person thinking about them, is emphasized. The mind is a blank slate waiting to receive and reflect images from the physical world. Consciousness is the awareness of experience in which objects and organisms are related. Realism is exhibited anywhere from an expression such as "Just take a look" to an insistence that reality is mediated by meaning. The latter viewpoint expresses that the real is judged to be true on the basis of personal experience.

A clear orderliness in the universe is recognized by realists, and for this reason they may describe the world much in the same way as naturalists. Unlike the naive naturalist however, realists do not see a substance or an energy as the primary core of the universe. Two values are primary in the realistic school of thought: (1) values are elements that are experienced as one experiences them and (2) values are dependent on the emotionality of those experiencing them.[8] Thus, ethically, good is often defined as a quote from John Stuart Mill, "the greatest happiness to the greatest number."[8] This is not a hedonistic type of view; rather it is a communal one. The pleasure of society is more important than that of the individual.

Realists perceive in primary and secondary qualities. Primary qualities reside within the object; secondary qualities are defined by one's own perceptions, which can be false.[25] If one believes that there is a future in which individuals will be more fully developed, then one will recognize an obligation to fulfill that potential. "Because there are permanent possibilities of happiness, they should take precedence over any transitory happiness which 'corrupt' them."[27]

EXAMPLE: Sister Antonia was from a very wealthy family. Her position in business and humanitarianism resulted in a tour of a prison. After the tour, she felt compelled to upgrade the conditions of the prison. Although married, she visited the prison often. Her marriage deteriorated, she moved to San Diego, and divorced. Eventually she lived in a women's prison so she could be near. Her stance was that she did not condone what the prisoners did, but she felt that someone must care for them, because they were human beings. She conducted many community health activities for the prisoners such as increasing medical and dental care, decreasing scurvy and rickets by obtaining better nutrition, and having tattoos removed so that when the prisoners were released they would not be labeled. Her belief is that she receives more from the prisoners than she gives to them.

It is not difficult for realists to develop a consistent ethical framework because decisions must be based on cold hard facts. Situations in which realists find decision-making easier are when actions are necessary to keep persons alive in differing circumstances.

EXAMPLE: A young person in respiratory arrest may be put on a respirator instead of an older person. The older person will likely die on the respirator, whereas the younger person will likely recover. To whom should a donated kidney be given if the US President and a 1-year-old child need the kidney? Who gets the only Intensive Care Unit (ICU) room available if two people come into the emergency room, one is a benefactor of the hospital and the other is a bleeding posttonsillectomy child?

A weakness of realism is that by relying on pragmatics there is sometimes no foundation for making a decision without a further ideological framework outside of "the highest good to the highest number" or the longest lasting good.

Utilitarianism

The principles of utilitarianism, as stated by John Stuart Mill, are that "Actions are right in proportion as they tend to promote happiness, wrong as they tend to produce the reverse of happiness." This philosophy focuses on the consequences of actions rather than on the actions themselves. Thus good intention could be considered morally wrong if the outcome proves disadvantageous. Utilitarianism is not based solely on what is good for the decision-maker alone; rather, the focus is on the best interest of all involved.[20] Utilitarian moralism seeks to enhance the amount of pleasure experienced by the majority of individuals to the greatest possible degree.

An example of utilitarianism in practice might be a national push for organ donors and a donor networking system to get the organs to those individuals who can best use them. Nurses are encouraged, sometimes even required by their employer institution, to pursue organ donation with families of brain-dead patients before removing life support systems. All ramifications must be considered from the utilitarians' point of view. First, the needs of potentially healthy individuals (organ recipients) and their potential service to the community must be weighed against the donor's family needs (religious beliefs, emotional status at the time of the donor's death). Health professionals involved should expect that their personal values and beliefs count also.

Utilitarian theory is divided into two schools of thought. These schools apply the same utilitarian principles but the focus of their principles differ. The "act" utilitarians believe that each situation should be assessed individually. "Rule" utilitarians believe that policies should be determined based on validated principles of utility and acted on whenever a situation occurs that falls into that category.

"Act" utilitarians take a different position. They look at each case before determining what, if anything, needs to be done. The act utilitarian does not completely disregard the appropriateness of rules, but feels that they should be general guides for actions and not firm and fast laws.

The following hospital policy exhibits "rule utilitarianism." The example is an actual situation known to one of the authors.

EXAMPLE: Hospital policy states that staff are to "provide complete care for infants regardless of any malady or birth defect." It directs a nurse in procedure if a premature, congenitally imperfect (or grossly malformed) infant in an incubator experiences cardiac arrest. No thought need be given to questions such as who pays, how much will they pay, the pain the infant may experience, the quality of life the child will have, who will care for the child, and the ability to care for the child, as well as consideration of the nurse's own personal beliefs. In this instance, nursery costs-to-care for the infant were estimated at $247,000 after less than 2 months. Future improvements in the infant's condition would have to be significant for life outside the institution to be a possibility. Thus, the dilemma (should this infant be kept alive) continues with no apparent ending, as nurses continue to administer care.

Strengths and Weaknesses. The major strength of utilitarianism is that the majority is considered when policies are made. Without this principle, current studies that include artificial hearts, organ transplants, medical versus surgical treatment of various illnesses, and testing of drugs that may be future healers (such as the polio vaccine was in the past) might not become a reality. Some may argue that other philosophies address this issue. However, utilitarians believe this tenet is the major focus of their philosophy.

The major weakness of utilitarianism is that this view does not consider individual rights: a nurse could be held accountable for the reputation of the hospital in the event of a malpractice suit, experimental drugs could be given to an indigent population without prior consent, or prisoners on death-row could be injected with the AIDS virus so that researchers could study the effects and find a cure for the disease that may become the twentieth century plague.

Rationalism

"I think, therefore I am" is the basic tenet of rationalism. Rationalists believe that knowledge is obtained solely through deductive reasoning based on inborn tenets. They contend that the mind was initially provided with a number of faculties that only needs reason to decide future knowledge and truths. Reason itself, without the benefit of observation, provides true knowledge.[20]

Through this concept, known as *a priori,* the mind is perceived to be active. It prescribes what it knows with regard to forms and conditions as they appear. Kant, for example, states that the reason *a priori* is a reality is because the same knowledge has been at work in the formation of all that appears. Thus we understand the world because of what we know, and the world as we know it is conversely a product of our understanding. Based on this tenet, rationalists will accept as true only that which is clearly and distinctly in existence. This occurs via various stages of determination dealing with what is true and what is false. It is believed that knowledge is gained and reason achieved if memory of all earlier steps are accurate and true. Ideas do not exist because of an individual but exist on their own, based on clarity and the logical pattern that they follow. It is believed that sensory perceptions lead to error because of distortions.

Strengths and Weaknesses. One of the strengths of rationalism is that it is a logical sequencing, it is adaptable to each situation, and it is equally shared by any individual. There need be no argument about whose observations are more accurate or more important. With the same rational process applied, conclusions should be the same.

A question of the rationalist position is whether it is possible, in fact, to have *a priori* knowledge without experience. Furthermore, what was "knowledge" 50 years ago may no longer hold true today, and basing decisions on that knowledge is facetious.

EXAMPLE: Tuberculosis is treated far differently from the method of treatment 50 years ago. If treatment today were based solely on knowledge of the disease known 50 years ago, there would be no change in the method of treatment and the quality of care would not be improved. The archaic methods of blood letting, surgical lobotomies, and various kinds of shock therapy for mental disorders are a few examples of what no longer should be done. Modern medical advances came about not through reason alone but by referencing the material world through scientific research.

Pragmatism

Pragmatism is basically a method of clarifying ideas objectively.[19] Pragmatists believe that facts must be assessed as they are. This requires recognition of a problem, formulation of hypotheses, collection and observation of data, and testing of the hypotheses. This allows an individual to determine the correct way to respond in a particular situation and affords a value to any given action. When an action occurs, change results and the change, over time, can be a positive response. Pragmatists believe that no general rule is appropriate for every situation and ethics is needed as it is possible or applied.[12] The world is characterized by this process of change. It is continually incomplete and has ends only within its own process. Man is not the cause for the world's existing, and despite change, our world does not guarantee success.[8] The pragmatist believes that the past cannot be changed and the future is yet to be formed. Therefore a "here and now" orientation is stressed. Individuals must assess every situation encountered and deal with it in the best way possible, attempting to decrease conflict among its various components and to control for future successes.

Because nursing is grounded in the physical and biological sciences, it too used the same approach to integration of knowledge as the pragmatic ethicists did in the past. In order for nurses to incorporate pragmatism in practice it is necessary to understand the profession as simply one facet in the large scheme of things.

Existentialism

Existentialism is largely a revolt against traditional eighteenth century European philosophy, which considered philosophy a science. Existentialists argue that objectives are universal and certain knowledge is unattainable. They investigate what it is like to be an *individual* human being living in the world. For existentialists, every individual is a human being who must face important and difficult decisions with only limited knowledge and time. This predicament lies at the heart of the human condition.

Existentialists conclude that human choice is subjective because the individual must make choices without recourse to external standards such as laws, codes of ethics, or traditions. The individual is *free*. However, the individual is completely responsible for choices made. Because man is forced to choose for himself, both freedom and responsibility are thrust on him.

The realization that one is completely responsible for one's decisions, actions, and beliefs is the cause for existential anxiety. Yet, a major tenet of existential thought is the need for authenticity. To live meaningfully and authentically a person must become fully aware of the true character of the human situation and accept it. The situation is that of an uncertain and purposeless world.

Existentialists believe that death is a part of one's own self-hold. It happens to an individual regardless of what a person does and comes into existence at the time of birth. Nothingness is a part of all and we return to nothingness. Sartre said that one exists as others perceive one to exist. There is no place that man can be comfortable, because he is not wholly a part of the existing world. Outside of man's creative activity, there are two options: that of possibility (holding on to life) and the other of factility (giving up, despair).[23]

Strengths and Weaknesses. Existentialism's major weakness is that it denies reference to codes of ethics and codes of behavior in general. Therefore it is impossible to discuss ethics in the framework of a profession or an institution. Ethical decision-making is solely the responsibility of the individual. It is subjective and not built on a concrete framework.

A strength of existentialism is that it promotes committing oneself to social and political issues. For that reason, at least, existentialists believe one must become involved in ethics, and are often more ethically conscious than others. However, they tend to have a form of floating anxiety about everything in general, but nothing in particular.

Theory of Justice

A unique modern moralistic theory that evolved from the 1970s and 1980s is Rawl's Theory of Justice. Rawl combined utilitarianism with the views of Kant and Ross in an attempt to answer modern moralistic dilemmas. He believes that every person has a right to equal use and applications of liberty as it is stated in the US Constitutional Preamble.[30]

He further asserts that social and economic inequalities should evolve in such a way that the greatest benefit is assessed to the least advantaged and attached to positions that are open to all in an equal and fair exchange. This in turn will lead to a just society where opportunities are not based on whom one knows or how much material gain is obtained. In this society man has natural duties. One must support justice, assist others who are in need, abstain from harm or injury to oneself and others, and always keep promises. Rawl's theory would greatly support socialized medicine.

Strengths and Weaknesses. A strength of Rawl's theory is that it proposes equal treatment to all. For example, if a disaster occurred, a nurse on a med-surg unit would not determine who had a Blue Cross-Blue Shield card and a hefty bank account, but rather would look at who needs the most care. The nurse in the military, applying this theory of justice, would minister to soldiers on the battlefield based on medical condition and urgency of treatment. Whether the soldier were white or black, male or female, a colonel or a private, would not affect the nurse's triage assessments.

If nurses apply this philosophy, they would be dependable, comply with the angel-of-mercy image of nursing, and act to do good or not to harm others. These are admirable qualities, but how realistic are they? For example, how does one determine allocation? Is money given to those who are disadvantaged? Is it more fair to give the money to the disadvantaged than to the bright and ambitious? Who decides what is fair? Does a 60-year-old male get a kidney before a 9-year-old child?

How does the theory of justice differ from that of utilitarianism? Both look at the best for the greatest number and try to be fair in assessing what is given or what is withheld.

PATIENT RIGHTS

In 1975, the American Hospital Association (AHA) published a document entitled "A Patient's Bill of Rights" (see box).[1] This statement is not the source of patient rights but rather a formal recognition of their existence. The twelve principles in "A Patient's Bill of Rights" may be summarized under the following four headings:

1. The right to adequate health care (Principles 1, 7, and 10). The AHA bill recognizes the patient's right to "considerate and respectful" care, to "reasonable continuity of care" and to a "reasonable response" for the patient's request for service. These words, however, are vague and subject to different interpretations. They do not address directly the more basic question, that is, whether health care is a right or a privilege. This question will be addressed in greater depth later in the chapter.

2. The right to information (Principles 2, 3, 8, 11, and 12). Principle two seems to limit the patient's rights to information by excluding what is not "medically advisable." Principle three enunciates the information necessary for giving informed consent. Principles 8, 11, and 12 discuss informing the patient of relationships between the physician and others, between the hospital and other institutions, information about the patient's bill, and information about hospital rules and regulations.

3. The right to privacy and confidentiality (Principles 5 and 6). Physical privacy and

PATIENT'S BILL OF RIGHTS*

1. The patient has the right to considerate and respectful care.
2. The patient has the right to obtain from his physician complete current information concerning his diagnosis, treatment, and prognosis in terms the patient can be reasonably expected to understand. When it is not medically advisable to give such information to the patient, the information should be made available to an appropriate person in his behalf. He has the right to know by name the physician responsible for coordinating his care.
3. The patient has the right to receive from his physician information necessary to give informed consent prior to the start of any procedure and/or treatment. Except in emergencies, such information for informed consent, should include but not necessarily be limited to the specific procedure and/or treatment, the medically significant risks involved, and the probable duration of incapacitation. Where medically significant alternatives for care or treatment exist, or when the patient requests information concerning medical alternatives, the patient has the right to such information. The patient also has the right to know the name of the person responsible for the procedures and/or treatment.
4. The patient has the right to refuse treatment to the extent permitted by law, and to be informed of the medical consequences of his action.
5. The patient has the right to every consideration of his privacy concerning his own medical care program. Case discussion, consultation, examination, and treatment are confidential and should be conducted discreetly. Those not directly involved in his care must have the permission of the patient to be present.
6. The patient has the right to expect that all communications and records pertaining to his care should be treated as confidential.
7. The patient has the right to expect that within its capacity a hospital must make reasonable response to the request of a patient for services. The hospital must provide evaluation, service, and/or referral as indicated by the urgency of the case. When medically permissible a patient may be transferred to another facility only after he has received complete information and explanation concerning the needs for and alternatives to such a transfer. The institution to which the patient is to be transferred must first have accepted the patient for transfer.
8. The patient has the right to obtain information as to any relationship of his hospital to other health care and educational institutions insofar as his care is concerned. The patient has the right to obtain information as to the existence of any professional relationships among individuals, by name, who are treating him.
9. The patient has the right to be advised if the hospital proposes to engage in or perform human experimentation affecting his care or treatment. The patient has the right to refuse to participate in such research projects.
10. The patient has the right to expect reasonable continuity of care. He has the right to know in advance what appointment times and physicians are available and where. The patient has the right to expect that the hospital will provide a mechanism whereby he is informed by his physician or a delegate of the physician of the patient's continuing health care requirements following discharge.
11. The patient has the right to examine and receive an explanation of his bill regardless of source of payment.
12. The patient has the right to know what hospital rules and regulations apply to his conduct as a patient.

*Published by the American Hospital Association, 1975.

confidentiality concerning the patient's condition are recognized. It is in this area, however, that the limitation of rights becomes an issue. Other people have legitimate rights that limit patient rights in these areas. However, considering the special relationship that exists between nurse and patient, the presumption may be that the latter's rights to privacy or confidentiality prevail, unless there is clear evidence to support the contrary.

4. The right to self-determination (Principles 3, 4, and 9). Principles 4 and 9 recognize the patient's right to refuse treatment and to refuse to participate in research. Principle three, dealing with the right to information, also has relevance here because informed consent is a necessary component of self-determination or autonomy.

The right of an individual to control one's own destiny is perhaps the most basic right that a human possesses. One of Wellman's definitions of a right is "a system of normative autonomy." But to exercise the right of self-determination, the patient must have all the pertinent information to make an informed choice.

The doctrine of informed consent is relatively simple. It includes two elements: information and consent. The information element requires that the information is presented, and that it is presented in a way that is understood by the patient. The consent element requires voluntariness (freedom from coercion and undue pressure) and competence (the ability to consent).

One final observation about the limitation on rights is that not only are the rights of one person limited by the rights of other persons, but a specific right can be limited by another right possessed by the same person. Thus a patient's right to adequate health care might limit the right to information in those cases in which the former would be adversely affected by the latter. However, caution should be exercised in making this kind of judgment. Always presume, in the absence of overwhelming evidence to the contrary, that the right to be informed takes precedence, because this is necessary for the exercise of autonomy.

THE NURSE AS ADVOCATE

The practice of nursing inherently requires clinical knowledge and expertise. This does not mean that patients are passive recipients within the health care process. The American Nurses' Association (ANA) Code for Nurses (see box) is the guide the student and professional are expected to use in ministering to the needs of their clientele; their needs and desires are of utmost importance for the caregiver. If the ANA Code is not upheld, the nurse loses the respect of coworkers, as well as patients. One of the principles addressed in the ANA Code for Nurses is that of patient advocacy.

Kohnke defines advocacy as "the act of informing and supporting a person so that he can make the best decisions possible for himself."[24] As advocate, a nurse has two primary functions: (1) to inform patients of their rights and see to it that they have all the

PREAMBLE

The *Code for Nurses* is based on belief about the nature of individuals, nursing, health, and society. Recipients and providers of nursing services are viewed as individuals and groups who possess basic rights and responsibilities, and whose values and circumstances command respect at all times. Nursing encompasses the promotion and restoration of health, the prevention of illness, and the alleviation of suffering. The statements of the *Code* and their interpretation provide guidance for conduct and relationships in carrying out nursing responsibilities consistent with the ethical obligations of the profession and quality in nursing care.

ANA CODE FOR NURSES

1. The nurse provides services with respect for human dignity and the uniqueness of the client unrestricted by considerations of social or economic status, personal attributes, or the nature of health problems.
2. The nurse safeguards the client's right to privacy by judiciously protecting information of a confidential nature.
3. The nurse acts to safeguard the client and the public when health care and safety are affected by the incompetent, unethical, or illegal practice of any person.
4. The nurse assumes responsibility and accountability for individual nursing judgments and actions.
5. The nurse maintains competence in nursing.
6. The nurse exercises informed judgment and uses individual competence and qualifications as criteria in seeking consultation, accepting responsibilities, and delegating nursing activities to others.
7. The nurse participates in activities that contribute to the ongoing development of the profession's body of knowledge.
8. The nurse participates in the profession's efforts to implement and improve standards of nursing.
9. The nurse participates in the profession's efforts to establish and maintain conditions of employment conducive to high quality nursing care.
10. The nurse participates in the profession's effort to protect the public from misinformation and misrepresentation and to maintain the integrity of nursing.
11. The nurse collaborates with members of the health professions and other citizens in promoting community and national efforts to meet the health needs of the public.

From American Nurses' Association: Code for nurses, Kansas City, 1978, American Nurses' Association.

information necessary to make an informed decision and (2) to support them in the decisions they make.[24]

In an ethical system that emphasizes the primacy of patient rights, and rejects the traditional paternalistic view that "the doctor (or nurse) knows best," "patient advocate" is an excellent way of describing the role of the nurse. When accepting the role of advocate, a nurse should be prepared to cope with opposition.[37] Opposition may come from the physician who views the relationship with a patient as paternalistic, or from a hospital administrator who doesn't want anyone to "rock the boat."

Application of Ethics and ANA Code for Nurses

EXAMPLE: Ms Blake reported for charge duty at 6:30 am on a 24-bed medical unit of a local hospital. The charge nurse on the adjacent medical unit had called in sick. Two licensed practical nurses (LPNs) were assigned on the unit, but Ms Blake was given the responsibility for being charge nurse of both units for the day. She discussed her concern about the added assignment with her nursing supervisor. The response of the supervisor was, "I understand your concern, but I have no RNs to assign to that unit. It is your duty to the hospital and to the patient to supervise the LPNs so that care can be given to patients on both units. You see, I did assign an additional aide to assist you with patient care."

EXAMPLE: Student nurse McDonnaugh was asked to care for an OB-GYN patient in critical health status until the private duty nurse arrived. When she requested assistance from the nursing staff, the head nurse told her, "When I was in nursing school, I cared for the entire labor area on the 11 to 7 shift. What is wrong with you nursing students today?" The student was especially upset over the dilemma because she wanted to work in the hospital after her graduation.

EXAMPLE: A nursing researcher was working with an interdisciplinary team that received private grant monies to study causal relationships in lung disease within a large American city. The research funds were received from a corporation facing allegations that their manufacturing plant was emitting copious amounts of polluting agents into the air. The researcher was approached by the chief research investigator and asked to report only data that was favorable to the company. He was told that further grant monies were dependent on a favorable outcome.

EXAMPLE: A student nurse in a community health clinic was assigned to a home health care agency. One patient, Mr Geraldi, was a 70-year-old stroke victim. The student nurse saw the patient over a period of 6 weeks and was elated about the progress made with Mr Geraldi's decubiti and nutritional status, knowing that this was a result of his teaching efforts with the family. All was recorded, as he had been taught, in the agency's progress notes. The student nurse was confronted by his agency nurse preceptor regarding his charting, and was informed that charting on Mr Geraldi's progress would result in discontinuation of payment by state and federal agencies. The rationale for this statement was based on the fact that the client may be "too well to qualify for care." He was encouraged to keep his positive progress notes on Mr Geraldi in his student file away from the eyes of state and federal inspectors. The rationale for using the student file was based on his preceptor's knowledge of the student's dedication to the care of the patient. The preceptor and the student were aware that a pattern of reduction of funds would ultimately result in staff reduction. With a decrease in funds, there would be little chance in the agency for a position to offer new graduates. The student nurse planned to apply for a nursing position there in the spring after graduation.

   Each example reflects real-life work situations. The ANA Code for Nurses, (see box, p. 197) addresses these and similar dilemmas that nurses face daily. One can readily pull from this Code a few statements that relate to the issues stated in the four situations and serve as the ideal for nursing practice in any setting.

Article 4 states, "The nurse assumes responsibility and accountability for individual nursing judgments and actions." This means that nurses are responsible for the care clients receive, and for their own practice as both student and professional nurse.

Article 9 states that "the nurse participates and maintains conditions of employment conducive to high quality nursing care," which means that nurses must address conditions of their employment that allow for the practice of nursing within the guidelines and standards set for nursing practice.

Ms Blake and instructor Jones are caught between abiding by the ethical code to which they ascribe and giving in to their supervisor's assignment, which would alleviate conflict for the moment and also not jeopardize job security. It would not, however, alleviate them from accountability for any actions they choose to take or judgments they make with regard to patient care.

Articles 10 states "The nurse participates in the profession's effort to protect the public from misinformation and misrepresentation, and to maintain the integrity of nursing." Nurses are responsible for warning the public against the use or exposure to any product that could lead to illness. The nurse should not abuse professional communications to make deceptive claims to further individual or business gains. The nurse researcher and the home health nurse are caught between furthering the client/public good by speaking out and altering the truth to serve their employer's need, and thereby affording themselves job security.

How is it possible that nurses are faced with these discrepancies? The field of nursing is composed largely of women, and has had secondary power only by complying with the demands of others.[7] This social role was reinforced by the hospitals' hierarchal system, which establishes that the physician orders and the nurse complies.[26] Because this was the accepted role of nurses for many years, many nurses continue to comply. In so doing, nurses provide themselves momentary alleviation of the stress that would occur should they challenge this role. Nurses should, however, consider the fact that, by doing nothing, they are doing something.

Dyck addresses this dynamic in his statement: "All of us make assumptions about the nature of ethical judgments; and even if we are not formally explicit, we still unwittingly represent one or the other of the existing metaethical options."[21]

Special Categories of Patients

Special groups of patients place them in special need of an advocate. The following four groups; children, the mentally ill, the elderly, and the dying will be considered.

Children. Ethical issues involve the treatment of children and their rights to information, autonomy, and privacy.

Information. Being a child does not take away the patient's need, or moral right, to truth and information. How and what, when and by whom is the child to be told are difficult questions. However, the right to know still exists, and the obligation to provide information cannot be avoided on the grounds that the child cannot understand.

"Children's supposed inability to comprehend is often more adults' failure to communicate effectively."[7] Obviously the pediatric nurse needs special skills to perform this difficult task effectively. The nurse should be aware that giving information to the parents does not satisfy the child patient's "right to know."

Autonomy. In autonomy, the rights of child patients are limited by the legitimate rights of their parents or guardians to make decisions on their behalf. Especially in view of the legal rights and responsibility of parents, pediatric nurses must be careful about how they exercise advocacy on behalf of their patients. However, the rights of parents are not the same as the rights of their children. There are potential areas of conflict (as when a parent does not want the child to be told that he is dying). In situations such as this, the nurse may be caught in the middle. While always remaining sensitive to parental concerns and desires, the nurse must maintain, as the primary concern, the rights and welfare of the child.

The law distinguishes between "emancipated" minors and those lacking such status.[4] Although the legal distinction must be given serious consideration by the nurse (and, indeed, can serve as a legitimate basis for making an ethical distinction) it is evident that the mature "unemancipated" child should not be denied decision-making rights simply on the basis of being legally "unemancipated."

Privacy. Principles 5 and 6 of the AHA's "Patient's Bill of Rights" (see p. 195) affirm the right of the patient to privacy and confidentiality. However, if the consenting party, the parent must be given the necessary information to make an informed decision regarding treatment for the child. In this case, it can be argued that the child's right to privacy is overridden by the parent's right to know.

If the child is the consenting party, the conflict is between two rights of the child: the right to privacy versus the right to adequate health care.

In some cases (e.g., drug abuse) adequate health care might not be possible without parental notification, given the child's condition. The nurse should ask herself, "Does *this* child, under *these* circumstances have a right to privacy as far as the parents' right to know is concerned?" Only if the answer is "no" may the nurse inform the parents.

The Mentally Ill. In many respects, the ethical issues facing those caring for the mentally ill are similar to those involving children. The right to information, autonomy, and privacy are crucial issues also. But in cases involving mentally ill adults, the presumption (legal as well as ethical) is that the individual has the right to make personal decisions. Any judgment to the contrary requires a clear indication that the patient's condition is one of incompetence.

Autonomy. Because some mentally ill patients are considered dangerous, either to themselves or to others, they are sometimes committed to institutions against their wills. Certainly, the right of others to protection from harm limits the right of potentially dangerous people to walk the streets. But who is to decide who is a threat to others? There is little or no evidence to support the belief that the mentally ill, as a group, are any more dangerous than the "sane" population.[14] And how qualified are psychiatrists and other mental health personnel to determine who is potentially dangerous? Several studies question this supposed expertise.[14] The major ethical issue, then, is not whether the right of others to protection limits the rights of potentially dangerous mentally ill people, but rather, who is to decide who is "potentially dangerous" and on what basis.

When the involuntary commitment is a result of the patient being considered a threat to himself, the conflict is between one's right to autonomy and the right to adequate health care. In recent years, the courts intervened to insure that the civil liberties of the mentally ill are protected, sometimes thereby putting the individual's physical health and safety at risk.[7] The general principle that the mentally ill should be treated in the "least restrictive environment" capable of taking care of them seems ethically sound. However, an overemphasis on civil liberties at the expense of adequate care can result in thousands of the mentally ill roaming the streets; homeless, ill-clothed, and ill-fed, many "dying with their rights on."

Privacy. The general principle is the same, one person's right to privacy is limited by others' right to know. But with the mentally ill, the "right to know" often extends to many more people than in the case of children. This is especially true in situations in which there is potential danger to others.

Third party insurers are included in the "right to know" category. Patient privacy may adversely affect adequate coverage. Employers and fellow workers may also belong to the "right to know" group. Insofar as the condition of the patient admits participation, the patient should always be involved in decisions about disclosure of personal records.

Another aspect is the privacy rights of other people. Often, the testimony of family, friends, and others will be part of a patient's record. Does the patient have a right to know what others have said? The traditional right to privacy versus right to know conflict is reversed in this instance and can create serious problems for the mental health professional. The question is this: does *this* patient, under *these* circumstances, have a right to *this* information? Only if the answer is negative should the information be withheld.

The Elderly. Those over 65 years of age comprise the fastest growing segment of our population today. Not surprisingly, they are also the group with the greatest need for health care. With modern technological advances, the ability to prolong life and the ethical questions accompanying this progress have grown dramatically. Two questions, that of euthanasia and the just allocation of health care, will be considered later in this chapter. The focus here is on ageism and paternalism versus autonomy.

Ageism. Ageism, according to Butler, who coined the term in 1968, is another form of prejudice, similar to racism and sexism. It is a process of systematically stereotyping and discriminating against older people because of their age.[9] It classifies them as ugly, rigid, senile, garrulous, and largely useless, a negative description with which many elderly come to view themselves.[10]

Ageism is a natural outgrowth of a culture that equates human worth with productivity. One is identified by what one does, or perhaps with how much one earns. As the elderly's ability to produce diminishes, their "usefulness" declines, and with it a decline in society's (and their own) estimation of their value. This attitude threatens two of the elderly patient's rights, the right to respect and the right to adequate health care.

The role of patient advocate for the elderly is important not only in a hospital setting, but also for the 5% of the elderly population in nursing homes and for the home-bound aged. In each of these cases the nurse is the main source of health care and is responsible for coordinating nursing services with diagnostic and therapeutic services. The two functions of the advocate, to inform and support, are invaluable if the rights of this very vulnerable population are to be respected.[35]

Paternalism versus autonomy. Dworkin defines paternalism as "interference with a person's liberty of action justified by reasons referring exclusively to the welfare, good, happiness, needs, and interests or values of the person being coerced."[5] Paternalism then, is a consequentialist position, justifying the violation of an individual's right to decide on the grounds that one will be "better off," or that "The end justifies the means."

Paternalism toward the elderly is exercised by the state and by individuals. Medicare and Social Security programs are examples of state paternalism. Placing an unwilling elderly parent in a nursing home to receive better care is an example of familial paternalism. A nurse or physician dealing with an adult child about treatment for an elderly parent, rather than with the patient, is an example of medical paternalism. In all of these cases, the welfare of the elderly person motivates the behavior of all concerned. The best intentions, however, are not sufficient to justify an action if that act achieves its results through a violation of an elderly person's right to self-determination.

Again, the question that the patient advocate must ask is "Does *this* person in *these* circumstances have the right to make decisions?" If the answer is "yes," advocacy requires that the patient be supported in that choice. The answer is complicated by a factual question "Does this individual have the *ability* to exercise autonomy?" Autonomy is possible only when one can comprehend and decide. Senility, confusion, drugs, pain, etc. adversely affect the ability of the elderly patient and, at times, may render him incapable of exercising autonomy. Such judgment, however, should not be hastily made. Especially objectionable is the conclusion that if the patient's decision is different from that of the nurse, that fact in itself is an indication of mental incapacity. Autonomy implies the right to disagree as well as to agree, to refuse as well as consent.

The Dying. The question of the right to refuse life-sustaining treatment will be addressed in a later section, as will questions concerning brain death, advanced directives, and assisted suicide. Here, following Barry's format, discussion will be limited to three issues: telling dying patients their condition, determining where one is to die, and administering drugs for pain relief.[7]

The right to be told one's condition. Of the two major arguments for *not* telling dying patients their condition, one is nonconsequentialist, the other is consequentialist. The nonconsequentialist argument is that the dying do not want to know. If this is true, because rights are permissive of their possessor, they can forego this right to information. This argument, however, is not supported by the evidence, which indicates that the vast majority of dying patients *do* wish to be told.[7] And certainly, if they wish this information, the fact that physicians, nurses, or family members feel uncomfortable in discussing it with the patient does not relieve them of their obligation.

The consequentialist argument is that the dying patient, if told, will lose all hope, cease fighting to live, and thus will be physically and emotionally harmed by knowing.

Again, there is evidence to question the validity of this contention.[7] But, even if it is true that in a particular case the consequences of withholding the truth from a dying patient will be better than informing, there is still the question of one's right to know. A patient advocate must decide whether the right to health care limits the patient's right to information. The presumption, especially in view of the strong factual doubts about whether health care is adversely affected by the patient's being told, seems to be that the right to information prevails.

To maintain that a patient has a right to be told and that this right places an ethical obligation on others does not, however, solve the question of who is to do the telling, or of when and how this is to take place. Because one always has the obligation to act to minimize the danger of harm, these questions require sensitive and careful consideration by all concerned, health care professionals and family members alike.

The right to decide where to die. Until recently, the percentage of people dying in hospitals rather than at home steadily increased. In recent years, at least two factors, tighter controls by government and private insurers on financing hospital care and the increased influence of the hospice movement, have begun to reverse this trend. Still, the great majority of deaths in the United States occur in hospital settings. Most people, however, state that they would prefer to die at home.

Why the discrepancy? Are the rights of people who wish to die at home, but who nonetheless spend their last days in a hospital, being violated? If so, what can the nurse advocate do?

Frequent reasons for placing unwilling dying patients in hospitals are (1) the family cannot provide adequate health care at home and (2) children should not be exposed to the experience of a family member's death. Although these reasons (especially the first) have some validity, neither, in the majority of cases, poses an insuperable problem.

The patient advocate can be helpful in addressing the family's reservations about home health care. The nurse can help determine whether adequate health care is realistically possible at home and she can educate the family in how to provide this care, reassure them that they can do it, and provide support services. One effective way to exercise advocacy for the patient and for the family is to put them in contact with local hospice volunteers, who provide a variety of services to those wishing to die at home.

Hospice workers also are skilled in helping minimize the negative effects exposure to death might have on children. With proper support from family and others, children can be psychologically strengthened, rather than harmed, by such an experience.[7]

Administration of drugs to the dying. Studies show that "fifty percent of the terminally ill have unrelieved pain; twenty six percent have severe or serious pain; and sixteen percent have continuous severe pain."[7] Failure to relieve pain, when relief is possible, seems a violation of the patient's right to adequate health care. Reasons often given for failure to administer sufficient drugs for adequate pain control are the fear of addiction, the adverse effects that drugs may have on the patient's decision-making capacity, and the fear that certain powerful drugs may shorten life. None of these reasons, at least for the natural law ethician, is compelling. This is a clear-cut case of the principle of double effect, in which the intended good is a relief of severe pain and the unintended, but foreseen, evil effects are those just mentioned. If the pain is severe, and if there are no alternative means for relief that would not include these negative effects, there is a "proportionate reason" for permitting them.

One might ask just how great an evil it is for a dying person to become physically or psychologically addicted to a pain-killer. Certainly it would be a lesser evil than intractable pain. One might question whether drugs inhibit autonomous decision-making abilities to any greater extent than the pain they are relieving. As a true advocate for the dying patient, the nurse should do everything possible to ensure that the weeks, days, and last moments are as pain-free as possible. Anything less constitutes a violation of the patient's right to adequate health care.

SELECTED BIOETHICAL ISSUES

In addition to the ethical problems arising from special categories of patients, other bioethical issues are of concern to the nurse who wishes to function as a patient advocate. Although limitations of space prevent any comprehensive treatment of these issues, a selective number of them will be examined.

Personhood

An important and difficult question facing the nurse is not an ethical question at all, but rather a metaphysical one, "what is a person?" Is every being with biologically human qualities a person, or is personhood an additional perfection? On the presumption that only persons have rights, these questions are of utmost importance. Is the fetus a person? The anencephalic or other severely malformed infant? What about the individual in a persistent vegetative state or irreversible coma? One's position on these and other related cases will profoundly influence ethical decisions in several areas.

Theories of personhood may be divided into *absolutist* and *process* views.

Absolutist View

An absolutist position equates person and human being. Personhood is founded in nature, in the kind of thing that something is. An individual substance of a rational nature is a classical definition of a person, attributed to the philosopher Boethius in the sixth century. Characteristics of an absolutist view of personhood include the following:

1. All humans are persons.
2. There are no degrees of personhood. No one is more or less a person than another.
3. Personhood is acquired and lost instantaneously. Although the process leading up to the acquiring and loss of personhood is gradual, one becomes and ceases to be a person instantaneously. Death, then, is an event, not a process.
4. Personhood is rooted in nature.

Process View

A process view of personhood distinguishes a person from a human being. Personhood is founded in powers, in certain abilities that the individual possesses. Joseph

Fletcher is a noted proponent of the process view. He lists several tentative "indicators of humanhood" that he suggests are necessary before an individual can be deemed a person. Among these are minimal intelligence, self-awareness and control, a sense of the past and the future, and consciousness of an ability to relate to and communicate with others. This "cardinal indicator," which is at the basis of all the others, is referred to by Fletcher as *neocortical activity*.[16] A process view of personhood includes the following:

1. Not all humans are persons.
2. There are degrees of personhood. Some people are more fully persons than others.
3. Personhood is gradually acquired and (in many cases at least) gradually lost. Death is a process.
4. Personhood is rooted in powers.

One's view of personhood, then, will certainly be a significant factor in a consideration of patient rights. If the criteria for personhood are accepted, those qualifying presumably have the same rights as any other patient.

For most advocates of an absolutist view, the fetus is a person, an individual possessing the kind of nature that has the potential, given the proper circumstances, to develop into a baby, a child, an adult. The human sperm and ovum in this view are potentially a person; the fetus is a person with potential.

Process advocates deny personhood to the fetus. Certainly many of Fletcher's necessary criteria are lacking in the fetus (as well as in the newborn). Warren is a typical proponent of this view. "...a fetus is a human being which is not yet a person, and which therefore cannot coherently be said to have full moral rights."[34] Because process advocates see personhood as a gradually developing quality, they should presumably consider a fetus at a later stage of pregnancy to be "more of a person" than one at an early stage. Full personhood, however, does not occur until well after birth.[34]

The patient with anencephaly, in the absolutist view, is a person. The defect does not alter the nature of the individual, but rather prevents that nature from exhibiting the powers found in one without this defect. As a person, then, the patient with anencephaly is the possessor of rights.

For the process advocate, patients with anencephaly are not persons. "Defective human beings, with no appreciable mental capacity, are not and presumably never will be people."[34] Because, unlike the normal fetus, they do not have the potential for becoming persons, whatever consideration accorded a potential person would not be due them.

The same may be said for those in a permanently comatose or persistent vegetative state. The absolutist views them as persons, albeit incapable of functioning in many basic ways as such. In the process view, they have ceased to be persons. As their powers diminish and become nonfunctional, so does personhood gradually cease. This leads to a radically different view of what constitutes "brain death." In the process view, a cessation of neocortical activity signals the death of the person, although the human is still capable of breathing, etc. on his own.

The absolutist, however, considers the presence of self-initiated and self-sustained physiological activities to be an indication that the person is still alive. Death is indicated only when there is total cessation of all functions of the brain, including the brain stem. For the absolutist, Karen Ann Quinlan, lying in a vegetative state for the years subsequent to her removal from life-support systems. remained a person; in the process view, she was long since dead.

Reproductive Issues

Abortion. Abortion is a bioethical issue that divides people into opposing camps and provokes emotional controversy. In the celebrated *Roe v. Wade* decision of 1973 (410 US 113) the US Supreme Court declared that a fetus is not a person in the legal sense, guaranteed protection under the Fourteenth Amendment. Thus the legal right of a woman to have an abortion, with certain restrictions as outlined by the Court, was assured. The ethical issue, however, remains the subject of controversy.

Ethical considerations are contingent on one's view of the antological status of the fetus. If the fetus is not a person, or only a potential person, any ethical objections to abortion would be based on something other than the protection of rights. However, if the fetus is a person, as most absolutists maintain, then from an ethical perspective, its rights deserve protection on the same basis and to the same degree as those of any other person. Given the personally helpless and legally defenseless status of the fetus, the argument could logically be made that, if it is a person, it is more in need of a patient advocate than any other.

If ethically opposed to abortions, the nurse is usually excused from participating in activities considered morally repugnant. The nurse should also realize, however, that the woman having an abortion has ethical views on the issue that may differ from that of the nurse, and as a person and a patient, deserves respectful care.

The acrimony associated with the abortion issue could be lessened if the two sides would accept the following:

1. "Pro-life" advocates should limit their judgments about abortion to the act and refrain from judging the people who obtain or perform abortions. To call abortion "murder" and those responsible for it "murderers" is to make a judgment of responsibility and imputability about another that no human being has the right to make.

2. "Pro-choice" advocates should refrain from comments such as "If you think abortion is wrong, then don't have one; if I don't see anything wrong with it, then what I do is none of your business." A similar argument was made by slave-holders to those who opposed them. Such an argument fails to recognize the fact that, if opposition to a practice is based on the conviction that human rights are being violated by that practice, those who hold this conviction have no ethical alternative than to oppose it. It is their business.

In Vitro Fertilization. One aspect of the in vitro fertilization (IVF) issue is identical to that of abortion: does the fetus become a person at fertilization. If so, many zygotes and embryos are destroyed or discarded in this process and human persons are being used as a means to an end.

Apart from the question of the destruction of fertilized ova, several ethical issues remain. One, which concerns natural law advocates, involves separation of the generative from the sexual act. Natural law, which sanctions the use of scientific knowledge to enhance bodily functions, judges as "unnatural" the separation that eliminates the need for sexual intercourse. For consequentialists and Kantians, this would probably not present a serious problem. The Kantian is more concerned with the rights of children conceived through such a process. What if a defective child is born? Is there a likelihood that a child conceived in this way would be the subject of excessive curiosity, ridicule, and even rejection by society? Would such a child be more likely than one conceived "naturally" to be looked on as a mere possession, rather than as a person?

For the consequentialist, the ethical issue centers around the effects of IVF on the parents, the child, the marriage, and society. Certainly within the narrow context of a barren couple's desire to have a child, the results if successful, are beneficial. But within the broader context of the uncertain effects on the child, the family, and society, many consequentialists question whether the overall consequences are desirable. Those concerned with the most equitable use of society's limited resources question whether this approach to infertility is a project to which research methods of science and medicine should be directed.[34]

Surrogate Parenting. Surrogacy adds its own special problems to those of IVF. Chief among these are the severing of the mother-child relationship when the surrogate surrenders the child to the biological father, the "baby-selling" aspects of paid surrogacy, and the "child as a product" implications of most surrogacy contracts. In the celebrated "Baby M" case of 1987, for example, the surrogate mother, Mary Beth Whitehead, signed a contract in which she agreed to the following:

1. To undergo amniocentesis and if the fetus were found to be abnormal, to have an abortion. Refusal to abort would relieve William Stern, the contracting father, of all legal obligations.
2. To accept a $1000 fee for a fetus aborted at Stern's demand or for a stillbirth or miscarriage after the fifth month of pregnancy. (She would receive no compensation for a miscarriage before the fifth month.)
3. To give a live child to Mr Stern for a fee of $10,000.

These factors raise serious questions about whether the money paid is for a *product* rather than for services.[3] Add to these questions those concerning the effects of surrogacy on the family, on the traditional marital relationship of husband and wife, plus the total separation of sexuality from procreative reproduction, and urgent ethical caution flags are necessarily raised. Then, when the surrogate mother refuses to "give up" the child to the contracting father (as happened in the "Baby M" case) or when the father decides he doesn't want the baby because it isn't "normal" (as in the case of Christopher Stiver, born in 1983) the legal complications, with their resulting dangers for the well-being of the child, result in many ethical and legal authorities becoming critical of the whole process.[3]

More and more, as technology makes many previously impossible reproductive procedures reality, the ethical question "it *can* be done, but *should* it be done" becomes crucial. It is critical that every nurse have an awareness of what the ethical issues are, and a clear understanding of her own ethical values.

THE NURSE AND THE ORGANIZATION

As a professional, the nurse belongs to a specially educated group with its own licensing procedures, professional associations, system of peer review, and code of ethics (see ANA Code for Nurses, p. 197). The nurse is committed to a certain set of values, anchored in a dedication to the rights and well-being of the patient.

Even though nurses are professionals, they often function in a bureaucratic setting. The values of a bureaucracy are often at odds with those of a profession. (Nurses, of course, are not alone in this type of situation. Teachers, for example, have to work within the bureaucracy of the university or school system.) Bureaucracy emphasizes efficiency, division of labor, quantitative criteria for judging success and a structured hierarchial system. Professionalism, however, entails more flexibility and individual attention (the nurse who can administer medication to a certain number of patients in a shorter period of time is not necessarily doing a better job than another who takes longer). Also, collegial decision-making and a peer review system of accountability mark the professional outlook.

Perhaps more basic is the different attitude toward health care itself. For the nurse, health care is a service. The good of the patient is the underlying goal; economic constraints are unfortunately necessary secondary considerations. In a bureaucratic system, however, health care is a commodity, an economic good like any other, subject to the same values that dominate any other good business.

A nurse in a bureaucratic setting, then, can become caught up in a conflict between different value systems. This can be further complicated by the dual roles in which nurses often find themselves when they function both in an administrative or supervisory capacity and deliver patient care. The problem of the primacy of loyalties can become an acute ethical dilemma for the conscientious nurse.

In addition to the professional-bureaucratic conflict, the nurse may also encounter problems in relationships with physicians. Barry[7] mentions the following differences that can cause problems:

1. Sex differences—although this is changing, most physicians are still male, most nurses are female.
2. Differences in educational background—this, too, is gradually changing. Physicians, however, still have more formal training.
3. Differences in career patterns—most physicians are self-employed; most nurses are not.
4. Differences in social class—physicians make more money, have more prestige, associate with those higher in authority, and are more likely to come from upper/upper middle class families.
5. Differences in authority—physicians have special status in hospitals, especially because they are the ones who admit patients.
6. Semantic differences—words (e.g., cooperative) may have different meanings for physicians and nurses.

7. Differences in patient orientation—the nurse is oriented to caring for patients, the physician to curing. The nurse spends more time with the patient, often knows the patient better than the physician.

These differences can cause conflicts that undermine morale, destroy team unity, and threaten welfare of the patient. For this reason, they constitute an ethical issue.

In an attempt to counteract dissonance, some administrators may attempt to push nurses back into the traditional setting by using ethics to support or validate their statements and beliefs. One way to accomplish this goal may be through various forms of "game playing." A few of the major strategies that can be used will now be mentioned.

One strategy is called "crumbs for meatloaf." To facilitate the dynamics of this strategy, an administrator offers a pittance in return for passing excessive workload expectations. In the earlier example (p. 198) of Ms Blake's patient load increase by an entire unit, her supervisor gave her an additional aide to accomplish the job. But could the aide supervise the LPNs, administer the RN's medications and treatments, and check IVs? These issues were not addressed.

Another strategy of employers is to offer flattery in return for compliance. This is seen in the case of Instructor Jones who, when given an overload assignment, is told, "I figured you wouldn't mind because you are so competent and efficient in performing your duties as a nurse." Flattery does not decrease the nurse's responsibilities for insuring that clinical components of nursing objectives are met and patient safety is maintained.

When all else fails, the infliction of guilt is a last resort in the art of using persuasive tactics. This was seen in the example of the home health nurse (p. 198) who was presented with the possibility that his patient's care would be decreased if a substantial improvement in his patient's condition were known. Masked threats serve as further reinforcers.

The home health nurse was told that continuation of care for the patient and his job security were dependent on hiding the facts from those who may act negatively on them. The nurse researcher also was faced with the dilemma of reporting the whole truth or only those parts which best served his employer's needs. Again, job security was used as an incentive to comply. The saddest part is that these coercive statements are more fact than fiction.

The dynamics described here have more profound results than appear at first glance. The impossible is often asked of the nurse but when the situation backfires and negative consequences result, the Professional Practice Act and the Nurses' Code of Ethics are used to point the finger of blame back at the nurse. The nurse is then left with no support from peers, administration, or the public. Fearing consequences of professional behavior when contradictory action is taken, nurses are often faced with the dilemma of following the internal ethical mind-set, which is based on ideals into which they were professionalized, or comply with what is being asked. This results in professional limbo. Feelings of helplessness and hopelessness are the result. The continual pull of this perpetual process on nurses results in depression and despair.

The potential for conflict increases dramatically when commitment to patient rights impels the nurse to engage in reporting a physician or another nurse.

EXAMPLE: Ms Parker, a new graduate nurse was to give a PRN injection of morphine for pain to a patient with metastasized cancer. When checking the order and the Physician's Desk Reference, Ms Parker noted the physician had ordered a dosage of morphine 50 mg higher than the safe standard level indicated. The nurse reported her findings to the head nurse on the unit. The head nurse responded angrily, "Dr. Bradley *doesn't* like her orders questioned. If you want to worry about something, worry about the patient who's in pain while you stand questioning the order. The medication orders are OK. Why don't you just go ahead and give the shot?"

In this case the nurse risks being ostracized by friends and confreres, being considered a troublemaker by superiors, or even being terminated of employment. Despite these dangers, however, the ethical nurse has no choice. It is imperative to insure the rights of the patient. It should be done, however, in a way least damaging to the institution, other health care professionals, and the nurse's own welfare. When there is conflict between any of these and the rights of the patient, the nurse's role as patient advocate requires the welfare of the patient first.

During the past 10 years this has changed significantly. Judicial decisions repeatedly support the nurse, not for doing what the physician ordered or what a hospital expected, but rather, for reporting any obvious inadequacy or irregularity of treatment, regardless of the nature of the patient illness or circumstance. To determine the nature of a nurse's responsibility in such a situation, for example, one must review the third code in the ANA Code for Nurses which states, "The nurse acts to safeguard the client and the public when health care and safety are affected by incompetent, unethical, or illegal practice of any person.[7] To eliminate double bind situations, it is important for nurses to: (1) develop strategies and outline dynamics of interactions encompassing ethical components and (2) use the Code for Nurses as a guide for resolving situations dealing with ethical dilemmas.

The first step requires evaluating nurses' abilities to work within an organizational framework. This requires a definition and assessment of unwritten procedures in the organization. It is also imperative for nurses to determine their own individual ethical values and beliefs. Incongruencies between these need to be addressed, and strategies for coping with dilemmas that may flow from these incompatibilities need to be developed, so that nurses are not left in ethical crisis situations with nothing but denial or catastrophic responses to draw from.

Too often nurses deny what could easily become reality by thinking that a situation that is not within their own value system could never occur. By assessing the compatibility between organizational and individual value systems, the nurse avoids dealing with the possibilities of a highly stressful situation.

Situations involving ethics are usually complex; rightness or wrongness of any action is dependent on its consequences for all involved. Actions need to be based on knowledge of their multiple ramifications.

_____ RIGHTS OF THE NURSING PROFESSION _____

1. The right to find dignity in self-expression and self-enhancement through the use of special abilities and educational background.
2. The right to recognition for contributions through the provision of an environment for its practice, and proper professional economic rewards.
3. The right to a work environment that will minimize physical and emotional stress and health risks.
4. The right to control what is professional practice within the limits of the law.
5. The right to set standards for excellence in nursing.
6. The right to participate in policy making affecting nursing.
7. The right to social and political action in behalf of nursing and health care.

The Code for Nurses offers a guide when taking a professional stand, and needs to be used by the nurse in support of ethical responses to dilemmas.

Many factors in the foregoing discussions can contribute to a feeling of powerlessness on the part of many nurses. This powerlessness can contribute to a number of undesirable consequences, including burnout, job dissatisfaction, a diminished self-image, and ultimately, poorer patient care. To function optimally as a person and as a professional, the nurse's rights must also be respected. Fagin lists several rights as being basic to the nursing profession (see box).[15]

THE NURSE AND THE PATIENT
Models of Nurse-Patient Relationships

Veatch lists four major models of physician-patient relationships [34] (see box).

Veatch criticizes the engineering model because it denies the physician any moral integrity. The problem with the priestly or paternalistic model is that the freedom and dignity of the patient are destroyed. The collegial model espouses an equality and unity of goals that simply do not exist in reality. The contractual or covenant model, Veatch asserts, avoids the major flaws of the other three and best safeguards the rights and responsibilities of both parties.[33]

A similar analysis of models of nurse-patient relationships may also be made. Sheri Smith analyzed models based largely on an analogy with Veatch's models of physician-patient relationships.[31] She addresses three prominent views of the nurse-patient relationship: (1) the nurse as surrogate mother, (2) the nurse as technician, and (3) the nurse as contracted clinician.

The Nurse as Surrogate Mother. This view is marked by the nurse's total commitment to the patient. "It is the nurse's obligation to provide nursing care, to take care of the patient, and to act in his or her best interest at all times." The nurse "has an obligation to determine what constitutes the best care for the patient."[31] This commitment to patient

---

_____ MODELS OF PHYSICIAN-PATIENT RELATIONSHIPS _____

1. The engineering model—the physician is a scientist or technician, presenting the patient with all the pertinent medical information and letting the patient make all the decisions. The physician is a value-free medical repairman, following instructions in much the same way that a plumber would.
2. The priestly (paternalistic) model—the physician is the "new priest" or father figure; the patient is the child. All decision-making is in the hands of the physician, whose major ethical obligation is to "benefit and do no harm" to the patient.
3. The collegial model—the physician and patient are colleagues, pursuing a common goal. They are "pals," equal in dignity and value contributions.
4. The contractual model—the physician and patient are like partners in a marriage covenant, each with obligations and expected benefits, each willing to "go the extra mile," each maintaining moral integrity and proper sphere of influence.

---

welfare leads to the surrogate mother model when it is combined with the conviction that patients, because of their illness are "fearful, dependent . . . unable to exercise emotional control or to make important decisions and, in at least some respects, may be irrational." It is, therefore, the nurse's responsibility to make decisions for a patient as a mother would for her child.[31]

The Nurse as Technician. This view considers nursing a clinical science and the nurse's obligation to apply scientific methods to patient care. The nurse should be ethically neutral and not impose personal values on the patient. This assumes that sickness and hospitalization have not impaired the patient's ability to make decisions, and that the nurse should simply apply knowledge and skill to insure the patient's wishes. "She should not be concerned with the decisions which the patient might make about his treatment or health, even if her involvement in his decisions would be for the patient's own good."[31]

The Nurse as Contracted Clinician. This view assumes, as does the technician model, that the patient is capable of determining self-interests and that the rights of the patient determine the responsibilities of the nurse. The patient contracts with the nurse for certain care that the nurse is obligated to provide. If the patient desires care that would involve a violation of the nurse's ethical values, the nurse has the right to refuse to agree to the relationship. Although decision-making remains essentially with the patient, it is the nurse's role to aid in determining what the patient's best interests are.[31] This relationship forms the basis for what Sally Gadow calls *Existential Advocacy,* which, she maintains, constitutes the essence of nursing.[17]

Smith avows the contracted clinician model is best, specifying the rights and duties of both the patient and the nurse. In the surrogate mother model, the right of the patient to self-determination is taken away. In the technician model, the ethical values of the nurse are jeopardized, as is the right of the patient to the best care available, because the nurse leaves all decision-making about care to the patient. The contracted clinician model recognizes the primacy of the patient's right to self-determination, but also recognizes the responsibility of the nurse to maximize the patient's best interests within the limits imposed by the obligation not to violate patient rights.[31]

NATURE OF RIGHTS

Veatch's contractual model and Smith's contracted clinician model emphasize the importance of respect for patient rights. The obligations of nurses are specified by the rights of their patients.

What, then, is a right? Wellman argues that a right has at least the following three characteristics.[35]

1. It is permissive of its possessor—those possessing a right (e.g., to be informed about their condition) may choose *not* to be told.
2. It implies a duty on the part of others—the nurse does not have the option of withholding information from a patient who wishes it.
3. It ought to be protected by society or secured by law—laws exist, in part, to insure that people's rights are protected. The right exists, however, even in the absence of societal or legal protection.

Wellman then defines a right as "a sphere of decision that is, or ought to be, respected by other individuals and protected by society."[36] In a later edition, Wellman defines a right as "a system of normative autonomy."[37] Although this concept of a right may be criticized, it has considerable value in a discussion of the rights of patients.

Because moral rights are rooted in the basic dignity of the human person, they are not unlimited. At least two limitations exist: (1) They are limited by the final end of the person. No one has a right to frustrate the attainment of someone else's end. In other words, no one has a right to commit an ethical evil, and (2) they are limited by the rights of other people. One popular expression is "your right to swing your arm ends where my nose begins."

This limitation obviously results in disagreements about whose rights prevail in specific cases. The rights of an AIDS patient to confidentiality are limited by the rights of others to know; the rights of an individual to health care are limited by society's rights (and responsibilities) to provide care for others. Civil law and the courts are often required to identify the limit of rights and adjudicate conflicts. This is proper as long as the basic dignity, which is the source of rights, is recognized. At other times, however, the nurse must judge who actually has a right in a specific conflict situation.

• • •

Ethical dilemmas often result from crisis situations. Thus, they need to be thought through in advance and analyzed. Nurses can anticipate ethical problems that could conceivably arise with patients under their care, in much the same way as they think of medical problems that could occur when caring for their patients. Although ethical components of situations that materialize may not mimic the dilemmas that were envisioned, three outcomes result from practicing this strategy, as follows:

1. Students see themselves as active participants within the health care team, and accept the responsibilities that come with it
2. Many situations may closely resemble those planned for, and the student nurse is more prepared for them if thought were devoted to ethical perplexities beforehand
3. Working through situations affords the student the opportunity to practice ethical decision-making outside of the bounds of glaring emergencies

No nurse can think or process information for another, nor can one react in another's behalf. There are no magic answers or pat solutions. To accomplish effective ethical decision-making, it is necessary that each aspiring professional nurse search for background data on which to build an ethical repertoire. This can be found in literature in ethics and health care, and documentation, such as actual cases in legal libraries, and ethical review board decisions.

Also, it is imperative that the ANA Code for Nurses[2] be read and understood. As patient advocates, student and professional nurses need to adhere to guides that foster optimal health choices.

Although a strong theoretical framework is imperative to nursing, greater demands and an expanded role require more from the nursing profession. Nurses today need to be accountable for and have the freedom to react within their own value system. To support this, one needs to study philosophers and theologians for statements regarding ethics and values within one's life.

Regardless of one's opinions and thoughts about ethics, all nurses encounter perplexities in deciding what is right or wrong. Some state that ethics is a relative matter, others point out the absolute necessity for applying Christian ethics in the modern world, and still others emphasize a need to look at one's motivations and to subsequent consequences. Students should participate in ethical rounds and address ethical dilemmas in postconferences with instructors. This allows the student opportunity to apply what was learned in didactic course material. With "practice," students are offered a framework and peer support. This decreases the aloneness felt by many when they attempt to use ethics in delineating their practice.

To further support its importance to nursing, ethics should be included in nursing care plans, to reinforce a student's use of ethical behavior after graduation. In addition, students must understand and appreciate the role of their professional organizations to this end. Reinforcement may occur if professional seminars and issues classes are conducted for student-instructor discussions.

Ethical dilemmas need also to be included in nursing shift reports, rounds, and care conferences. This is necessary so that nurses in their one-to-one contact with patients consider the moral and ethical ramifications of their actions; this leads to genuine humanistic nursing care.

Professional student organizations join legal, ethical, and social systems in support of professional behavior. Student organizations facilitate exchange of communication between members regarding actual clinical situations and how they were resolved. This too is a fertile ground to foster growth in ethical decision-making. The end result serves to reinforce the fact that students cannot expect "cut-and-dried" answers from texts, faculty, and individual practitioners.

Although these sources and role models are important, students need to be responsible for developing a personal and professional framework through individual processing, and through membership with their peers in their own professional organizations. Furthermore, the concern for ethical practice needs to be evidenced daily on all levels, to ensure that ethics committees and other formal hospital and community groups are successful in practicing ethics with their patients.

Ethics committees are forming in response to the difficult ethical decisions faced by patients, families, and health care providers. Technological capability, the escalating costs of health care, and the lack of unification in legal opinion result in the need of in-house resources to assist in the facilitation of decision-making. Ethics committees generally consider ethical issues involving quality of life, terminal illness, and use of scarce resources. Committees should be composed of ethicists, nurses, physicians, social workers, clergy, lay people, and possibly, the institution's legal advisor. The committee must be multidisciplinary to provide the broadest expertise and range of perspective. Committee functions must be consultative, to assist patients and/or their families to face and resolve ethical dilemmas, and educational, to assist professionals in developing a systematic reasoned approach to ethical problem solving. A further function may be the development of policies and guidelines on such issues as implementation of cardiopulmonary resuscitation, treatment of handicapped newborns, organ transplants, and initiation and withdrawal of intravenous food and fluid. Needless to say, every committee should keep a record of all deliberations and recommendations with due protection of confidentiality. In 1984, the ANA adopted a motion to promote nurses' active participation in multidisciplinary institutional ethics committees to assure reasoned decision making in all health care settings.

To use the Code fully, nurses need to become cognizant of what they are doing to others and what others are doing to them. Otherwise, they may find themselves trapped by the very Code designed to support them in their professional ethics.

In support of nurses' evolving role, the ANA Code for Nurses lists criteria for functioning as a professional who can expect to enjoy professional rights and privileges as well. In order to assist nurses in addressing ethics in practice, professional and societal support is needed. Nurses need to band together and speak as one voice on all fronts. This can be accomplished through professional organizations that ascribe to the Code. These professional organizations in turn have a moral responsibility to assist nurses in their attempt to synthesize ethics into practice.

STUDY ACTIVITIES

1. What school of ethical thinking most parallels the beliefs of the reader?
2. Describe situation(s) concerning family and/or friends in which ethical decision-making was involved in planning health care, or decisions of life/death were made.
3. How do you think life/death and other serious health care decisions should be made for patients/clients?

4. What are the major points in the Patient's Bill of Rights?
5. What are the major points in the ANA Code for Nurses?

REFERENCES

1. American Hospital Association: A Patient's Bill of Rights. 1975, American Hospital Association.
2. American Nurses' Association: Code for Nurses. Kansas City, 1978, American Nurses' Association.
3. Annas GJ: Baby M: babies and justice, Hastings Center Report, 17(3), June 13-15, 1987.
4. Annas GJ: The rights of hospital patients, New York, 1975, Avon Books.
5. Bandman EL and Bandman B: Nursing ethics in the life span, Norwalk, Conn: 1985, Appleton-Century-Crofts.
6. Barrett C: Philosophy, New York, 1935, MacMillan Co.
7. Barry V: Moral aspects of healthcare, Belmont, Calif, 1982, Wadsworth.
8. Butler JD: Four philosophies and their practice in education and religion, ed. 3, New York, 1968, Harper and Row.
9. Butler RN: Why survive? Being old in America, New York, 1975, Harper and Row.
10. Butler RN and Lewis MI: Aging and mental health, ed. 2, St. Louis, 1977, CV Mosby Co.
11. Calkins MW: The philosophical credo of an absolutist personalist. In Adams GP and Montague WP: Contemporary American Philosophy, vol. 1, 1930, MacMillan Publishing Co.
12. Dewey J: Creative intelligence, New York, 1917, Holt, Reinhart and Winston.
13. Dwarkin G: Paternalism. In Beausuchamp TL and Pinkard TP, eds.: Ethics and public policy, ed. 2, Englewood Cliffs, New Jersey, 1983, Prenctice Hall.
14. Ennis BJ and Siegel L: The rights of mental patients, New York, 1973, Avon Books.
15. Fagin C: Nurses' rights, Am J Nurs 75, 84, Jan 1975.
16. Fletcher J: Indicator of humanhood: a tentative profile of man, Hastings Center Report, 2(2), 3, Nov, 1972.
17. Gadow S: Existential advocacy: philosophical foundation of nursing. In Specker S and Gadow S eds.: Nursing: images and ideas, New York, 1980, Springer Publishing Co, Inc.
18. Halverson WH: Concise introduction to philosophy, ed. 4, New York, 1981, Random House.
19. James W: Pragmatism: a new name for some old ways of thinking, New York, 1976, Johns Hopkins University Press.
20. Joad CE: Guide to philosophy, New York, 1957, Dover Publication.
21. Kant I: Foundations of the metaphysics of morals, New York, 1959, Liberal Arts Press.
22. Kant I: The fundamental principles of the metaphysics of ethics, New York, 1938, Appleton-Century-Crofts.
23. Kierkegaard S: Sickness unto death, New York, 1941, Doubleday and Co.
24. Kohnke MF: The nurse as advocate, Am J Nurs November, 1980.
25. Locke J: An essay concerning human understanding, New York, 1959, Dover Press.
26. McConnell TC: Moral issues in health care: an introduction to medical ethics, Monterrey, Calif, 1982, Wadsworth.
27. Montague WP: The way of things, Inglewood Cliffs, New Jersey, 1940, Prentice Hall.
28. O'Rourke K and Bradiur D: Medical ethics: common ground for understanding, St. Louis, 1986, The Catholic Health Association of the United States.
29. Perry RB: Present philosophical tendencies, New York, 1912, Longmans, Green and Co.
30. President's commission for the study of ethical problems in medicine and biomedical and behavioral research: securing access to health care, Vols. I and II, Washington, DC: 1983, Superintendent of documents.
31. Rawl JD: A theory of justice, Cambridge, Massachusetts, 1981, Harvard University Press.
32. Smith S: Three models of the nurse-patient relationship. In Arras J and Hunt R, eds.: Ethical issues in modern medicine, ed. 2, Palo Alto, Calif, 1983, Mayfield.
33. Steele SM and Harmon VM: Values clarification in nursing, ed. 2, New York, 1983, Appleton-Century-Croft.

34. Veatch RM: Models for ethical medicine in a revolutionary age, The Hastings Center Report, June 1972.
35. Warren, MA: On the legal and moral status of abortion. In Arras J and Hunt R, eds.: Ethical issues in modern medicine, ed. 2, Palo Alto, Calif, 1983, Mayfield.
36. Wellman C: Morals and ethics, Glenview, Illinois, 1975, Scott, Foresman & Co.
37. Wellman C: Morals and ethics, ed. 2, Englewood Cliffs, New Jersey, 1988, Prentice-Hall, Inc.
38. Winslow GR: From loyalty to advocacy: a metaphor for nursing, Hastings Center Report, June 1984.

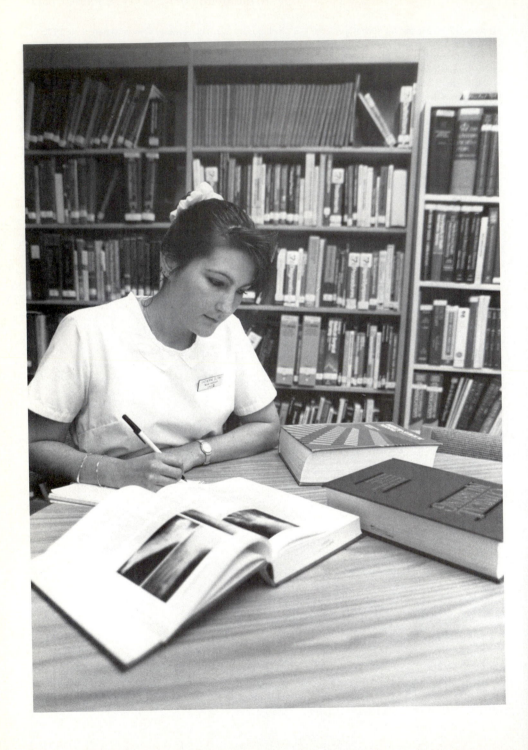

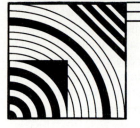

C H A P T E R 8

NURSING EDUCATION

Diane M. Billings

OBJECTIVES

After completing this chapter the reader should be able to:

- Discuss changes in society that affect nursing education today

- Describe how government, especially at state level, sets standards and regulates nursing

- Describe how the federal government has affects on nursing education

- Discuss evolution of nursing education, beginning with the Goldmark Report to the present, in particular, development of education for nurses in academic settings

- Describe the difference between LPN, ADN, diploma, and baccalaureate nursing education programs

- Discuss the Master's Degree program of study in nursing and what the graduate from such a program may expect to do

- Discuss various approaches to doctoral education of nurses and what those graduates are prepared to do in practice

- Discuss educational mobility and how these strategies work

- Describe what is meant by the statement: the common base of nursing education and practice must be *scholarly nursing practice*

Health care needs of the 1990s and beyond will require increasing numbers of nurses prepared as generalists and specialists for a variety of roles. Nurse educators are responding to this challenge by developing nursing programs and curricula that meet the needs of the learner and prepare nurses for the changing and varied demands of nursing practice. The purposes of this chapter are to recognize the dynamic context in which nursing education programs develop, differentiate types of nursing programs, explain mechanisms for educational mobility, and identify alternative curriculum patterns created to meet the needs of a changing population of nursing students. The chapter concludes by raising issues for further dialogue about the future of nursing education.

EDUCATIONAL PREPARATION FOR NURSING PRACTICE
Context of Nursing Education

Nursing programs are an outcome of a dynamic relationship with social, educational, legislative, economic, and professional forces in contemporary society. Nursing and health care in the 1990s will emerge in forms and patterns unlike those of the 1980s. Nurse educators must therefore be responsive to contextual change and develop and revise nursing programs to prepare graduates as citizens and professionals.

Social Context. The social context in which nursing programs are embedded is changing. In the United States, for example, there is an increase in the number of older adults and a decrease in the birth rate. There are increasing numbers of Hispanics and Asians, but the numbers of black Americans and Caucasians are decreasing. Furthermore, the epidemiology of health problems is changing as an aging society copes with increasing chronic diseases, new communicable diseases such as AIDS, and other health problems caused by a polluted and shrinking environment.

Educational Context. A discussion of the context of nursing education must address the current issues facing post-secondary education and nursing education. Post-secondary education, and particularly higher education, is criticized for graduating students unprepared for the future and maintaining curricula that perpetuate a lack of purpose and learning.[9] In response to public criticism and a demand by state commissions for higher education for assessment of outcomes and accountability, colleges and universities are revising curricula to prepare liberally educated individuals with an area of study in depth, as well as informed citizens and graduates able to contribute to an information-based society.

Nursing education programs must accommodate to the curriculum revolution of the institution of higher education and the mandate for change in nursing curricula.[5,18,37,59] Regardless of debates about professional versus technical education and preparation for entry into practice, schools of nursing are raising questions about what is learning, what should be taught, how should it be taught, and how can performance and outcomes be assessed. As nurse educators question historical models of curriculum development and urge reform of both undergraduate and graduate education, new patterns in nursing curricula are emerging to integrate theory and practice, to redefine learning, and to use teaching-learning strategies that facilitate learning as nurses move from novices and beginning practitioners to expert clinicians.

Legislative Context. Nursing education is influenced by legislation at local, state, national, and international levels. Such legislation defines nursing practice and nursing education and sets standards for determining who will be the practitioners. At the state level, for example, state boards of higher education have responsibility for planning and recommending numbers and types of programs, whereas state boards of nurses registration and education establish standards for licensure and quality of nursing education programs, qualifications of faculty, and curriculum requirements.

State legislation also enables nurse practice acts. Legislation in North Dakota, for example, has separate licensure for two categories of nurses, the technical and the professional nurse.[39] This same legislation specifies two types of nursing education programs, associate and baccalaureate, to prepare graduates for entry into practice.

Federal legislation, however, influences nursing education at the national level. Examples include funding nursing research, providing student financial assistance, and funding innovative nursing education programs.

Economic Context. Closely related to legislative forces, economic forces affect nursing education by influencing supply and demand for nurses, salaries, and health care delivery systems. Staffing patterns, utilization of nurses in differentiated practice, and employment opportunities can contribute directly to recruitment into educational programs, as well as numbers and geographic location of these programs.

Professional Context. Also important are the professional forces and organizations that are shaping the direction of nursing education programs and curricula. These forces are related to the marketplace, practice environment, and strategies for effective use of nurses with varied educational preparation. The work of two nursing organizations can be traced to demonstrate the relationship of nursing's professional organizations and the development of nursing education programs.

In 1965 the American Nurses' Association (ANA) proposed two entry levels for the practice of nursing; the technical nurse, with an associate degree as educational preparation, and the professional nurse, with the baccalaureate degree as educational preparation. In 1984 the ANA reaffirmed its position on the baccalaureate degree in nursing as entry for practice, and in 1985 voted to support two categories of nurses, the technical and the professional with education in associate and baccalaureate programs.[3] At the same time, the National Commission on Nursing Implementation Project (NCNIP), composed of a governing board representing a variety of nursing and health care organizations, including the American Association of Colleges of Nursing, American Organization of Nurse Executives, the National League for Nursing (NLN), and the ANA, was established for the purpose of implementing recommendations of earlier studies[58] by identifying trends and establishing consensus for action to effect the future of nursing.[45] In 1987 NCNIP identified characteristics of professional and technical nurses of the future and established a timeline for changes in the educational system, developed a model for describing nursing care systems that are cost effective and assure quality, explored how nursing research can be used to influence public policy, and advocated an information system to assure timely access to data for education, practice, and research.[17,44]

Nursing specialty organizations affirm the ANA position and the direction established by NCNIP. For example, in 1989 the American Association of Critical Care Nurses identified competence statements for the technical and professional nurse in differentiated practice.[32] It is in these contexts, then, that nursing programs are designed to prepare graduates with the knowledge, skills, and values to practice in a complex and changing health care arena.

Nursing Programs

Nursing educators develop nursing curricula to ensure adequate numbers and categories of nurses to meet current and future societal needs. In the United States, nursing programs meet this need by preparing nurses as technical nurses (practical nurse and associate degree programs), and professional nurses (baccalaureate degree, masters degree, and doctoral degree programs). The programs differ in type of client, roles, and practice settings. They also differ in educational base, curriculum, educational setting, accrediting agency, and professional organizations that advocate their interests. Each program is described below.

Practical nurse programs

Practical nurse programs prepare students to become licensed practical nurses (LPN) or licensed vocational nurses (LVN). The graduates give patient care under the direction of a registered nurse or other licensed health professional.

The first practical nurse program was offered in 1892 as a 3-month training program by the YWCA in Brooklyn, New York; others followed in the 1900s. Later, world wars created a demand for nurses that could be quickly trained and the number of practical nurse programs increased. In 1941, the schools formed an Association of Practical Nurse Education and began accrediting schools of practical nursing in 1945.

Educational Setting. The practical nurse program is typically offered by a trade or technical school. The program may also be sponsored by high schools, hospitals, or community colleges.

Entry Requirements. Requirements are a high school diploma or demonstrated high school equivalency. Other requirements may be stipulated by the educational institution.

Educational Base. The curriculum builds on introductory content in the biological and social sciences. These courses may carry college credit, or may be integrated into the curriculum.

Curriculum. The course of study is 12 to 18 months and includes courses with a focus on acute and chronic illness, rehabilitation, maintenance of health, and prevention of disease. Heavy emphasis is on clinical practice.

Graduates from LPN/LVN programs are prepared to give care, under the direction of a registered nurse or licensed physician, to patients whose care plan is well established, and in structured settings such as long-term care or acute care hospitals, homes, outpatient settings, or physician's offices.

Licensing Examination. After graduation from the LPN/LVN program the graduate is eligible to write the National Council for Licensure Examination-Practical Nursing (NCLEX-PN) examination. The LPN/LVN is licensed for employment as a practical/vocational nurse.

Accrediting Agencies and Professional Organizations. The Council on Practical Nursing of the NLN is responsible for accrediting LPN programs. Other accrediting agencies may be involved in the accreditation process for the technical school in which the practical nurse program is located. Several professional organizations such as the National Association for Practical Nurse Education and National Federation of Licensed Practical Nurses are active in advocating quality education and informing the public about the role of practical nursing in nursing service.

Diploma programs

Diploma programs prepare students to become registered nurses. The programs are typically associated with a hospital, but more recently are affiliated with a college or university. The programs prepare graduates for technical nursing practice.

Diploma schools of nursing were the primary educational agency for educating nurses during the 1800s and early and mid-1900s. The schools were patterned after the Florence Nightingale training school model. The first school in the United States was the New England Hospital for Women and Children. Linda Richards was its first graduate in 1873.

As a result of studies, commissions, and position papers,[3,45] the setting for nursing education programs shifted to colleges and universities. The number of diploma schools and entrants in diploma schools has steadily declined since 1960. As of 1988 there were 177 diploma schools accredited by the NLN, with 21 scheduled to close.[19]

Educational Setting. The hospital is the educational setting for the diploma program. Cooperative arrangements may be established with a community college or university to provide general education courses in the biological and social sciences. The focus of the diploma program shifted from using students for service to the hospital to establishing a learning environment for the student and preparation for nursing practice in a variety of health care agencies.

Entry Requirements. A high school diploma is required for entry into a diploma school. Some schools use scholastic aptitude tests such as the SAT and nursing aptitude tests as admission guidelines.

Educational Base. The diploma program is based on a foundation of general education courses in the biological and social sciences. Generally, these courses are offered by a college or university with credit transfer arrangements with baccalaureate or masters degree programs.

Curriculum. The curriculum is designed to prepare nurses for direct patient care and includes courses in nursing management and home health care. The curriculum can be completed in 2 to 3 years. Heavy emphasis is on clinical practice.

Licensure. Graduates from diploma programs take the NCLEX-RN. Graduates are licensed as registered nurses.

Accrediting Agencies and Professional Organizations. Diploma programs are accredited by the Council of Diploma Programs of the NLN. Professional organizations representing the interests of diploma programs are the NLN and ANA.

Associate Degree Programs

Associate degree programs prepare students to become registered nurses. The curriculum is offered in a community college or senior university and prepares the graduate for technical nursing practice.

The associate degree program originated in the early 1950s. The development of the program was influenced by (1) the need for additional nurses in the work force and (2) experience from the cadet nurse training program that indicated that registered nurses could be educated in less than the 3 years of the typical diploma program. The first associate degree nurse (ADN) program was conducted in the Cooperative Research Project in Junior and Community College Education at Teacher's College, Columbia University, under the direction of Mildred Montag.[43] The purpose of the program was to prepare technical nurses who could assist professional nurses. The curriculum was designed to increase the science base and decrease the practice base, which was to be provided in the employment setting. Although originally intended to serve as a terminal degree, most ADN programs now serve as a base for RN Mobility programs.[52]

Educational Setting. Associate degree programs are offered primarily by community and junior colleges. They may also be offered in vocational colleges, senior universities, or as free-standing degree-granting institutions.

Entry Requirements. Applicants to associate degree programs must meet the entry requirements of the college or university in which the program is located. These requirements typically include graduation from high school or the equivalent college preparatory curriculum and evidence of scholastic aptitude. Entry requirements for LPN to ADN programs may include licensure as an LPN and clinical practice experience.

Educational Base. Associate degree education is based in general education courses. The courses meet degree requirements of the college or university and include biological and social sciences. Approximately one half of the curriculum (30 credits) is composed of general education courses.

Curriculum. There are two curriculum patterns preparing graduates for the ADN degree. The first is a generic or basic curriculum. The second pattern is a LPN-to-ADN program that provides mobility for graduates of LPN programs and accepts credit and experience for previous learning.

The ADN curriculum builds on the base of general education courses and includes nursing courses in adult and child health, maternity nursing, psychiatric and mental health nursing, legal aspects of nursing practice, ethical issues, and professional roles. The curriculum prepares graduates to practice nursing, under the direction of a professional nurse, in roles of care provider, communicator, client teacher, manager of care, and member of the profession. The curriculum can be completed in 2 academic years (60 credits).

The nursing practice of a graduate from an associate degree program is directed toward the following:

1. Clients who need information or support to maintain health
2. Clients who are in need of medical diagnostic evaluation and/or are experiencing acute or chronic illness
3. Clients' responses to common, well-defined health problems
4. Formulation of nursing diagnoses
5. Nursing interventions selected from established nursing protocols where probable outcomes are predictable
6. Individual clients, with consideration of the person's relationship with family, group, and community
7. Safe performance of nursing skills that require cognitive, psychomotor, and affective capabilities
8. Structured care setting but primarily occurs within acute- and extended-care facilities
9. Direct or indirect guidance by a more experienced registered nurse
10. Direction of peers or other workers in nursing in selected aspects of care within the scope of practice of associate degree nursing
11. Understanding of the roles and responsibilities of self and other workers within the employment setting[48]

Degree Granted. The degree is granted by the institution of higher education in which the associate degree program is located. The degree may be an Associate of Science in Nursing (ASN), Associate Degree (AD), or an Associate of Applied Science (AAS).

License. The graduate from an associate degree program is prepared to write the NCLEX-RN exam. In most states, the AD graduate is licensed as a registered nurse.[24] In North Dakota, however, the ADN graduate is licensed as a Licensed Practical Nurse under state legislation for differentiated education and licensure.[39]

Accrediting Agencies and Professional Organizations. Associate degree programs are accredited by the Associate Degree Council of the NLN. The institution of higher education may also be accredited by an appropriate technical or college accrediting agency.

Professional organizations promoting the interest of associate degree nursing are NLN, ANA, and NCNIP. The National Organization for the Advancement of Associate Degree Nursing was formed in 1986 to support associate degree education and nursing practice. The organization endorses registered nurse licensure for the associate degree graduate.

Baccalaureate Nursing Programs

Baccalaureate nursing programs, set in colleges and universities, are designed to prepare graduates as generalists in professional nursing practice. Baccalaureate graduates are care givers, client advocates, change agents, consultants, case finders, teachers, and leaders. Bachelor's of Science in Nursing (BSN) graduates care for individuals, groups, families, and communities and are prepared to give nursing care in structured and unstructured settings. The BSN degree may be earned in a 4-year college or university with a major in nursing, or after completing an associate degree or diploma and completing the post diploma/ADN baccalaureate nursing curriculum.

Baccalaureate programs began in the early 1900s; the University of Minnesota established the first nursing major in an undergraduate program in 1919. In the early years of baccalaureate education, programs were 5 years in length: 2 years for the college courses and 3 years for the nursing curriculum. Momentum for the program increased when an ANA paper in 1965 specified a baccalaureate degree in nursing as the minimum education for entry into the practice of professional nursing.

Educational Setting. Baccalaureate nursing programs are offered in senior (4-year) colleges and universities. Free-standing independent degree granting programs, usually supported by a health care agency in cooperation with a senior university, are alternative settings for the baccalaureate nursing program. These programs are affiliated with a college or university, but the degree is granted from the program itself.

Entry Requirements. Students entering baccalaureate nursing programs meet requirements of the college or university and the school of nursing that include high school graduation with college preparatory courses in English, chemistry, biological sciences, and mathematics. The college or university may also stipulate admissions tests such as SAT and specify a high school grade point average. Some schools of nursing admit or certify students only to the upper division major. In these instances students must complete and demonstrate success in lower division prerequisites.

Educational Base. The baccalaureate curriculum is founded on a strong base of liberal arts and sciences. These courses are selected to develop a liberally educated person and include inquiry, literacy, understanding numerical data, historical consciousness, science, values, art, international and cultural experience, and study in depth.[2,16,41] The liberal arts and sciences foundation composes approximately 60 credits of the 120 credit curriculum.

Curriculum. The two types of curricula preparing students for a BSN are the generic curriculum and the post associate or post diploma (two plus two, registered nurse baccalaureate, or second step) curriculum.

The generic curriculum builds on prerequisites in arts, sciences, and humanities.[54] Nursing courses offered in the last 2 years of the program (with a few courses in the sophomore year) include the following:

1. Theory
2. Research
3. Care of adults, children, and the child-bearing family
4. Psychiatric and mental health nursing
5. Interpersonal skills and group dynamics
6. Community health
7. Nursing management
8. Professional concepts with an emphasis on critical thinking, decision-making, and problem solving

The post associate/diploma programs build on the associate degree (or diploma) curriculum of the registered nurse. General education courses are supplemented by selected liberal arts courses and include senior level courses in nursing leadership and management, community health, group dynamics, interpersonal skills, professional concepts, nursing theory, nursing research, and health assessment.

The graduate from a baccalaureate program in nursing is prepared to perform the following[46]:

1. Provide professional nursing care, including health promotion and maintenance, illness care, restoration, rehabilitation, health counseling, and education based on knowledge derived from theory and research
2. Synthesize theoretical and empirical knowledge from nursing, scientific, and humanistic disciplines with nursing practice
3. Use the nursing process to provide nursing care for individuals, families, groups, and communities
4. Accept responsibility and accountability for the evaluation of the effectiveness of their own nursing practice
5. Enhance the quality of nursing and health practices within practice settings through the use of leadership skills and a knowledge of the political system
6. Evaluate research for the applicability of its findings to nursing practice
7. Participate with other health care providers and members of the public in promoting general health and well-being
8. Incorporate professional values and ethical, moral, and legal aspects of nursing into nursing practice
9. Participate in the implementation of nursing roles designed to meet emerging health needs of the general public in a changing society

Degree Granted. The degree granted is a BN (Bachelor of Nursing), BSN (Bachelor of Science in Nursing), or BA (Bachelor of Arts in Nursing).

License. The graduate from a baccalaureate program in nursing is eligible to write the NCLEX-RN examination. Registered nurse graduates from BSN programs have registered nurse licenses. At the fall 1988 meeting of the Baccalaureate and Higher Degree Council of the NLN, the council voted to support differentiated licensure.[14] This would create two licensing examinations, one for a baccalaureate degree with a major in nursing, and one for nurses educated with an associate degree in nursing.

Accreditation Agencies and Professional Organizations. Baccalaureate nursing programs are accredited by the Council of Baccalaureate and Higher Degree Programs of the NLN. Colleges and universities in which the program is based are accredited by higher education accrediting bodies. Professional organizations influential in baccalaureate nursing are ANA, NLN Council of Baccalaureate and Higher Degree Programs, NCNIP, and the American Association of Colleges of Nursing (AACN).

Master's Degree Programs

Master's degree programs in nursing prepare nurses for speciality roles in nursing practice. The programs also prepare nurses with a functional focus of educator, manager/administrator, clinical specialist, or nurse practitioner.

Master's degree programs in nursing originally developed to meet the need for teachers and advanced practitioners.[55] The first masters of science in nursing (MSN) programs were offered in the late 1800s in graduate programs at Yale, Harvard, and Johns Hopkins.

In the mid-1960s, a need for primary care practitioners was identified and certificate programs developed to prepare nurses as nurse practitioner, pediatric nurse practitioner (PNP), and family nurse practitioner (FNP).[12] The curriculum was 1 academic year and included 4 months of classroom content in primary care and extensive clinical practice.[30] Since 1975 these programs have moved into academic settings and are incorporated in MSN programs. Graduates of these programs now receive a certificate as a nurse practitioner and the MSN degree.

Educational Setting. Masters degree programs are offered in colleges and universities with graduate programs. The Masters program is usually located in schools with baccalaureate in nursing programs.

Entry Requirements. Requirements for admission to most MSN studies include graduation from a BSN program. Other admission criteria may include RN licensure and evidence of scholastic ability as measured on qualifying examinations such as the Graduate Record Examination and grade point averages from undergraduate study. For schools with a generic MSN program, admission requirements may include BS or BA degrees in a field other than nursing. RN-to-MSN programs require graduation from an associate or diploma program and licensure as a registered nurse, and in some instances evidence of professional accomplishments and demonstration of knowledge equivalent to a BSN degree.

Educational Base. The Baccalaureate degree in nursing is the educational base for the MSN degree. The base includes liberal arts and sciences courses of a baccalaureate degree and, depending on the curriculum, a baccalaureate in nursing degree or equivalent competencies.

Curriculum. There are three major curriculum structures for the MSN. The common structure is that of the post baccalaureate curriculum. Courses build on the liberal arts and sciences and nursing curriculum of baccalaureate programs. The curriculum consists of core courses in nursing issues, research, statistics, and nursing theory; courses in the speciality major (e.g., medical surgical nursing, critical care, psychiatry, maternal-child health); and courses in the functional role (e.g., education, administration, practitioner). The typical curriculum includes 30 to 45 credit hours.

The generic MSN is the first degree for entry into the practice of professional nursing. In this model, the curriculum builds on the arts and sciences background of a baccalaureate degree and includes nursing courses of the baccalaureate curriculum and that of the post baccalaureate masters degree. Students may or may not earn the BSN en route to the MSN.[28]

A third route to obtaining an MSN is becoming increasingly popular as nurses seek educational mobility. In this curriculum, registered nurse students with an associate degree or diploma enter the RN-to-MSN curriculum. Credit is awarded for previous knowledge in clinical nursing courses. Nursing research, professional concepts, issues, and statistics are taught at the MSN level with "bridging" content for the courses in the baccalaureate curriculum. The remainder of the curriculum is similar to the MSN curriculum.

The graduate from a MSN program is prepared to perform the following:

1. Incorporate theories and advanced knowledge into nursing practice
2. Demonstrate competence in selected role(s)
3. Identify researchable nursing problems and participate in research studies in advanced nursing practice
4. Use leadership, management, and teaching knowledge and competencies to influence nursing practice
5. Assume responsibility for contributing to improvement in the delivery of health care and influencing health policy
6. Assume responsibility for contributing to the advancement of the nursing profession[47]

Degree Granted. Graduates from masters programs receive the MSN or MA (Master of Arts). Several schools offer a MNSc, Master of Public Health, or Master of Education.[28]

License and Certification. Graduates from a generic MSN are prepared to write the NCLEX-RN; most graduates of MSN programs are previously licensed as a registered nurse. Some schools of nursing prepare graduates for a speciality practice, and graduates may write certification examinations or nurse practitioner examinations in the speciality as an outcome of the degree.

Accreditation Agencies and Professional Organizations. MSN programs are accredited by the NLN Council of Baccalaureate and Higher Degree Programs. NLN, ANA, and AACN advocate the interests of MSN curricula.

Doctoral Programs

Doctoral programs prepare nurses for roles as academicians, administrators, advanced clinical scientists, researchers, consultants, and independent practitioners. Doctoral degrees in nursing may be professional degrees (EdD, DNS, ND) or research degrees (PhD).

The first doctoral program in nursing was offered at Columbia University in 1924; the graduates received an EdD. Other doctoral programs developed slowly and the next school to offer a doctorate, a PhD, was New York University in 1934. During the 1960s doctoral programs in nursing science (DNS) were established in response to the need for nursing scientists and academicians. The professional degree (DSN) was developed at this time as a result of a lack of (1) prepared faculty, (2) a well-defined knowledge base, and (3) a research record required to establish research degrees.[40] In the 1970s there were four doctoral programs with a nursing major, expanding to 27 in the mid-1980s.[21] As of 1989 there were 44 schools of nursing with doctoral programs.[20]

Educational Setting. Doctoral programs in nursing are offered in colleges and universities with graduate programs in nursing. The school of nursing may be aligned with the university and follow an academic model for doctoral education, or be located in a health sciences setting with a professional model focus.[29]

Entry Requirements. Admission requirements to doctoral programs are set by the nursing program and the college or university. They may include completion of a MS program, evidence of scholastic achievement, and admission examinations such as the graduate record examination (GRE). Evidence of professional accomplishment and writing skills may also be required. Entry requirement for the nursing doctorate is a BS.

Educational Base. Doctoral programs in nursing build on the educational base of advanced arts, sciences, and nursing of the MSN program. Depending on the educational setting, the educational base for the program may follow an academic model or a professional model.[4,29]

Curriculum. There are four types of nursing doctoral programs, the Doctor of Nursing Science (DNSc, DSN); the Doctor of Philosophy (PhD), which is the most common;[4] the Doctor of Education (EdD); and the Nursing Doctorate (ND).[23,27,40,57] The curriculum design of the doctoral degree depends on the purpose of the program, program objectives, and the degree granted. A typical plan includes 90 credits with an inquiry component (statistics, research methods) of 15 to 18 credits, a concentration in the nursing major (theory development, substantive focus courses) of 30 to 35 credit hours, and an external cognate minor, related to the area of concentration in the major, of 12 to 15 credits. Other credits for the degree are obtained from elective and dissertation credits.

The doctorate may be combined with other fields of study such as the PhD-LLB degree combining nursing and law, or the PhD-MBA combining nursing and business. More than 90 credits may be required to obtain dual degrees.

The DNS is a professional degree that prepares graduates for practice. Core courses provide a base for advanced nursing knowledge and practice, clinical specialization, and interdisciplinary leadership. The research focus is on communication, use, and interpretation of findings of research rather than generation of new knowledge.

The PhD is a degree that prepares graduates to conduct basic research and develop and test nursing theory. The emphasis of the program is the discovery of new knowledge and ability to conduct research. Courses focus on clinical scholarship and the design and testing of theory.

The EdD, the least common type of nursing doctorate, is an applied degree. Graduates are prepared for scholarship and research, but the emphasis is on application of knowledge rather than generation or dissemination.

The generic doctorate, the ND, is a professional degree that is based on a baccalaureate education.[38] The curriculum prepares the graduate for generalist practice and interdisciplinary collaboration. The research focus is on interpretation or reinterpretation of nursing knowledge. Some educators advocate the ND as the degree for entry into practice.

Graduates from doctoral programs are prepared to function in advanced nursing roles. Educational outcomes depend on the type of program, although outcome differences are often negligible.[4,57]

Degree Granted. The degree granted depends on the type of educational program the student attends. The degree may be a PhD, DNS or DNSc, EdD, or ND.

Licensure. Graduates from the ND are eligible to write the NCLEX-RN. Graduates from nursing doctoral programs are already licensed.

Accreditation Agencies and Professional Organizations. As of 1989 there is no accreditation for doctoral programs in nursing. The graduate program of the university, however, is accredited by its higher education accrediting body. Nursing doctoral programs are monitored by peer review and judged by the quality of the faculty and graduates. The AACN has developed a position paper on The Indicators of Quality in doctoral programs in nursing to be used as assessment guidelines.[1]

Several professional organizations assume responsibility for advocating doctoral education. The doctoral forum was established in 1977 by deans and directors concerned with doctoral education. The group continues as a peer-operated committee and monitors and debates issues related to doctoral education. The AACN and the NLN also have committees supporting the interests of doctoral education.

EDUCATIONAL MOBILITY

As previously discussed, there are five types of educational nursing programs. Although each is designed to attain specific educational and professional outcomes, graduates from one program can, and are often encouraged, to seek degrees and career opportunities requiring subsequent education.[31] The movement to another degree program is referred to as *educational mobility.*

Educational mobility facilitates multiple points of entering the profession of nursing, as well as career advancement through additional education without loss of credits from previous education. For example, an individual may enter the nursing education system as an LPN in an associate degree program, exit with an ADN degree, and at a later date reenter the system in an RN to MSN program and obtain an MSN or doctorate in nursing (Figure 8-1).

Nursing programs have been developed for mobility from LPN to ADN, LPN to BSN, ADN to BSN, RN to BSN, RN to MSN, and BSN to doctorate. Nursing programs are also being developed to facilitate education for graduates with bachelor degrees in other disciplines into a MSN program (BS or BA to MSN).[33] Each mobility program is developed according to the philosophy of the school of nursing, employs a variety of curriculum patterns, and uses a variety of mechanisms to award credit for previous education. The concept of educational mobility is supported to recruit nurses into the profession and encourage preparation for advanced practice roles.

One major advantage of educational mobility is that there are a number of options for nursing education. The options fit student educational interests and abilities, career plans, and financial and work commitments. Another advantage of a mobile nursing education system is that students can graduate with one degree and be employed while earning another degree. Employers and many health care organizations support the concept of educational mobility because employees can be quickly prepared for the work force; additional education can be obtained while the employee is working.

Mechanisms for Educational Mobility in Nursing

Educational mobility can be promoted by articulation and advanced placement. Nursing programs may incorporate one or more of these strategies to facilitate mobility.

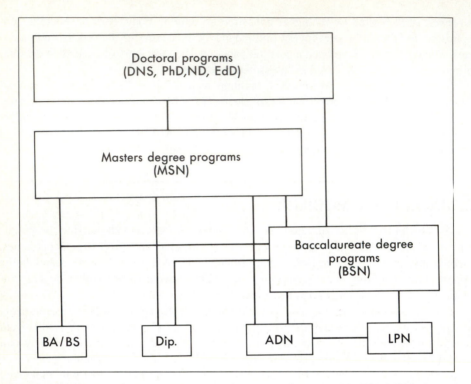

Fig. 8-1 Mobility in Nursing Education. *(Courtesy, Pontious M, RN, MSN, Associate Professor of Nursing, Indiana University School of Nursing.)*

Articulation. Articulation refers to a process in which nursing programs cooperate to plan programs to minimize duplication of learning experiences.[10] The curriculum is designed so that one program is a base for another. For example, a BSN program may be designed to build on the background of an associate degree or diploma curriculum.[52] The credits and course work for one program are included in the entry and degree requirements for the next program. In articulated programs there is little or no duplication of previous learning or loss of program credits.

Advanced Placement. Advanced placement is a procedure for recognizing previous learning.[49] Advanced placement can be accomplished by transferring credit, establishing course equivalency, and awarding credit for previous learning.

Credit Transfer. Credit transfer involves transferring credits from one nursing program into another. The credits in general, liberal, and nursing education are used as degree requirements in subsequent programs. Programs not based in a college or university, such as LPN programs or diploma programs, may have affiliation agreements with a college or university and incorporate these courses in the curriculum, with the intent that the credits would be accepted by a junior or senior university if the graduate wishes to continue education.

Credit transfer agreements may be established to assure mobility between specific programs. Although credit transfer preserves credits earned, it does not eliminate the need to complete other education and nursing credit required in the curriculum. Credit transfer for nursing credits is less common than for general or liberal education credits.

Educational mobility can also be facilitated by establishing *course equivalency*. Courses from one nursing program or college or university can be reviewed by the nursing program accepting the credits to determine that a course in one program is equivalent to a course in another program. Course equivalency can be established on a course-by-course basis or a blanket equivalency can be awarded for courses reviewed by faculty.

Credit for Previous Learning. When course comparability cannot be established by credit transfer, some nursing programs have developed mechanisms for validating previous learning and awarding comparable credit for advanced placement. Two ways of establishing credit for previous learning is by testing or portfolio.

Testing assesses knowledge, skills, and attitudes, and may be accomplished by administering standardized examinations developed for the purpose of promoting educational mobility such as those offered by the NLN* or ACT.[7] Schools of nursing may also use teacher-made examinations written by nursing faculty. These examinations may be developed for didactic courses, as well as to evaluate clinical proficiency. Passing the examination awards credit for the course.

The portfolio is another mechanism for awarding credit for previous learning. A portfolio is a compilation of evidence of achievement that provides a vehicle for assessment of competencies and educational outcomes.[34] The portfolio is presented to a faculty review board to review the materials to assure course comparability. Evidence may include the following:

1. Work experience
2. Formal courses
3. Examination scores
4. Continuing education experience
5. Letters of reference detailing competency

The portfolio is submitted as evidence of meeting course or program objectives, and is reviewed by faculty for verification of meeting of requirements. Portfolio acceptance confers credit for nursing or general education coursework.

Bridging Courses. When nursing curriculums are not designed for direct articulation, nursing programs have developed specific courses to provide content missing from previous learning to "bridge" the student into the program. These bridge, or transition, courses are developed specifically for each curriculum and for students in the mobility program. Bridge courses offer students opportunities to assess learning needs, obtain peer support, and prepare for nursing role transitions. On completion of the bridging

---

*NLN Mobility Profile I for the LPN to ADN, and the NLN Mobility Profile II for theRN to BSN.

courses, students may receive credit for nursing courses and then move into the additional content of curriculum.

Outcomes of Educational Mobility Programs

The evaluation of mobility programs indicate that curriculum designs are cost effective.[61] Mobility programs produce graduates who meet program outcomes, enlarge the pool for entrants into baccalaureate and higher degree programs,[52] and ultimately improve the quality of nursing care for the consumer.

ALTERNATIVE CURRICULUM PLANS IN NURSING EDUCATION

As the needs of employers change, and nursing students become older, have previous educational experience and degrees, seek educational mobility, and often live at a distance from the nursing program offering the degree, schools of nursing develop alternative curriculum plans to meet the needs. The alternative patterns of curriculum and instruction include flexible curriculum designs, creative delivery systems, and cooperative arrangements with nursing service and health care corporations.[26]

Curriculum Designs

Flexible curriculum designs are developed to facilitate diversity of educational opportunity and overcome barriers of distance and time.[22,26,42] These curricula are often competency based, focused on outcomes, and emphasize student involvement and responsibility for learning. These plans may include external degree programs, competency based programs, accelerated programs, and expanded programs.

External Degree Programs. An external degree is a degree awarded for study that does not take place within the typical structure of a classroom, but rather, takes place outside of the classroom and is self-paced. The outcome of learning is assessed through standardized criteria and referenced performance examinations, which may have cognitive, affective, and/or psychomotor components. One example of an external degree program is that of the New York Board of Regents, which offers both associate and baccalaureate degree programs in Nursing.[35] External degree programs have also been developed for doctoral programs.[51]

Proponents of external degree programs cite emphasis of professional practice, self-direction, use of adult education principles, accessibility, and match with learning style as advantages of this curriculum design. On the other hand, external degree programs are criticized for the decreased contact with faculty and student peers, lack of academic rigor, and unsupervised clinical practice.

Competency Based Curricula. Competency based education involves the definition of specific knowledge, skills, and attitudes (competencies) to be demonstrated. Instructional strategies are selected to facilitate learner attainment of competencies. Evaluation strategies are developed to indicate the criteria for successful performance, and are used to measure outcomes in multiple modes and contexts. Competency based curricula foster development of individual competence and can be self-paced for learners with varied needs.

Accelerated Programs. Accelerated programs offer the nursing major in a compacted time frame. These programs are developed to facilitate educational mobility and to expedite entry into the work force. Courses are offered in a sequence that is convenient for the learner and can be completed without delay of disrupted course sequence. Course work that might typically be completed in 2 calendar years (4 semesters) can be completed in 12 to 18 months.

Expanded Programs. Nursing programs have been developed to accommodate the needs of learners who wish to study at a slower pace. In expanded programs the learner can enroll in part-time studies over a longer period of time. The curriculum is developed to encourage options for students who are unable to enroll in the typical full-time course sequence.

Instructional Delivery Systems. Another alternative to traditional nursing programs is modification of the way instruction is made available to the student. Although the curriculum remains the same as that offered at the school of nursing, creative ways are sought to bring instruction to the student. These innovative instructional delivery systems include videoteleconference, correspondence courses, computer conferencing, and off-campus programs.

Videoteleconference. Videoteleconferencing uses television to broadcast courses to students at distant sites.[6,11] The course is broadcast from a studio classroom and received at one or more reception sites. The same class that is offered on campus is thus available to students at reception sites city, state, or worldwide.

Correspondence. Correspondence courses are described as *noncontiguous* communication between students and faculty, usually in the print medium, and using the postal service.[8] The courses are preproduced prepackaged courses in which there is active participation of the student through lessons, assignments, and examinations. The courses are the same as those offered on campus, but permit the student flexibility of time to complete the lessons and can be used when the student is at a distance from the school offering the course.

Computer Conferencing. The computer has opened new channels for delivering instruction to students. The computer can be used as an electronic telecommunications network to provide interactive instruction in the same way as correspondence instruction. The technology can also be coupled with audio and graphics, and used to provide instantaneous access to print material at remote sites.[62]

Off-campus Programs. Another approach to serving distant students is to bring the program to a geographically convenient site, often referred to as an *outreach site*.[36,60] This may involve developing nursing programs in an existing system campus, developing a local school site, or having faculty commute to the site. The curriculum offered on the parent campus is thereby offered at a time and place convenient to students who might otherwise be unable to attend the program.

Self-directed Learning. In the self-directed learning approach to course development, students and faculty advisors design a personal learning plan. The plan includes the content, how the content will be learned, the time period, and the criteria for evaluating outcomes.[50] The content is comparable to courses in the curriculum and carries equivalent course credit. Self-directed learning courses encourage flexibility and independence in meeting course objectives and fosters responsibility for self-learning. Self-directed learning is particularly useful as an instructional delivery system in mobility programs.[13]

Cooperative Programs

Cooperative programs refer to the integration of classroom study with practical experience.[22,56] Cooperative programs offer students opportunity for clinical practice, income or tuition reimbursement, and employment opportunities. These programs extend the nursing program to the practice setting and maximize use of clinical facilities and clinical preceptors. Benefits also accrue to the cooperating agency who gains student service and recruitment potential. Examples of cooperative programs include internships, preceptorships, and work-study.

Internships. Internships are based on a physician education model that bridges the gap between education and practice. Nursing internships involve an educational experience that provides a transition from student to practitioner. Internships are primarily offered by employing agencies and may last from 2 weeks to a year. The internship provides classroom experience, often in the area of nursing management, as well as clinical practice. Internships may be used as a recruitment tool for health care agencies and have benefits of a well-oriented and prepared staff nurse who is likely to remain at the agency for an extended period of time.

Preceptorships. Preceptorships are specially designed relationships matching a novice with an expert to facilitate acquisition of skills, knowledge, values, and orientation to the work environment. Like internships, preceptorships bridge the gap between education and nursing service. Although preceptorships are primarily offered by the employing agency, they may also be incorporated into senior courses in a nursing curriculum. Here, preceptors are matched with a senior student to facilitate the transition from student to staff nurse. When preceptorships were integrated into a senior practicum in a baccalaureate nursing program, students who had a preceptor experience demonstrated significantly different professional socialization and were better able to make the transition from student to staff nurse.[15]

Work-study. Work-study programs combine employment and education. The study and work may be alternated, that is students engage in a period of study, followed by a period of employment. The classroom experiences provide the theory base, and the employment period provides time for application and testing of the theory. Work-study arrangements may also be designed so that employment and study take place concurrently. Various mechanisms are used to grant credit for the employment experience, which may range from full credit to additional credit or partial credit. The advantages of work-study accrue to the employer and the student, and include self-paced education, recruitment and retention opportunities, and financial benefits for both parties.

•   •   •

Nursing education is embedded in a dynamic social, educational, legislative, economic, and professional context. Although there are currently five types of nursing programs to prepare nurses for a variety of nursing practice roles, opportunities for educational mobility, and flexible curriculum plans, nurse educators and consumers must continue to examine the issues affecting curriculum and instruction. The following issues are raised to stimulate discussion about the future of nursing education:

1. Students—who will be the nursing students of the future? Currently, there is a shrinking pool of potential nursing applicants because the number of college-age students is declining. Furthermore, there are increasing employment options for both men and women. What will attract future nurses to the profession? Costs in terms of time and money influence decisions about educational options. Will the cost of a nursing education deter future students? Where will funding to recruit and educate be found?

   It is anticipated that nursing students of the future will be older, married, have children, employed, have previous educational experience, and live at a distance from the institution of higher education. How will issues of access to nursing education be addressed? Will instructional delivery systems that support distance education be developed and funded? How can nursing education take advantage of educational technology that supports outreach for nursing curricula? There is currently strong support for educational mobility. Will nurse educators continue to develop curricula for multiple entry and exit from nursing education programs?

2. Nurse educators seek a curriculum revolution. Fundamental assumptions about learning, teaching, and curriculum are being challenged. Are nursing programs responding to the need for change? Should they? What does nursing education research reveal about effective and efficient teaching-learning strategies? How will student and program outcomes be evaluated? Do current accreditation models serve the needs of students, educators, and clients?

   Nurse educators are the leaders and developers of nursing programs of the future. As students' needs and curriculum patterns change, nurse educators must be prepared to teach in the information age of education and health care. What are the qualifications for nurse educators? How will nurse educators prepare for the challenges of teaching in future educational systems? Who will support funding for nursing education research and development of the high-tech teaching systems of the future?

3. The link between nursing education and nursing service is tenuous at best. If nursing is to influence health care and health policy, nursing education and practice must establish a common base of scholarly nursing practice. New models for both nursing education and practice are likely to evolve. Will curriculum patterns accommodate to these changes? Will graduates of varied programs and curricula be employed in settings that use the differences rather than the similarities of the outcomes of nursing education?

The issues facing nursing education pose challenges for students, educators, and the health care system. Dialogue regarding these issues is valued and contributes to nursing education programs and products responsive to the needs of the stakeholders.

STUDY ACTIVITIES

1. What is meant by technical and professional nursing? What educational programs prepare students for these two levels?
2. What is your ultimate educational goal in nursing and how might you achieve it, based on discussion in this chapter?
3. How do nursing programs fit in a college or university setting? Can you see ways to improve that fit?
4. What do you think it will take to establish nursing on an equal basis with other health professions?

REFERENCES

1. American Association of Colleges of Nursing: Indicators of quality in doctoral programs in nursing, J Prof Nurs 3:72-74, 1987.
2. American Association of Colleges of Nursing: Integrity in the college curriculum: a report to the academic community, Washington, DC, 1985.
3. American Nurses' Association, Board of Directors: Scope of nursing practice. (Report:Da-87). Kansas City, Missouri, 1987.
4. Andreoli KG: Specialization and graduate curricula: finding the fit, Nurs Health Care, 8(2):65-69, 1987.
5. Benner P: From novice to expert: excellence and power in clinical nursing practice, Menlo Park, Calif, 1986. Addison-Wesley.
6. Billings DM, Frazier H, Lausch J, et al.: Videoteleconferencing: solving mobility and recruitment problems, Nurse Ed 14(2), 1989.
7. Billings D, Jeffries P, and Kammer C: RN to BSN: review and challenge for RN mobility, Philadelphia, 1989. JB Lippincott Co.
8. Billings D, Marriner A, and Smith L: Correspondence courses: an instructional alternative, Nurse Ed 11(4):31-37, 1989.
9. Bloom A: The closing of the American mind, New York, 1987, Simon and Schuster.
10. Bowles JG, Lowry L, and Turkeltaub M: Backgrounds and trends related to nursing articulation in the United States. In Rapson MF, ed: Collaboration for articulation: RN to BSN, New York, 1987, National League for Nursing.
11. Boyd N and Baker CM: Using television to teach, Nurs Health Care 8(9):223-227, 1987.
12. Brower HT, Tappen RM, and Weber MT: Missing links in nurse practitioner education, Nurs Health Care 9(1):33-36, 1988.
13. Carroll TL and Artman S: Fitting RN students into a traditional program: secrets for success, Nurs Health Care 9(2):88-91, 1988.
14. CBHDP Acts on wide range of issues at annual meeting, Nurs Health Care 10(1):37-40, 1989.
15. Clayton G, Broome M, and Ellis L: Relationship between a preceptorship experience and socialization of graduate nurses, J Nurs Ed 28(2):72-75, 1989.
16. Coleman E: On redefining the baccalaureate degree, Nurs Health Care 7(4):193-196, 1986.
17. DeBack V: Competencies of associate and professional nurses. In Looking beyond the entry issue: implications for education and service, New York, 1986, The National League for Nursing.
18. Diekleman N: Curriculum revolution: a theoretical and philosophical mandate for change. In Curriculum revolution: mandate for change, New York, New York, 1988, The National League for Nursing.
19. Diploma Programs in Nursing accredited by the NLN, 1988-89, Nurs Health Care 9(7):393-395, 1988.
20. Doctoral Programs in Nursing, 1986-1987, New York, 1988, National League for Nursing.
21. Downs FS: Doctoral education: our claim to the future, Nurs Outlook 36(1):18-20, 1988.
22. Duffey ME: Innovation as a survival strategy. In Patterns in Nursing: stratetic planning for nursing education, New York, 1987, The National League for Nursing.
23. Edens GE and Labadie GC: Opinions about professional doctorate in nursing, Nurs Outlook 35(3):136-140, 1987.
24. Edge S: Appendix B, State positions on tutoring and licensure. In NLN, Looking beyond the entry issue: implications for education and service New York, 1986, National League for Nursing.

25. Essentials of college and university education for professional nursing, Washington, DC, 1985, American Association of Colleges of Nursing.
26. Farley VM: Strategic planning: an organizing framework for nursing education. In Patterns in nursing: strategic planning for nursing education, New York, 1987, National League for Nurses.
27. Fields WA: The PhD: the ultimate nursing doctorate, Nurs Outlook 36(4):188-189, 1988.
28. Forni PR: Nursing's diverse master's programs: the state of the art, Nurs Health Care 8(2):71-75, 1987.
29. Forni PR and Welch MJ: The professional versus the academic model: a dilemma for nursing education, J Prof Nurs 3(5):291-297, 1987.
30. Geolot DH: NP Education: observations from a national perspective, Nurs Outlook 35(3):132-135, 1987.
31. Hart SE and Sharp TG: Mobility programs for students and faculty. In Looking beyond the entry issue: implications for education and service (pp. 53-66), New York, 1986, National League for Nursing.
32. Hickey MR: Competence statements for diffentrated practice in critical care, Newport Beach, Calif, 1989, American Association of Critical Care Nurses.
33. Keating SB: Baccalaureate to MSN: an accelerated pathway for second degree students, Nurs Ed 14(1):35-36, 1989.
34. Lambeth SO, Volden CM, and Oechsle LH: Portfolios: they work for RN's, J Nurs Ed 28(1):42-44, 1989.
35. Lenburg CB: Preparation for professionalism through regent's external degrees, Nurs Health Care 5(6):319-325, 1984.
36. Lethbridge DJ: Independent study: a strategy for providing baccalaureate education for RN's in rural settings J Nurs Ed 27(4):183-185, 1988.
37. Lindeman CA: Curriculum revolution: reconceptualizing clinical nursing education, Nurs Health Care 10(1):23-28, 1989.
38. Lutz EM and Schlotfeldt RM: Pioneering a new approach to professional education, Nurs Outlook 33(3):139-143, 1985.
39. McCarty P: North Dakota educates under new rules, Am Nurs 21(2):8-9, 1989.
40. Meleis AI: Doctoral education in nursing: its present and its future, J Prof Nurs 4(6):436-446, 1988.
41. Miller C: Transforming the patterns of nursing education. In Looking beyond the entry issue: implications for education and service (pp. 67-77), New York, 1986, National League for Nursing.
42. Mitchell CA: Future view: nontraditional education as the norm. In Patterns in Nursing: strategic planning for nursing education (pp. 71-89), New York, 1987, National League for Nursing.
43. Montag ML: Community college education for nursing. New York, 1959, McGraw Hill.
44. National Commission on Nursing Implementation Project: An introduction to timeline for transition into the future nursing education system for two categories of nurse and characteristics of professional and technical nurses of the future and their educational programs, Milwaukee, WI, 1987, NCNIP.
45. National Commission on Nursing Implementation Project: Overview of the project, Milwaukee, WI, 1987, NCNIP.
46. National League for Nursing: Characteristics of baccalaureate education in nursing, New York, 1987, National League for Nursing.
47. National League for Nursing: Characteristics of master's education in nursing, New York, 1987, National League for Nursing.
48. National League for Nursing: Competencies of the associate degree nurse on entry into practice (Publication No. 23-1731), New York, 1978, National League for Nursing.
49. National League for Nursing: Methods for awarding credit for previously acquired nursing knowledge and competency, New York, 1987, National League for Nursing.
50. Peterson JM and Duda S: System theory facilitates student practice in self-directed learning courses, Nurs Ed 11(5):12-15, 1986.
51. Pickard MR: The nontraditional doctorate: an asset or liability in nursing education? Nurs Ed 11(6):33, 1986.
52. Rapson MF: Implications for nursing education and the nursing profession. In Rapson MF, ed: Collaboration for articulation RN to BSN, New York, 1987, National League for Nursing.

53. Rapson MF, ed: Collaboration for articulation: RN to BSN, New York, 1987, National League for Nursing.
54. Redman BK, Cassells TM, and Jackson SS: Generic baccalaureate nursing programs: survey of enrollment, administrative structure/funding, faculty teaching/practice role, and selected curriculum trends, J Prof Nurs, 1:369-380, 1985.
55. Reed SB and Hoffman SE: The enigma of graduate nursing education: advanced generalist? or specialist? Nurs Health Care 7(1):43-49, 1986.
56. Ross S and Marriner A: Cooperative education: experienced based learning, Nurs Outlook 33(6):177-180, 1985.
57. Snyder-Halpern R: Nursing doctorates: is there a difference? Nurs Outlook 34(6):283-285, 291, 1986.
58. Stull MK: Entry skills for BSN's, Nurs Outlook 34(3):138, 153, 1986.
59. Tanner C: Curriculum revolution: the practice mandate, Nurs Health Care, 9(8):427-430, 1989.
60. VanHoff A: An off-campus second step BSN program, Focus on critical care 10(3):50-53, 1983.
61. Williams C and Gallimore K: Educational mobility in nursing, Nurs Ed 12(4):18-21, 1987.
62. Winn B et al.: The design and application of a distance education system using teleconferencing and computer graphics, Ed Technol 26(1):19-23, 1986.

University

ean and Faculty of
hard School of Nursing
Master's Program

certificate to

so

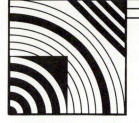

CHAPTER 9

LICENSURE AND RELATED ISSUES IN NURSING

Sharon M. Weisenbeck
Patricia A. Calico

OBJECTIVES

After reading this chapter the reader should be able to:

- Understand why licensure for nurses was begun, and how safe and effective nursing care was tied to the needs of society

- Discuss the time in history when regulation of nursing was begun and how it evolved into the system existing today

- Describe how licensure as a regulatory mechanism portrays/supports the advocacy role of nursing

- Verbalize understanding of the role of the federal government in occupational licensure through interpretation of the Constitution

- Discuss the composition of state boards of nursing and their specific duties and responsibilities

- Describe how a measure of uniformity in licensure requirements among states is maintained through the National Organization of Boards of Nursing

- Discuss future trends in licensure, particularly as they pertain to nursing

From the beginning of organized nursing, the establishment of standards was closely linked to societal needs. The goal that the ideals of the nursing profession would be practiced by every nurse strengthened efforts in mandating requirements. Nursing influenced legislation to provide safe and effective nursing care for the citizens of their respective states. Coupled with this altruistic goal was an acute awareness of society's needs and the contributions nurses could make in meeting those needs. Serving in an advocacy role, nurses spoke for those who had very little opportunity to make their needs known. Thus, nursing's sensitivity to societal needs and perception of ideal nursing practice underpinned the regulation of nursing.

The regulation of nursing, initiated in the 19th century, has evolved during the 20th century from a focus on sickness and custodial care to that of health and wellness in a highly technological environment. As in the past, issues facing the profession continue to concern (1) establishment of standards and requirements for initial licensure, (2) establishment and determination of continuing competence, and (3) expansion of scope of practice relating to educational preparation. In addition to the persistent need for autonomy and control of practice, efforts to achieve appropriate recognition and reimbursement are currently being addressed.

Many trends and issues surround the regulation of initial licensure, continuing competency, and the determination of scope of practice. The key to public protection is again the responsiveness of the nursing profession in establishing and maintaining standards. Although differing viewpoints exist regarding the most effective approaches to regulation of nursing, the licensure of nurses is consistently supported and carefully guarded by the profession. Yet, controversy continues on whether or not licensure, certification, registration, or other processes are ample protection of the public in dealing with specialty or advanced practice of nursing. The issue of regulation versus deregulation in efforts to control health care costs has affected nursing. The balancing of public protection with that of individual interests and the need for appropriate regulation by the state have raised antitrust concerns and procedural rights issues. The complexity of health care delivery systems, multiplicity of new providers resulting from advances in science and technology, increased involvement by the federal government, and "turf protection" by other licensed health care groups are all factors affecting the regulation of nursing.

Historical Overview of Nursing Regulation

The major drive for regulation of nursing by a legal body began in England. As early as 1867, Dr. Henry Wentworth Ecland of England sought credentialing of nurses. Ethel Gordon Bedford Fenwick continued his efforts in 1887. Ms Fenwick founded the British Nurses' Association, which worked to obtain a royal charter for the testing and registering of nurses. This group met substantial opposition, including that of Florence Nightingale, who believed that the focus should be on social and moral standards of the professional nurse rather than abilities of nurses.[2] While the British nurses struggled over the issue of "self-regulation" versus "legal regulation," other nurses in the world were successful in their efforts to enact laws governing nursing. Interestingly the nation in which women had the first right to vote, New Zealand, was the first country to enact an independent licensing law, in 1901. With those in New Zealand, nurses in the United States viewed registration of nurses by a legal entity as a primary way to establish recognition for nurses and to provide assurance for protection of the public health and welfare. There was some disagreement among nurses regarding the need for legal recognition, but the principal opponents included physicians and hospital administrators, who believed that such recognition by the state would lead to loss of control over nurses.

Isabelle Hampton Robb, who is credited with founding the professional nursing organization now known as the *American Nurses' Association* (ANA) believed that recognition by a legal entity was necessary for nursing to obtain "its full dignity as a recognized profession."[7] Another early leader in American nursing, Annie Damer, stated that nurses "should demand recognition as a profession through granting of a proper certificate by a state constituted and maintained board of examiners."[7]

In 1897, the Association Alumnae of Trained Nurses of the United States and Canada (now the ANA) was founded. One of its fundamental goals was to establish uniform standards for nursing education. Members of the Association Alumnae rallied support for registration laws in the United States. In just a 4-year period, 1898 through 1902, the Association Alumnae accomplished the formulation of state nurses' associations. It was the members of these associations that worked to enact registration laws for nurses.

The first state to enact a registration law was North Carolina in 1903. Also in 1903, New Jersey, New York, and Virginia enacted registration laws. By 1910, 20 states had established such laws and within 20 years after the first legislation had been introduced in North Carolina, all 48 states, Hawaii, and the District of Columbia had enacted laws regulating nursing training (see box).

These early laws included the following three basic provisions:
1. Use of the title "registered nurse" denied to untrained nurses
2. Mechanism for examining training school graduates
3. Mechanism to recognize individuals practicing as nurses (grandfathering mechanism)

A significant omission in these laws was a definition of the practice of nursing and a limitation of the practice of nursing to those who qualified. This omission is not surprising because the work of nurses at that time was considered primarily custodial in nature. What is surprising, however, is that nurses, in view of the position of women in society at that time, could influence state legislatures to enact bills that recognized them as nurses. The contributions made by these early nurses were valued and seen as significant to society.

Definitions of Nursing

Early regulation of nursing set forth a registration process that protected the title of those persons who met a minimum set of criteria for registration. These requirements include the following:

1. Completion of an educational program that met standards set by the first board of nursing
2. Successful completion of an examination that involved written and performance components
3. Evaluation of moral and character fitness appropriate for a nurse

In addition, a provision for "grandfathering" waived the training and testing requirements usually allowed for the registration of individuals recognized as nurses. The "waiver period" was often very short, sometimes a matter of months. Also for initial licensure, requirements were mandated early for renewal of licensure and for disciplinary action against those individuals who violated the law. Included in the law were provisions for establishing the board agency and structure, which operated autonomously.

Although the enactment of registration acts in the United States occurred with surprising rapidity, these early pieces of legislation were diverse and inconsistent from state to state. No definition of the practice of nursing or the scope of that practice was included in the first laws. Because only the title was protected, nursing organizations directed efforts at protecting the public and the profession from individuals who were not nursing qualified. To accomplish this objective it was necessary to define the scope of nursing practice. In 1938, New York was the first state to define the scope of nursing practice

---

ENACTMENT OF PRACTICE ACTS BY YEAR

Early 1903	North Carolina
1903	New Jersey, New York, Virginia
1904	Maryland
1905	California, Colorado, Connecticut, Indiana
1907	Georgia, Illinois, Iowa, Minnesota, New Hampshire, West Virginia, Washington, DC
1909	Delaware, Michigan, Missouri, Nebraska, Oklahoma, Pennsylvania, Texas, Washington, Wyoming
1910	Massachusetts, South Carolina
1911	Idaho, Oregon, Tennessee, Vermont, Wisconsin
1912	Louisiana, Rhode Island
1913	Arkansas, Florida, Kansas, Montana
1914	Kentucky, Mississippi
1915	Alabama, Maine, North Dakota, Ohio
1917	Hawaii, South Dakota, Utah
(at this time 45 states and 2 territories had nurse practice acts)	
1921	Arizona
1923	Nevada, New Mexico
(at this time 48 states, Hawaii, and Washington, DC, had nurse practice acts)	
1941	Alaska
1945	Virgin Islands
1952	Guam
(at this time 50 states and Washington, DC, had enacted nurse practice acts)	

and adopt a compulsory law. This type of law, known as a *mandatory licensure law* (versus permissive law), met both support and resistance in the various states. State legislators were slow in enacting such laws; by 1946 only 10 states had legislated a definition of nursing. Resistance was primarily from hospital administrators, who realized the economic effect of mandatory licensure for nurses. Further, World War II delayed implementation of mandatory licensure because of the corresponding acute nursing shortage. The shortage resulted in full recognition of practical nurses, and in the 1950s, laws included regulation of the "licensed practical nurse" or "licensed vocational nurse." Several other factors promoted efforts for mandatory licensure laws besides the recognition of the licensed practical nurse group. The publishing of a standard curriculum guide for schools of nursing in 1937 and the establishment of a national examination in the 1940s were significant influences as well. It was not until the mid-1960s that all of the states included law definitions of nursing that used the model definition adopted by the ANA in 1955.

This model definition prevented involvement of nurses in diagnosis or prescription of therapeutic or corrective measures. Although these efforts attempted to distinguish nursing from medicine, they unfortunately failed to clarify the difference in focus between the professions of medicine and nursing. As practice acts were revised to include these provisions, nurses progressed from a dependent role to varying levels of independence in increasingly technological and complex care. In addition, nursing roles and advanced clinical specialties evolved in health care. Obviously, definitions of nursing needed updating to effectively reflect practice. As the definitions evolved in the 1960s and 1970s, nursing was distinguished from medicine by the identification of components of nursing pratice. As the definitions evolved in the 1960s and 1970s, nursing was distinguished from medicine by the identification of components of nursing practice. Numerous jurisdictions attempted to accommodate the expanding role of nursing in health care by including in the definition the authorization of nursing acts of diagnosis and treatment. Language was also introduced that made the individual accountable for educational preparation and experience in rendering nursing care.

In recent years, the following provisions were introduced in the definitions of nursing practice and in other related state statutes or provisions:

1. Specific sections that dealt with specialized nursing practice
2. Blanket prohibitions against medical diagnosis and treatment, including prescription and dispensing of medications
3. Performance of additional acts by educationally prepared nurses who were recognized by boards of nursing

These provisions are unfortunate for the public and for nursing. They hinder nursing efforts to be recognized for reimbursement for services and to implement the full scope of nursing practice in contemporary settings. Thus needs of various populations are not being met. Additionally, the legal definition of nursing practice is now found not only in the statutes defining nursing, but also in administrative rules and regulations of boards of nursing. These variations in the legal definitions further compound the lack of uniformity in a definition of nursing.

Although nursing has made significant and heroic progress in its regulation, there remain severe problems in its efforts to be identified as a unique and specialized service to the public. Some of these problems will be discussed in the section that deals with the regulation of advanced practice.

The regulation of nurses in the United States has been troubled with conflict and controversy. Although there now appears to be a move toward congruency in the bodies that legally regulate nursing, these agencies were often in conflict with one another in the past; the multiple organizations for nursing had not accepted a universal professional definition of nursing, and there were serious concerns about control when the National Council of State Boards of Nursing (NCSBN) was established as a freestanding organization in 1978. Before then, boards of nursing were organized under a Council of State Boards of Nursing housed within the ANA. Faced with challenges by governmental groups of potential conflict, the ANA Council established a freestanding organization. Conflict was heightened because of the new organization's intent to develop a model nursing practice act. This activity heretofore had been the sole prerogative of the ANA despite the establishment of many other specialty nursing organizations.

NCSBN Model Nursing Practice Act and Definition of Nursing

The nursing practice and standards committee of the NCSBN began to develop a model nursing practice act shortly after the NCSBN was organized. The first task of this committee was to develop a definition of nursing, which they based on the 1977 definition by the US Department of Health, Education, and Welfare that defined licensure as follows[18]:

> The process by which an agency of government grants permission to an individual to engage in a given occupation upon finding that the applicant has obtained the minimal degree of competency necessary to ensure that the public health, safety, and welfare will be reasonably well protected.

In summarizing the work of this committee, its chairperson, Virginia Cleveland, stated, "...that distinctions between legal and professional definitions might become more apparent if an attempt is made to compare them in four ways: (1) origin of the definition, (2) its purpose, (3) content of the definition, and (4) implications."[3]

As an organized profession, nursing has a responsibility to define nursing to adequately describe the nature and components of the occupation. To define the occupational practice, the nursing profession must interact with the public to meet the needs of the public. Although a professional definition of nursing should originate from professionals and evolve with the practice as needed, a legal definition is influenced by (1) case law, (2) interpretation within the context of the existing nursing practice act, and (3) a determination of whether certain actions fall within the bounds of the legal definition. A legal definition is static and is limited to what is necessary or indispensable. The professional definition, however, should assure advancement, flexibility, and growth, and should outline the scope of nursing practice and communicate nursing's purpose and social significance. The legal definition determines the basis for licensure, sets essential standards of nursing education practice, and prohibits or removes unqualified and incompetent persons from the nursing practice.

In its statement on "The scope of nursing practice" published in 1987, the ANA addresses professional and legal regulation of practice. The ANA states that there are "parallel relationships of the component parts of professional and legal regulations of nursing practice."[1] Although the definitions differ in origin, purpose, content, and implications, they are related and interdependent in response to societal needs.

Recognition of Nurses

Acknowledging the need for guidelines, nurses sought governmental regulation as a means to implement standards and insure public safety. Through the leadership and influence of nurses in the early 1900s, laws were passed to provide for the registration of individuals who wished to practice nursing and to protect the public. Initially, any individual could practice nursing. However, this law ensured that the title of registered nurse could be used only by those individuals who had met the requirements. Thus a mandatory licensure process protected the title and the scope of practice, and nursing became a recognized entity in the health care delivery arena. Numerous health occupations continue to seek recognition by licensure to gain legal recognition that benefits both the public and nursing. With the advancement of technology and corresponding complexity of health care delivery, the trend toward more licensed occupations is not lessening.

Cost of Mandatory Regulation

Opponents of licensure use the cost of mandatory regulation as an argument for deregulation. Traditionally, the cost of nursing regulation was borne by nurses through fees paid by the licensees. This self-supporting regulation focused attention on cost factors and resulted in promulgation of "sunset laws" in the 1970s. These laws reexamined the concept of licensure and the inherent regulatory costs by using state-developed criteria for determining the needs for continuing regulation of all types of licenses. This process expended exorbitant funds in evaluating whether or not the licensure of various groups should continue. Throughout 10 years of "sunsetting" during the late 1970s and into the 1980s, the regulation of nursing was carefully examined and, in a number of states, was lauded for its regulatory procedures and effectiveness.

Despite all the efforts to deregulate health care professions, little change in the basic structure for licensure has occurred. Legislative and judicial branches of government conclude that governmental regulation of occupations is self-serving, anticompetitive, and costly to the public without corresponding benefit for the protection of the public. In the foreseeable future, it is likely that increased regulation will be imposed due to the complexity of the rapidly expanding technology involved in delivery of health care.

Mandatory licensure of all individuals practicing nursing has continued to evolve. Currently, only Texas has a permissive law that merely protects the title. Educational standards are the pivotal point around the regulation of nursing. Schools of nursing were required to meet approval standards set by boards of nursing. Such approval by a governmental entity is unique to nursing. The regulatory focus remained on educational preparation, but practice continued to be institutionally and medically controlled. Although nurses practice independently in response to societal needs, practice was effected by the dependent role of the nurse in the institutional care setting in which the schools of nursing were housed. Hospitals were controlled by medicine; therefore, nursing education was controlled by medicine. The legal definition of nursing practice placed the performance of nursing acts under the supervision of the physician. Further, nurses were the employees of the medically controlled hospital. It was in the area of public health that nurses practiced with more freedom, and despite the perennial physician dominance, performed services for the public in both times of war and peace.

Progressiveness of Nursing Advanced Practice

The development of nursing theory and more precise definition of the scope of nursing practice began in the late 1950s and 1960s. Educational preparation of nurses at the baccalaureate level flourished. At the masters and doctoral levels the same trend existed, although at a considerably slower pace. Nurses applied such terms as "nursing diagnosis" and "nursing process" to practice, and they demonstrated expanding skills.

The advanced nurse practitioner brought controversy when legislation was introduced to recognize this "new" nurse. Legislators, health care administrators, and physicians expressed concern about public protection. Nurses persisted, and in the late 1970s legislation was passed that recognized the advanced preparation and skills of individuals who were known as "nurse practitioners" or "nurse specialists."

Critical elements in the regulation of nursing persisted and interfered with expansion of the scope of nursing practice. These critical elements, which were carefully guarded by the medical profession and later by the pharmacy profession, involved the concepts of diagnosis, prescription and dispensing of drugs, and treatment. Medical and pharmacy groups maintained that their practice laws reserved the acts of diagnosis, prescription, dispensing, and treatment exclusively to licensed doctors and pharmacists. These groups proposed the creation of still other health care providers such as physician assistants, registered care technologists, pharmacy technicians, and clinical pharmacists. Such efforts emphasize control, rather than provision, of adequate cost effective care for all populations.

Interestingly, over 20 states have legislation that authorizes "nurse practitioners" to prescribe and treat patients within given protocols in collaboration with a physician. This situation is perplexing, because it demonstrates that nurses, with appropriate preparation and experience to diagnose and treat within certain parameters, are safe and effective practitioners.[17] The ethical, social, and economic issues are complex when populations are in need of such competent services as those provided by nurses and at the same time the availability and accessibility of physicians to these populations is minimal to nonexistent.

Determination of Competence

Governmental regulatory agencies have the authority to issue and deny licenses and to remove those individuals deemed incompetent to practice. Determination of continuing competency for renewal of licenses became the focus in the 1960s. Peer review, self evaluation, mandatory continuing education, reexamination, and several other mechanisms were discussed and tested. Currently, approximately 17 states require continuing education for renewal of licenses for registered nurses, licensed practical nurses, and/or advanced practitioners. Although the goal of mandatory continuing education is to ensure competence, it is not adopted as a viable regulatory mechanism. A combination of various mechanisms appear to be more acceptable, because costs associated with mandatory continuing education are substantial and its effectiveness is difficult to document. Additionally, individual responsibility and accountability of licensees and the role of the employer are constant arguments in discussions against mandating continuing education. The problem persists as states continue to seek alternatives to assure their citizens that licenses are issued only to individuals who are competent to practice.

The 1980s saw widespread growth in the issuance of practice opinions by boards or other governmental entities responsible for the regulation of nursing. In some states, the standards for practice were in regulatory form, which is law; others issued opinions based on specific questions or issues raised. In those states in which rules or regulations are not in effect for governing practice, the opinion statements are considered just that, an opinion. These statements do not have the force and effect of law. However, because the opinions are issued by a peer review process, they are expected to influence litigious circumstances.

CONSTITUTIONAL LAW AND THE REGULATION OF NURSING

Granted by the US Constitution and state constitutional parameters, each state has jurisdiction over its affairs. It is the obligation of state legislatures to protect their citizens. This is done by the enactment of laws that govern any occupation that meets criteria set by the state, which regulates requirements for protection of its citizens. Bearing this jurisdictional authority in mind, Toni M. Massaro, in response to an inquiry from the NCSBN, cites the following three principles of occupational law that provide guidance in setting such requirements.[11]

1. The more restrictive a regulatory scheme is on the right to practice nursing, the more vulnerable that regulatory scheme becomes to legal challenges on constitutional grounds, and to resistance from the profession. As such, the objective basis for increased regulation should be clear and documented.

2. The more subjective the regulatory requirements are (e.g., peer review versus an objective written examination) the more vulnerable the requirements are to charges of unlawful arbitrariness, discrimination, or unreasonableness. Correlatively, subjective requirements must be accompanied by greater procedural mechanisms to protect against unfairness or discrimination. These procedures, which may include evidentiary hearings, involve time and money.

3. Increased regulation of the profession may have anticompetitive effects. Special licensure, relicensure, certification, or other restrictions on the right to practice nursing will create a special group of nurses who have met the qualifications or have been "grandfathered." This group may charge higher rates for their special services, or may enjoy an advantage in the employment market generally. Increased regulation also may extend the time necessary for individuals to enter the new field and reduce access to the field. These anticompetitive effects may violate the federal antitrust laws (15 USC §1 [1975]), unless the regulation is expressly authorized and actively supervised by

the state. This means that the state legislature must expressly authorize any regulation that restrains competition, must participate actively in establishing the terms of the regulation, and monitor and enforce the regulation. The state cannot safely delegate general authority to the state board members to adopt regulations with anticompetitive effects; nor can the board cede its regulatory authority to private entities. In either situation, a court may conclude that the regulatory scheme violated the antitrust laws and enjoin enforcement of the regulations, or award money damages.[11]

Further, Massaro stated that, "The United States Constitution limits the state's authority to regulate the professions in two ways: (1) the regulatory scheme must bear a rational relationship to a valid state purpose and (2) the regulatory scheme must provide a person who is denied the right to practice the profession, or specialty within that profession, certain procedural rights, such as notice and an opportunity to be heard about the denial."[11]

Rational Relationship Test

The "rational relationship" test is satisfied when two conditions are met: (1) the intent of regulatory law to protect the public from licensees that are incompetent or unfit to practice an occupation and (2) regulation deemed to be a "reasonable means" of accomplishing the goal of public protection. When the state empowers a board of nursing to set new requirements for the licensing of the nursing occupation, additionally imposed regulation on current licensees must be an "accurate measure of relevant, job-related skills, and thus... rationally related to a legitimate state goal."[11]

In addition, caution against discrimination must be taken when new regulations have an adverse impact on minorities. Because the memberships of boards of nursing are predominantly licensed nurses, any regulation that decreases competition can lead to accusations that new regulations are for the benefit of the profession versus the public good and that they may increase costs as well. Massaro states that boards of nursing, due to their composition, "... are particularly vulnerable to allegations of self-interested motives in making decisions that exclude or expel individuals from the profession."[11]

Currently state boards of nursing have not experienced challenges to the licensure of registered nurses and licensed practical nurses. However, the regulation of advanced nurse specialists or practitioners have been challenged, by groups such as medicine. Thus caution is required by the regulatory boards of nursing when setting requirements for advanced practice.

New regulations not expressly authorized by statute have the potential for closer scrutiny by the judiciary system. As Massaro said, challenges to licensure examinations have been unsuccessful and there is a widespread acceptance of most regulation of the nursing occupation by boards of nursing. With the initiation of new regulations, courts are expected to closely review such regulations and demand that the reasonableness of the new regulations be documented. It is incumbent on the state or the regulatory agency that new requirements for entrance or for continuing in the profession are directly related to a documented need for public protection. Solid rationale must exist for the new regulation, and the end result of the new regulation must bear evidence of meeting the identified need.

Due Process

States are obligated by the US Constitution to develop procedures that ensure due process in enforcement of requirements imposed on applicants or licensees. Such procedural rights provide the framework for making decisions that are unbiased, sound, and fair. Notice and an opportunity to be heard are two basic requirements of due process. A subjective requirement is more likely to be inadequately documented and subject to challenge. A psychometrically sound and legally defensible examination is an objective requirement. On the other hand, evaluation by peers is considered more subjective in nature than an examination that is carefully constructed and validated. Because of the more subjective nature of peer evaluation, increased costs need to be born by a licensing board in producing meticulous safeguards that protect the individual's right to practice or to gain entry to the profession. An individual licensee's right to notice involves notification and time to meet requirements, or time for defense in a disciplinary action.[11]

The adoption by many states of uniform administrative procedures acts and the elaborate reviews in promulgation of new regulations by boards of nursing and other agencies, though costly, protects agencies and provides for input before regulations become effective. The former detail procedures that protect agencies when taking disciplinary actions or when denying licensure to applicants. Regardless of the type of regulatory schemes adopted by a board of nursing, a critical feature of active state supervision must be implemented. In other words, a board of nursing may not delegate the responsibility for enforcement of requirements to private entities or to accept the administration of the requirements by bodies outside itself without active participation.

New requirements imposed for specialty designation, for continuing licensure, or for new entrants to a given profession may be required if the legitimate state goal of public protection is documented and procedural safeguards are provided. However, regulatory agencies must be aware of the possible effect of new regulations to avoid challenges of unfairness, discrimination, and issues of antitrust that involve unlawful restraint of trade or anticompetitive behavior. As stated previously, it is incumbent on boards of nursing to be diligent in responding to societal needs by assuring that licensees are competent.

STATE GOVERNMENT ORGANIZATION AND REGULATION OF NURSING

The administration of the nursing practice acts in 62 jurisdictions of the United States is vested in an agency of the executive branch of state government (see box). The 62 jurisdictions are the 50 states; six states with separate boards for practical/vocational nurse licensure (Georgia, Louisiana, West Virginia, Texas, Washington, and California); the District of Columbia; and the territories of Guam, the Virgin Islands, American Samoa, the Northern Marianna Islands, and Puerto Rico. The statutes or nurse practice acts of these jurisdictions authorize the agency, usually the board of nursing, to promulgate rules and regulations that are necessary for implementation of the statute.

ADMINISTRATION OF NURSE PRACTICE ACTS IN THE UNITED STATES
———————————— BY JURISDICTION ————————————

Jurisdiction	Number of agencies*
The United States	50
States with separate boards for LPN/RN	6
Washington, DC	1
Territories: Guam, the Virgin Islands, American Samoa, the Mariana Islands, Puerto Rico	5
TOTAL	62

---

*Agencies of the executive branch of government.

Responsibilities of Boards of Nursing

The general responsibilities of the board of nursing in each jurisdiction are presented in the box.

Initially, boards of nursing were established as independent and autonomous agencies in state government, reporting directly to the office of the governor. Subsequently, there were attempts to place the boards of nursing under already existing state departments such as the health department. As state government bureaucracy expanded, some boards were placed under centralized agencies. Before 1930, five of these agencies existed, in New York, Illinois, Washington, Pennsylvania, and California. The centralization of similar agencies within state government occurred rapidly. Reorganization of the executive branch of government resulted in only 17 of the 50 states retaining autonomous boards, whereas the remaining 33 have some form of centralization. Despite the centralization, most boards of nursing, as well as other occupational boards, maintain control of professional licensing issues and matters dealing with disciplinary action. The concept of peer review and control is maintained.

The merits of centralization versus decentralization are debated in the political arena. In some states such as New Mexico occupational boards recently centralized are petitioning to resume an autonomous role when defined criteria have been met.

A review of the publication of The Council of State Governments entitled, "State Government Organization Charts" reveals the complexity of state level bureaucracy. Only two of the charts present specifically listed occupational boards. These two boards are pharmacy and medicine.

A recent development in state governmental activities that relates directly to boards of nursing is legislative oversight in the promulgation of rules and regulations. During the past 20 years, state legislatures assumed close scrutiny of rules and regulations primarily because these codes possess the force and effect of law. This development resulted in complex procedures that are costly and time consuming. The disadvantage of such complex procedures raises questions about the balance of powers between the executive and legislative branches of government.

BOARDS OF NURSING: RESPONSIBILITIES

Determination of the eligibility of applicants for licensure
Adoption and administration of examinations to applicants for licensure
Issuance of licenses to qualified applicants
Setting procedures for relicensure of previously licensed individuals
Establishing minimum standards for approval of prelicensure educational programs of nursing
Approval of mandatory continuing education in some jurisdictions
Investigation of complaints against licensees
Imposition of disciplinary action as authorized
Promulgation of rules that regulate nursing
Issuance of opinions and rulings on safe nursing practice
Overall enforcement of the provisions of the statute as promulgated in regulation

---

AUTHORITY OF REGULATORY BOARDS

Rule making authority—provides for setting of standards, as well as for due process requirements
Quasi-judicial authority—provides for enforcement of standards, and outlines procedures for adjudication of contested matters
Administrative authority—provides for elements needed to enforce standards such as agency budget, personnel, and office management

---

EXAMPLE: In 1986, in the Commonwealth of Kentucky, the legislature voted to codify all administrative regulations into law. After 2 years of exorbitant costs and efforts to draft thousands of administrative regulations into bill form, the 1988 Kentucky legislature rescinded the law to codify administrative regulations. In its place, a second legislative committee review was established.

To accomplish the mission of public protection, regulatory boards were charged with establishing requirements to be met by applicants before being issued licenses.* Another responsibility of regulatory boards is the enforcement of prescribed standards. Implicit in these two major responsibilities for upholding public protection are (1) rule making authority, (2) quasi-judicial authority, and (3) administrative authority (see box).

Accomplishments in Regulation

Significant accomplishments in the regulation of the profession included in this discussion are prelicensure programs of nursing education, adoption and administration of

---

*Licensure is a privilege to practice bestowed on an individual who has met legally prescribed requirements and standards.

licensure examinations for use on a national scope, provisions for handicapped candidates to take the examination, rigorous monitoring of licensees through reporting requirements, implementation of methods for dealing with impaired professionals, differentiation of nursing from medical care, the establishment of a freestanding organization for boards of nursing, and revision of definitions of nursing.

The comparison of nursing regulation in the early 1900s with the regulation of the occupation today shows vast differences. Initially, most states were concerned with registration of the individuals who were presenting themselves as nurses. Another concern was the setting of educational standards. Establishment of educational standards has remained an issue throughout the history of the regulation of nurses, and still is unresolved. Although educational standards were a primary focus of boards of nursing, the setting of standards for practice was left to the professional associations. Because these organizations have no legal enforcement powers, disciplinary actions against licensees were implemented by the boards of nursing. Legal standards of practice were promulgated within the past 20 years.

Disciplinary action against licensees was rare until the 1970s. Other societal influences or employer action removed unfit or incompetent individuals from practice. In the area of misappropriation or abuse of drugs, there is a drastic change in the processing of disciplinary cases in reporting and action taken by the boards. Nursing practice acts have been revised to include mandatory reporting of licensees suspected of violating the law. They also provide sanctions against individuals possessing knowledge of facts who fail to report suspected violations. The number of actions against licensees reported by boards of nursing has increased in cases of drug-related problems. This trend in disciplinary action parallels the increased use and abuse of chemical substances in society today.

The definition of nursing was first included in the law during the 1930s and evolution of the legal definition continues. Nursing evolved as a discreet service that was health-oriented versus illness-oriented. Definitions of nursing still include provisions that put nurses under the direction of licensed physicians. Currently, progress is being made to delineate specific dependent functions in the broader independent nursing-based definition for practice.

Another important accomplishment is the use of licensure examinations on a national scope. Beginning in the 1940s, nursing was the first occupation to establish a mechanism whereby all of the states recognized and used the same examination to facilitate interstate mobility of the licensees.

There is a significant change in the regulation of licensees in regard to disciplinary action of those persons who are reported for substance or chemical abuse. The term used is *impaired professional*. Trends show that boards of nursing no longer merely dispose of licensees by revoking their licenses; they are actively assisting these individuals to meet standards and to resume practice as contributing members of society. Provisions are being made for admittance of handicapped individuals to the profession. Current regulations provide limited licensure for both disciplined and handicapped individuals.

Changes are occurring that indicate "minimum safety standards" may no longer be acceptable. Words such as "essential" or "effective" are used in regulatory language for nursing. Methods to determine continuing competency are studied extensively to find solutions that assure the public that individuals who possess licenses are safe and effective practitioners. No measure has been developed to determine whether or not current licensees do in fact possess continuing competency, a determination that likely will be an issue of the 1990s.

A major issue facing boards and all governmental bodies is the cost of regulation. There is a direct relationship of costs to that of health care in a society that has become extremely technologically oriented. Setting and enforcing standards and determining competency incur costs that are directly reflected in the cost of health care.

FEDERAL GOVERNMENT INVOLVEMENT IN OCCUPATIONAL REGULATION

Federal agencies have recently become involved in scrutinizing effectiveness of state licensure and disciplinary practices. The increase in expenditures by the federal government in such programs as Medicare and Medicaid has escalated federal efforts involving health care licensees. The Office of Inspector General of the US Department of Health and Human Services and other federal agencies quickly point out that licensure and discipline of professionals is a traditional function of state government. Nevertheless, this state authority is being examined at the national level. As the largest purchaser of health care in the United States, the federal government examines and implements ways to ensure that only services provided by competent licensees are reimbursed. Although the federal government is appropriately concerned about quality care that is cost effective, some of the initiatives currently in effect give the appearance of developing "federal credentials."

EXAMPLE: Certain provisions of the Omnibus Budget and Reconciliation Act of 1987 (PL 100-203) include mandates for training, competency evaluation, and registration of nurse aides and home health aides. Medicare- and Medicaid-approved agencies must meet the requirements of this legislation or risk losing their funding for nursing home and home health care.

The establishment of a National Practitioner Data Bank enacted by federal legislation (PL 99-660) is a key federal initiative that mandates reporting and releasing of information on members of the health professions. This law is aptly entitled, "The Health Care Quality Improvement Act." Physicians and dentists were the first groups included in the data bank. Amendments to this Act (PL 108-177) include nurses and other health professionals. The purpose of the data bank is to track licensees who are found to be the following:

1. Incompetent
2. Disciplined by a state licensing board
3. Involved in malpractice lawsuits
4. Have adverse actions taken against them by professional societies or by health care entities in regard to clinical privileges

Although the Federal Trade Commission (FTC) has not directed major efforts toward nursing, it continues to review and evaluate rules to ensure that trade restrictions are not occurring by the promulgation of licensing requirements. Most of the FTC's interest is focused on advertising rules, but nursing must be alert to the possibility of such investigation.

The Office of Inspector General carefully scrutinizes the licensure and discipline of chiropractors, optometrists, dentists, and podiatrists. Again, because of the exorbitant increases in Medicare/Medicaid expenditures, the attention of the federal government is on those groups of licensees who bill the federal government for millions of dollars each year.

Another issue under investigation by the federal government is the possible discrimination against foreign medically trained physicians who attempt to move from one jurisdiction to another in the United States. Little uniformity exists among the state boards of medical licensure in requirements for licensure of this group.

A recent study by the Institute of Medicine (IOM) entitled, "Health services: avoiding crises[9] was mandated by Congress in 1985. The study addresses the following issues:

1. The role of allied health personnel and health care delivery
2. Future needs for each allied health group
3. Current practices of licensing, certification, and accreditation
4. Changes in allied health education and service delivery
5. The role of government, education, and health care institutions in meeting allied health needs

Finding potential future shortage of health care workers and the need to balance health care costs and quality, the IOM study recommends statutory certification rather than licensure for individuals in allied health fields, if it is determined that they need to be regulated.

Efforts to exempt health professionals from the jurisdiction of the FTC are routinely attempted by the strong lobbying forces of the medical profession. Although they have not been successful, this group will likely not abandon such efforts in the near future. If such an exemption were granted, unbridled control by medicine may well go unchecked at the expense of the public and the advancement of the nursing profession in its struggle for rightful recognition and place among health providers.

As discussed previously, the federal government is involved in regulating health personnel and the provision of health services. It also affects health care workers by the way it defines covered services. The Medicare and Medicaid programs contain regulations issued by the US Department of Health and Human Services that define required qualifications for individuals who provide services for reimbursement. These services include those rendered by registered nurses, licensed practical nurses, and nurse aides, as well as services such as speech therapy and physical therapy. Although the federal government does not directly regulate health occupations (regulation is in the jurisdiction of the states), it does have significant influence on state regulatory policy through the various avenues of supporting evaluation and research, sponsoring policy analyses, and promoting information dissemination.

The FTC conducts and sponsors research on the effects and outcomes of regulation and has aggressively prohibited anticompetitive practices and requirements promulgated by regulatory boards. In the 1970s, significant studies, research, and analyses conducted by the US Department of Health, Education, and Welfare (now the Department of Health and Human Services) and the Labor Department drew attention to problems created by state regulation of the health occupations. Resulting recommendations gave new directions and assisted the state in dealing with conventional health occupations such as nursing and medicine and aided new health care workers in allied health areas in setting standards for entry and practice. Partnerships with other groups are advocated by the federal government by its support of the Clearinghouse on Licensure, Enforcement, and Regulation of the Council of State Government and the National Commission for Health Certifying Agencies (NCHCA). The latter serves as a primary source for dissemination of information on state regulatory agencies, whereas the former sets standards for organizations that certify allied health personnel. The purpose of NCHCA standards is to assure that certifying agencies offer sound certification programs for accountability to individuals desiring certification, to employers and health care payers for services provided by such individuals, and ultimately to the public.

LICENSURE AND ALTERNATIVE METHODS OF REGULATION

The purpose of licensure laws is to protect the public. Because of restrictions that licensure laws impose on who may provide a service and the cost of the services provided by licensed persons that are passed on to the consumer, licensure of health professions is under continued scrutiny. The scrutiny is intensified by the shortage of health care workers to meet population needs, the cost of health care, and the increasing technological complexities of health care. In addition, increasing groups throughout the country are seeking licensure laws or some form of legal recognition.

Because of these factors, various groups study the need for state regulation and develop criteria for determining whether a health occupational (professional) group should be regulated (see box).[5]

Many jurisdictions attempt to apply such stringent criteria as listed above, but various states continue to license or grant legal recognition to new groups of health workers such as occupational therapists, mental health counselors, physician assistants, respiratory therapists, and acupuncturists.

Although licensure is the predominant mode for regulation of the nursing profession, other modes of occupational regulation such as registration designation and certification are used by the states. Goldman and Helms list the following six predominant modes of occupational regulation.[9]

1. PRACTICE STANDARD
   Without special enforcement
   Through the adoption of statutes and rules, this mode can establish restrictions on the practice of an occupation with civil or criminal penalties enforceable through the courts. This type of regulation requires no inspections, registration, or special enforcement staff. Rather, it relies on action by the harmed parties or by a consumer affairs office.

CRITERIA FOR REGULATION

CRITERIA I*:   The unregulated practice of an occupation will harm or endanger the health, safety, and welfare of the public. The potential for harm is recognizable and not remote or dependent on tenuous argument.

CRITERIA II: The practice of an occupation requires a high degree of skill, knowledge, and training, and the public requires assurances of initial and continuing occupational competence.

CRITERIA III: The functions and responsibilities of the practitioner require independent judgments and the members of the occupational group practice autonomously.

CRITERIA IV: The scope of practice of an occupation is distinguished from other licensed and unlicensed occupations.

CRITERIA V: The economic impact on the public of regulating this occupational group is justified.

CRITERIA VI: There are no adequate alternatives to regulation (i.e., licensure, statutory certification or registration) that will protect the public.

---

*Prerequisite for a health occupational group to be regulated.
(From the Commonwealth of Virginia Policy Review: the regulation of the health profession, Richmond, Virginia, 1983, Department of Health Regulatory Boards.)

With special enforcement
Through statutes or rules, or both, this mode can establish restrictions on the practice of an occupation in addition to establishing inspections, enforcement mechanisms, and penalties. However, this mode does not require registration, certification, or any assessment of the practitioner's credentials or competency.

2. REGISTRATION
Without standards
Through regulation, a state agency can require persons in an occupation to register and supply certain information without requiring any standards, testing, or enforcement.
With standards
It is also possible to have a registration requirement in combination with minimum practice standards that are set by a designated agency. Although registration would not be exclusionary, it would subject registrants to minimum standards and thereby provide some protection to the public.

3. STATUTORY CERTIFICATION
With state standards and state enforcement
Through regulation, occupational members can be required to meet certain state standards; only those who meet these predetermined qualifications may legally use the designated title of the occupation. This mode entails standards, testing, codes of practice, possible inspections, and enforcement.
With private standards and assessment and state enforcement
Through regulation, an agency of the state may require members of an occupational group to meet certain standards established by a private testing or assessment center or organization

(reviewed by the state), with the state handling the certification and any enforcement required. Legally, the state is responsible for the standards set and for monitoring the process.

4. STATUTORY CERTIFICATION AND PRACTICE STANDARDS

A state may establish, by rule, certification for an occupation and also request the legislature to pass a law that would establish practice standards for that same occupation. This combination would establish a system of title control for those meeting certain required standards of competency, as well as establishing standards of practice for anyone who practices the occupation.

5. REGULATION THROUGH SUPERVISION BY AN ALREADY LICENSED PRACTITIONER

Certification with standards

Through statutes and rules, an occupation can be certified and required to work under the supervision of an already licensed occupation; standards for practice can also be established.

Through standards of practice but without certification

It is also possible to regulate by providing that the occupation be performed under the supervision of a licensed professional with certain standards set forth but without requiring that the individual be certified.

6. LICENSURE

Licensure is the most restrictive form of occupational regulation, providing for both title control and an exclusive area of practice. It requires standards of practice, education, knowledge or minimum competency, and inspection and enforcement with civil and criminal penalties.

The complexity of the regulation of nursing is better understood when these six modes are applied to the current regulation of nursing. The setting of practice standards by the adoption of statutes and rules is not applied to the regulation of individual nurses, because of the licensure laws that exist for registered nurses and licensed practical nurses. However, an example of setting such standards are the requirements that health care facilities must meet for Medicare/Medicaid reimbursement. These standards are federally enforced and are detailed in state rules that affect care determinants and provision. Registration as defined by Goldman and Helms can be applied to certain states that use a similar process for recognition of advanced or specialty nurse practitioners. Federal reimbursement mechanisms for agency providers of health care also use this type of process and require minimum standards to be met by the registrants. Another example is the recent requirements of the federal government for employment of nurse aides in nursing homes and in home health care for Medicare/Medicaid reimbursement.

Again, the two modes: statutory certification, and statutory certification and practice standards, are applicable to the regulation of advanced or specialty nurse practitioners. There is title control and also the requirement to meet certain standards such as additional educational preparation and clinical experience. The recognition of certification processes conducted by nongovernmental groups and varying standards set by the state or by the federal government fall into these two categories.

A number of states require an advanced nurse practitioner to be supervised by a physician. This regulatory approach is included under the supervision by an already licensed practitioner. Another example is that of the licensed practical/vocational nurse where state nursing practice acts require that an individual so designated work under the supervision of a registered nurse, licensed physician, or dentist.

Finally, licensure in its purest form limits the practice of nursing to only registered nurses and to licensed practical/vocational nurses with limitations. Legal definitions of nursing still include provisions for supervision by other licensees (i.e., physicians) and, because of overlap in functions, even this method of regulation is problematic for nursing. Nonetheless, licensed nurses are accountable for safe practice and are frequently the subject of litigation involving malpractice suits. In summary, licensure of nurses involves a set of minimum standards for public protection, whereas certification is usually reserved for specialization or excellence in practice beyond minimum licensure standards. Multiple regulations by state and federal agencies, the use of unlicensed persons, and a proliferation of new workers are all influencing nursing in its efforts to provide safe care.

Certification

A review of the literature regarding certification processes for nursing shows a vast array of programs and organizations. A primary purpose of these certifying organizations is to evaluate members who wish to enter, continue, and/or advance in a nursing specialty, through a certification process that results in the issuance of credentials to those nurses who meet the required qualifications and level of competence. In nursing, 16 different national organizations certify approximately 100,000 nurses in about 36 areas of specialization.[15] Such certifying bodies assist in providing credentials for public information and they may make state regulation unnecessary, if they are not seen as a restraint of trade, because they are merely giving their opinion as to whether an individual possesses qualifications for being "certified." Under discussion, however, is whether or not private credentialing bodies such as nursing specialty organizations should escape all antitrust scrutiny.

In addition to state and federal regulation, there are private control mechanisms that can offer assurances of competence to the public. Numerous national nursing organizations have requirements for individual membership by licensed practical/vocational nurses or registered nurses. These organizations set qualifications for membership and also adopt codes of ethics that provide self-regulation and guidance to the members. Other forms of voluntary regulation include private accreditation. Although most state boards of nursing have exclusive authority for approval of the establishment and operation of any prelicensure program of nursing, forms of private accreditation also exist and are used to assure a degree of quality. These kinds of quality assurance mechanisms include private organizations such as the National League for Nursing (NLN). The NLN has four councils that set standards and processes for granting public recognition to licensed practical nursing education programs, associate degree programs in nursing, hospital-based diploma programs of nursing, and baccalaureate and higher degree programs in nursing. This type of accreditation is a peer review and is accepted as a standard of excellence.

Private forms of accreditation for institutions such as hospitals and nursing homes that affect the practice of nursing by setting standards and qualifications include the Joint Commission on Accreditation of Health Care Organizations. The NLN also has an accreditation program, recognized by the federal government, for the accreditation of home health care agencies.

Licensure as a mode of occupational regulation is criticized because of the restrictions it places on the individual licensee, and on individuals or agencies who employ such licensees. Because licensure limits practice of the occupation to only licensees, opponents argue that consumer costs are increased, there is reduced access to health care services, and less flexibility for managers. The idea of institutional licensure espoused in the past by the federal government is not acceptable to the states and is vigorously opposed by the profession of nursing. The recent study by the IOM, which cites potential for future shortages of health care workers and the need to balance health care costs and quality, recommends statutory certification "because this form of regulation offers most of the benefits of licensure but few of the costs."[9] Although this study did not focus on nursing per se, it looked at regulation in general and made other recommendations.

These recommendations include that regulation be as flexible as possible without undue risk of harm to the public. Multiple pathways to licensure or overlapping scopes of practice for some licensed occupations is suggested. The study also addresses the need for the public to be better informed of the scope of practice, entry requirements, and basic data on licensees, including disciplinary actions, board memberships, and procedures, especially complaint procedures. In addition, the study recommends that an advisory body be formed to objectively assess evidence and jurisdictional issues between and among health occupations, and that research programs be carried out to weigh issues of risk, cost, quality, and access in the regulation of the various health occupations. The recommendation that is certain to affect boards of nursing is that at least half the members of licensing boards should be from outside the licensed occupations. Such membership for licensing boards according to IOM should be drawn from a variety of areas, including health administration, economics, consumer affairs, education, and health services research.[9]

A NATIONAL ORGANIZATION OF BOARDS OF NURSING

In 1978, a freestanding organization was formed for boards of nursing. (Before 1978, boards of nursing were included as members in a council of the ANA.) This new organization, named the National Council of State Boards of Nursing (NCSBN), is composed of 62 members, consisting of state boards of nursing or agencies that regulate nursing in the 50 states. Five states have two boards of nursing, and the National Council membership includes American Samoa, Guam, the Northern Mariana Islands, Puerto Rico, and the Virgin Islands (see box on p. 254).

Several objectives of the National Council apply to a discussion on trends and issues in the regulation of nursing. The pertinent objectives include the following[13]:

1. Identify and promote desirable and reasonable uniformity in standards and expected outcomes in nursing education practice as they relate to the protection of the public health, safety, and welfare
2. Assess trends and issues affecting nursing education and nursing practice as they affect licensure of nurses

3. Identify continuing competence for practitioners of nursing and assist in efforts to promote the same

Other objectives deal with facilitation of effective communications; the collection, analysis, and dissemination of data on statistics relating to nurse licensure; provision of consultative services to Council members; the development of policies and procedures; and regulation of the use of the licensure examinations for nursing.

One task of the National Council was the production of a Model Nursing Practice Act. This document, first published in 1983 and revised in 1988, is intended to serve as a guide to states in considering revisions to their nursing practice act. As defined by the Council of State Governments a model act is a piece of legislation that seeks to address, in comprehensive fashion, a determined need. Model bills are often reformed legislation intended to provide order in an area where existing legislation is out of date, internally inconsistent, too broad or too narrow, or for some reason inadequate to implement state policy.

Considering the sovereign authority jurisdiction (states) possess, differences may need to exist with some variation resulting in nursing statutes. The national need to have some degree of uniformity among the nursing practice statutes can be met by the use of model acts so that a common, nationwide understanding of what constitutes the legally recognized practice of nursing will be insured. This type of uniformity furthers the concept of nurses and nursing as valuable national resources. In addition, the geographic mobility of nurses to meet needs and interest is facilitated.

Model nursing practice legislation is developed by professional associations and by organizations composed of regulatory boards, such as the NCSBN. Each organization has a different perspective on its proposed legislation and such varying perspectives can be useful for those contemplating needed changes. It must be recognized that model acts are suggestions. Because each state is a sovereign jurisdiction, its laws must be written in accordance and within its constitutional framework. Other laws influence the regulation of nurses such as the administrative procedures acts and public health acts; therefore, persons are always urged to seek legal counsel and a review of state laws before attempting to apply any provision of a model act.

TRENDS AND ISSUES IN REGULATION

Some of the major issues and trends facing nursing today include the following:
1. Determination of continuing competency
2. Recognition of advanced registered nursing practice, including mandatory registration or licensure
3. Scope of practice for licensees, including prescription privileges
4. Due process
5. Rights of licensees, including concepts of grandfathering or "grandparenting"
6. Establishment of requirements for entry to practice
7. Regulation of unlicensed nursing personnel
8. Payment mechanisms for nursing services

9. Influence and credibility of nurses
10. Administrative aspects of boards of nursing
11. Strengthening of legal standards included in statutory provisions relative to violations and reporting of violations
12. Impaired nurse professionals

Definition of Nursing

Some states are developing legislation that expands the scope of practice for licensed practical nursing. The new definition would give licensed practical nurses considerably more latitude by authorizing performance of acts commensurate with required educational preparations. Further, it would make the licensed practical nurse accountable to the consumer for the quality of care given by the licensee. Functions considered to be practical nursing would be broadened to include the teaching and supervision of auxillary personnel, not heretofore considered a part of practical nursing. In some of the proposals for expanded scope, the definition continues to require that the licensed practical nurse function under the direction of a registered nurse or physician. Some states are eliminating the language in both definitions, RN and LPN, that prohibits performance of acts of medical diagnosis or prescription of therapeutic or corrective measures. Language is being introduced to define the scope of services as being commensurate with the educational preparation of the individual, to allow for an expanded scope of practice for those with more nursing education.

Inherent in legislation for prescription and treatment privileges for advanced nursing practitioners is a change required in the definition of registered and licensed practical nursing practice. As prescription privileges continue to be granted for advanced nursing practice, the language in definition of practice in nursing acts needs to include that prescriptions and orders from advanced practitioners may be implemented by registered nurses and licensed practical nurses.

Continued Competency

Although the trends to require mandatory continuing education for renewal of licenses is waning, the issue of determination of continuing competency has gained emphasis. Seventeen states require mandatory continuing education for renewal of licenses, and/or designation of advanced practitioners. Different tactics to arrive at continuing competency are being attempted. Requirements for refresher courses for nurses who have not practiced within a given period of time are being implemented. Another requirement is documentation of a number of work hours in a given period and/or also requiring continuing education documentation.

EXAMPLE: The Florida Board of Accountancy statute was amended to require that in addition to continuing education requirements, licensees must pass an examination on Florida accountancy law and the board's rules before renewal of their licenses. To date, no nursing board has such legislation in process. In fact, Florida is one of the few states to require an examination for renewal of any professional license.

The NCSBN position paper on continued competency includes the following[13]:

Boards of Nursing have the responsibility to assure the health, safety, and welfare of the public by verifying that nurses practice competently. Although current research does not support any single method of insuring continued competence, the National Council recommends that individual boards continue efforts to establish mechanisms that validate continued competence.

In so doing, each board of nursing should provide regulations that are based on the following principles[13]:

1. That the mechanism be reasonable, applied in a nondiscriminatory manner, and include procedural safeguards for the licensee
2. That the mechanism provide for the inherent difference between the RN's and PN's legal scope of practice
3. That evidence of current knowledge, skills, and abilities be required after a significant period of lapse in nursing practice
4. That the mechanism be tied to the board's disciplinary process

Approximately 30 states require some form of continuing competency determination for RN or PN licensure renewal. In addition to mandatory continuing education, 2 states use peer review, 14 states require refresher courses for reentry into nursing practice, 3 require a competency examination, and 10 have a minimum practice time requirement.

Composition of Board Membership

In the past several years, many nursing practice acts included revisions in the composition of the members composing the board of nursing. Trends include a citizen or consumer member on the board. Several states have pending legislation that would increase the number of consumer or citizen-at-large members to as much as 50% of the board membership. Involvement of consumer members on regulating boards results in less frivolous and more essential requirements for licensure of individuals.[8]

Another issue relating to composition of board membership is the mechanism for appointment of members to the board. A number of states have board members appointed by the governor, with various groups submitting nominations for consideration for appointment. In those states in which nomination lists are submitted exclusively by various professional groups there is potential for challenge.

EXAMPLE: The Supreme Court of South Carolina in 1986 struck down a statute of that state's medical licensure board that allowed nominees for consideration for appointment to be submitted only by the state medical association. The statute was considered unconstitutional and unfair in that due process was not afforded when the state medical association membership was composed of approximately only 60% of the medical doctors licensed in that state.

Influences on Credibility of Nurses

With advanced practice prescription privileges, there is increased activity regarding legislative actions on payment mechanisms for reimbursement of nursing services. States that enact reimbursement legislation usually exclude payment for nursing services in hospitals, nursing homes, and doctors offices. Another area of concern is that of malpractice insurance for nurses. In addition to increasing costs for all nurses, premium rates have increased far higher than salaries. The costs for specialty groups such as anesthetists and midwives have not been justified by numbers of lawsuits and monetary damages awarded.

Entry Into Practice Requirements

Pressure to increase educational requirements for entry into various professions persists. Groups such as accountancy, social workers, and nursing are advocating increased educational preparation as a requirement for entry into the profession. Such efforts have often encountered disagreement among members of the profession involved, (i.e., objections from employers and educators, reluctance of state legislators to overregulate, and research questioning the validity of additional requirements). Nursing has had educational preparation requirements for licensure under discussion for over 25 years.

Due Process, Immunity

Boards of nursing and state regulatory agencies review procedures to insure due process rights of individuals. Significantly high numbers of disciplinary actions are taken by boards of nursing against licensees. The constitutional rights of individuals may be violated without adequate procedural safeguards. Individuals denied licensure or those individuals who are disciplined by the board use various procedures to appeal denials and other actions by boards of nursing. Although boards of nursing differ in structure and organization within the various states, the states that have uniform administrative procedures acts often will have procedures prescribed to assure due process.

Another consideration is immunity. Clauses are being introduced into nursing practice acts that provide for immunity of individuals who report suspected violations of the law, for staff and for board members. This may become a constitutional question. Some state constitutions provide that no individual may be deprived of the right of recovery in the event of harm done to them. An individual cannot be deprived of the right to sue. Recovery of an award is another matter.

Administrative Aspects of the Board of Nursing

Provisions in nursing practice acts establish boards of nursing; their structure, size, and qualifications for board membership; and powers and duties granted by statutory authority. The result is a variety of composition and size of boards of nursing, and their placement in the structure of state government. A number of boards function autonomously and several boards serve only in an advisory capacity. A concern of the past decade is the centralization of licensure functions in state government structures. Often, authority was removed from the board of nursing and vested in another state government agency.

Centralization of Regulatory Agencies

Centralization of regulatory agencies in the various states has advantages in the provision of routine administrative matters. However, the loss of control of funds generated by nursing boards is not advantageous to the nursing board agency. Often, money generated by the regulation of nursing subsidized other occupations with fewer numbers that were insufficient to support their regulatory functions. An argument for centralizing regulatory boards is that the public protection mission was not being implemented by professional expert boards. Arguments stated that the interest of the individual licensee was forwarded and that public protection was not carried out adequately by such boards. These arguments remain a dilemma. Expert composition of boards is needed to apply full due process rights of individuals so that they may be judged by a panel of peers who know and understand safe practice, as well as to protect the public. However, the determination of character fitness and continued competency are issues that must not be abused for self-interest. Boards composed of nurse licensee members have a license to practice a given occupation but they also have a license to license. As a member of a board, there must be separation from the work place, friendship, and professional vested interest. Members of regulatory boards of nursing must support persons who report incompetent practice, and actively encourage appropriate reporting as well. A board of nursing as a corporate body must take action with the best interest of public protection in mind. In addition, boards of nursing must be aware that their objectives and standards are different than that of the judicial system and must not depend on court actions as disciplinary guidelines. All too often, judges do not grasp the full significance of actions taken by licensees and do not understand where public protection may be jeopardized.

Increasing Educational Requirements

The question of increasing educational requirements for initial licensure is being discussed widely. Statutes in the various states are studied to determine whether or not current language authorizes a board of nursing to set new requirements by regulation. Several states seek attorney generals' opinions for guidance in this matter.

EXAMPLE: Opinions of the attorney generals in Minnesota and in West Virginia indicate that the nursing practice acts in those states did not include statutory authority for the boards of nursing to promulgate new educational requirements for licensure. However, the state of North Dakota received a favorable opinion from its attorney general, in that the law as written in North Dakota did in fact give authority to the North Dakota Board of Nursing to set new educational standards for applicants as licensure as nurses. The opinion of the North Dakota Attorney General was upheld when the North Dakota Board of Nursing was sued by two hospitals that operated diploma programs of nursing. Currently, the North Dakota Board requires a 2-year preparation, or an associate degree, in nursing to qualify for licensed practical nurse licensure, and a 4-year, or baccalaureate degree, preparation for eligibility for licensure as a registered nurse. Although a number of attempts have been made, Maine is the only state to legislate a change in educational requirements for future nurses. The Maine nursing practice act authorizes a study of the need and impact of requiring 2- and 4-year academic preparation for nurses.

Licensure Examinations

The successful completion of an examination before licensure has widespread acceptance in nursing, as it has in other professions. If the state specifically mandates the examination requirement and actively supervises its implementation, the state protects itself from challenges regarding anticompetition. Thus in the development of licensure examinations it is critical that the examination be job-related to demonstrate that the examination is a necessary measure of competence.

The NCSBN, which produces the National Council Licensure Examinations (NCLEX) used by all the states and jurisdictions, routinely completes incumbent job analysis surveys to validate licensure examinations. Often various groups mistakenly think that the licensure examination should be a test of competencies that are expected on graduation from a program of nursing. The licensure examination must be based on what is required of a new licensee on entrance into the occupation or profession. In addition, in the past 10 years, the National Council initiated procedures to monitor adverse effects on minority groups. If adverse effects exist, an examination may be acceptable if it can demonstrate that it is specifically job-related. Before 1982 the licensure examination was scored by using a normative reference system. Since then, a criterion reference scoring system was adopted that establishes a passing point for the licensure examination based on minimum competency requirements. Consistent with the new scoring system, the results of the licensure examinations beginning in 1988 are reported by "pass" or "fail" instead of a numeric score. Because the primary purpose of the licensure examination is to provide determination of those who are and those who are not competent, according to a minimum requirement, it is appropriate that numeric scores not be released. Too often numeric scores are misinterpreted as achievement. Cognizant of the scoring and pass point issues in constructing a legally defensible and psychometrically valid examination, the NCSBN is conducting research to provide computer-based testing for the licensure examinations by the middle of the 1990s. Computer-adaptive testing and computer-simulated testing are methods predicted to offer refinements in the determination of competency for new nurse licensees.

Demographic Variables

Demographic variables and the implications for the regulation of nursing practice are issues of concern to nursing. Basically, because of distribution of licensees, it is appropriate for other individuals in a community to perform the same kinds of services that are performed by better prepared or qualified persons in geographical areas where distribution is lacking. This again raises the need for the state to consider setting essential standards for effective care that is available and accessible to all citizens. It is incumbent that the state set standards that are effective for all the citizens and not just for a selected few.

The "graying" of the American population is given a great deal of attention, as has indigent care and the projected AIDS epidemic. The care requirements for an aging population, for the increasing number of medically indigent individuals, and the victims of

AIDS is estimated to burden an already costly health care delivery system in the United States. The role of nursing will be essential in meeting these demands that no doubt will place new requirements on nursing licensees, particularly as they relate to educational preparation and the needed competencies.

Violations—reporting

Nursing practice acts are being revised to clearly state what is considered a violation of the law that gives cause for investigation of licensees or applicants. The revisions include the following:

1. Clarification of documentation on essential records
2. Using fraud to obtain a license
3. Misrepresentation as a nurse
4. Convictions (misdemeanors or felonies) that are related to the practice of nursing
5. Action taken in another licensure jurisdiction on a nursing license

Remember that legal and professional standards are used for different purposes and they originate for different reasons. Often, investigations of nursing practice and competence find that professional standards are stated too broadly to be enforced. Regulatory boards are subjected to challenge when the law is not specific enough to alert a licensee as to what is unfitness or incompetence in practice. Therefore more specificity is being added to nursing practice acts to clearly define violations or incompetence in practice.

Nursing practice acts are changing rapidly and it is anticipated that this trend will continue. The basic purpose of licensure must be the guidepost when changing the laws and there must be evidence of a rational relationship for requirements that are imposed. Without careful consideration of due process, boards of nursing will be increasingly challenged in regard to restriction of trade, antitrust issues, and constitutional rights of individuals.

Regulation of Advanced Nursing Practice

There is an old adage: "History repeats itself." In the regulation of the new specialty usually referred to as *advanced nursing practice,* this adage appears to be true. With the growth of specialty or advanced preparation of nurses, controversy within nursing persists over whether or not this new group of nurses should be regulated by the legal entity or by self-regulation through an evolutionary and professional process. This controversy is not unlike that which existed in England at the turn of the century, discussed earlier in this chapter.

The NCSBN completed a comprehensive survey of its members on the statutory and regulatory requirements for advanced nursing practice.[12] Because of the diversity of regulations for titles, requirements, qualifications, and bodies outside nursing involved in the regulation of advanced practice, it is difficult to summarize the survey information with any brevity. A few high points to describe the regulation of advanced practice in the United States will be presented.

There is a mix of statutory and regulatory authority for the definition of advanced practice and for the definition of scope of advanced practice in the states. Forty-two states indicate some type of authority existing in the statute or regulation for authorization of advanced practice of nursing by registered nurses. In some states, the authority is granted under the medical practice act; in others the public health code accommodates specialty groups, or authority is granted by a categorical licensing board responsible for the regulation of a number of the health professions and occupations. Twenty-four states have no definition for advanced practice beyond the basic nursing definition. Twenty-nine states have definitions in statute whereas eight have definitions in regulations. An even greater diversity exists for the definition of the scope of advanced practice with 19 states not having any definition for the scope of practice and 18 using a variety of approaches to define the scope according to role specialty description, standards and educational requirements, or by description of a general role. The scope of advanced practice is defined in statute for four states and in regulation for 22 states.

It is interesting to note that the data relates to advanced practice titles. Thirty-eight titles were used for the recognition of advanced practitioners by boards of nursing. Nine states include the title descriptions in statute and 23 include the title in regulation, whereas one state accepts the titles described by the state nurses' association.

Recognition of national certification to authorize advanced practice is the credentialing mechanism most frequently used (23 states). Five states confer individual certificates, nine states provide additional licensure, and 13 use no credentialing mechanism to authorize advanced practice. Again, a variety exists.

As stated earlier, each individual state or jurisdiction has specific processes and procedures for promulgating regulations based on enabling statutory language. In the instance of promulgating regulations for advanced practice, the mechanisms used include additional procedural features. Nine states were required to promulgate regulations for advanced practice jointly with medical boards; eight states were required to obtain consultation/collaboration with medical boards before promulgation of regulation; and 14 states indicate autonomy or unilateral capability in the promulgation of regulations. Twelve states have no mechanism to promulgate such regulations. In addition to the mechanisms just cited, nine states use task forces, state nursing associations, statutory practice councils made up of pharmacists, physicians, and advanced practitioners, and categorical licensing boards or consultation with the state board of pharmacy on prescription privileges for nurse practitioners. Further, several states issued only guidelines for practice, which are not enforceable.

There is little consistency for educational requirements for advanced practice. Eight states require a baccalaureate of science in nursing, five require a masters of science in nursing for certain categories of practitioners, and 14 states have no specification for educational requirements. Again, as with titling, 20 states report a wide variety of mechanisms for educational requirements and approval processes for evaluating such requirements. The requirements for postbasic education programs for advanced practitioners and the approval authority of such programs by boards of nursing varies significantly. Seventeen states report approval authority of postbasic educational programs, whereas 20 indicate that the board of nursing did not have approval authority. The types of programs often found acceptable or board-approved were certificate programs and collegiate programs.

The legal recognition of advanced nursing practitioners resulted in specified relationships between advanced nurse practitioners and physicians. This relationship can be a positive effort to practice in collaborative roles. Fifteen states require supervision of the nurse practitioner by a physician, eight require direction from a physician, and 17 require collaboration with a physician. Fourteen states did not indicate a need for a specified relationship. The relationships involve consultation and referral or are as formal as a written agreement between the advanced nurse practitioner and the "supervising" physician. Twenty states require the latter and 18 do not. Eight states report that a written agreement is not specified. These types of arrangements consist of protocols, specified procedures, or relationship agreements. The protocol developed jointly by the nurse and the physician is a frequent type of arrangement. Again, there is no uniform approach in the regulation of advanced nurse practitioners as reported by the states.

Interestingly, 20 states require some type of written agreement, 32 states permit independent practice, and only six specifically prohibit independent practice. Nine states did not specify whether the individual nurse practitioner may practice independently.

The issue of prescription authority for advanced nurse practitioners is one that raises legal challenges and concerns. Twenty states authorize prescription authority, twenty do not, and seven do not have such authority specified. Limitations on prescription authority include nurses writing prescriptions only for drugs listed in a formulary, specified by written agreement, by protocol and/or for no controlled substances. Seven states have provisions for prescription authority with varying approval processes for drugs identified in rules or regulations. Twelve states indicate that advanced practitioners have dispensary authority whereas 27 indicate none. Six states did not specify. Limitations on dispensary authority include over-the-counter drugs only, by formulary, specific written agreements, protocol and/or no controlled substances. A number of states require that the prescribed medication be prepackaged as unit dose.

More states require mandatory continuing education for advanced nurse practitioners for recertification or relicensure than they did for registered nurses or licensed practical nurses. Thirteen require mandatory continuing education and 31 indicate acceptance of requirements by national certifying bodies. (As a point of information, 17 states require mandatory continuing education for nurses who are not advanced nurse practitioners.) Other mechanisms to assure continuing competence for advanced practitioners were reported by 10 states. These mechanisms include recertification by national certifying bodies, letters of reference from professional team members, complaint processes, minimum hours worked for each renewal period, and professional performance review by peers.

Issues in the regulation of advanced practice given attention by organized nursing and regulatory entities include the following:

1. Deletion of collaborative relationship agreements
2. Consideration of a generic scope of practice to cover all specialty areas
3. Increasing the educational preparational requirement to a masters in nursing for all specialty practice areas

4. Statutory and regulatory provisions for prescription authority
5. Requirements for periodic recertification by all national certifying groups
6. Abolishment of continuing education requirements and tightening of peer review processes
7. Implementation of some method to recognize advanced practice, although not through a licensure process

The status of regulation of advanced nursing practice is a potpourri of requirements, qualifications, titles, and approval processes. Although there is no consensus on the legal recognition, the fact remains that there are 42 jurisdictions that give some form of legal recognition to advanced nursing practice. Boards of nursing have not initiated this recognition for new areas of specialization in practice but respond to influences brought by nurses to the legislative process. Obviously there is no prevailing method for regulation of advanced practice; however, there exists four major methods: registration/designation, recognition, certification, and licensure. NCSBN in its Position Paper on advanced clinical nursing practice comments on three of these methods as follows[12]:

As boards consider alternate methods of regulating advanced clinical nursing practice, there are three major choices: designation/recognition, certification, and licensure.

The least restrictive of these is designation/recognition. This alternative would not limit the right of any nurse to practice. Rather, it would provide the public with information about nurses with special credentials. Under this approach, nurses with state-recognized credentials in a specialty could receive permission from the Board of Nursing to represent themselves as specialists. The designation/recognition alternative would not involve state inquiry into competence.

Certification as a regulatory mechanism is used to signify that an individual has met state established requirements that include an investigation of competence in an area of advanced clinical nursing practice. Under this mechanism, practice would not be restricted as long as noncertified nurses do not represent themselves as state certified.

The most restrictive alternative would be to issue a special license to practitioners of advanced clinical nursing. This method limits practice within the specialty to those nurses who hold such a license. It would have the potential for restricting generalist practice and the normal evolution of basic nursing practice.

According to the position of the NCSBN, "The preferable method of regulating advanced nursing practice is designation/recognition because it is the least restrictive means for assuring the public health, safety, and welfare.[12] The least restrictive form of regulation insulates the regulatory entity from exposure on grounds of impingement on constitutional rights of individuals and violations of antitrust laws. In addition, a consistent use of designation/recognition decreases limits to mobility of the practitioner and costs to the regulatory body and ultimately to the consumer. Other effects include support for the evolution of nursing practice, lack of impediments in relationships between nurses and other health professionals, and the potential for conflict with statutes and regulations promulgated by other administrative agencies.

States that have experienced challenges to the regulation of nursing practice and expanded roles include Kansas, Louisiana, and Missouri. In these states, state medical societies initiated challenges based on the interpretation of nursing practice acts and nurses practicing in the expanded role.

EXAMPLE: In the case of *Sermchief v. Gonzales,* the Missouri Supreme Court set precedent by affirming a broad interpretation of the Nursing Practice Act in Missouri to include advanced practice rules. In Kentucky, the Kentucky Board of Medical Licensure proposed rules requiring direct supervision of advanced registered nurse practitioners by physicians. The tables turned and nursing challenged the medical board at a hearing before promulgation of the regulation. Subsequently, the proposed regulation was withdrawn.

A principle to keep in mind when regulating a given occupation is that of the public's right and need to know. A historic statement published by the ANA entitled, "Nursing, A Social Policy Statement," emphasizes the obligation and responsibility of a professional group to the society it serves. To that end, the adoption of uniform standards on a national scope is urgently needed so that the public will be better served and the talents and skills of nurses who have excelled in speciality or advanced practice will be recognized.

Practice of Nursing by Unlicensed Individuals

State and federal authorities, boards of nursing, and the nursing profession have expressed rightful concern over the proliferation of health care providers who are being introduced into various health care settings. Questions are raised on whether or not the duties of such workers as respiratory therapists, surgical technicians, dialysis technicians, and the ever increasing duties of nurse aides, constitute practicing nursing without a license. This concern is not new. Individuals performing nursing acts have been a concern to the nursing profession since the regulation of nursing in the United States in the early 1900s. At the turn of the century, nurses believed that the regulation of nursing would curb indiscriminate practice by unlicensed persons who were, for the most part, trained on-the-job. The early regulation of nursing did in fact assist in setting standards; however, all nursing was primarily custodial in nature and was not technologically oriented. The introduction of additional workers into health care delivery settings increased with technology. The knowledge, skill, and abilities needed to provide safe and effective nursing care requires academic preparation that equips an individual with the ability to intellectually make judgments in patient care. Although the complexity of patient care in today's health care delivery system is acknowledged, the role of nursing functions under shadows of misconception about the expertise needed to practice nursing. In a "Statement on The Nursing Activities of Unlicensed Persons," the National Council of State Boards of Nursing indicate that the use of unlicensed persons was encouraged by many health care businesses in an effort to control cost. Another justification cited for the employing of unlicensed persons is a shortage of licensed nurses. The use of unlicensed persons for the delivery of health care more than likely will increase.

Boards of nursing are concerned that nursing care be performed under the supervision of registered nurses. Registered nurses who delegate selected nursing functions or tasks assume the responsibility and accountability for safe care. In response to this situation, boards of nursing develop opinion statements to give guidance to registered nurses and licensed practical nurses in the delegation of nursing acts to unlicensed persons. A number of boards of nursing issue administrative rules that state what tasks may or may not be delegated and under what conditions delegations may be made. The burden of determining the competency of the person who will perform the task and of evaluating the situation rests with the licensed nurse.

NCSBN found in 1986 that 44 boards of nursing reported concern over unlicensed personnel administering medications and performing treatments and other activities in a multiplicity of settings. After studying this issue, the National Council of State Boards of Nursing wrote their conclusions (see box).[14]

These conclusions and the problem in which unlicensed persons are being substituted for licensed nurses indicate that a critical challenge exists for organized professional nursing to control the scope of nursing practice of licensed nurses and those individuals who assist them in delivering care.

Of recent concern to nursing are the provisions in the Nursing Home Reform Act of

---

NCSBN STATEMENT OF THE NURSING ACTIVITIES OF UNLICENSED PERSONS

1. Performance of non-nurse delegated and non-nurse supervised nursing activities by unlicensed persons constitutes practicing nursing without a license and is not in the interest of the health, safety and welfare of the public.

2. Language in nursing practice acts that allows poor supervision of nursing activities by non-nursing persons is inappropriate.

3. The interpretation of physician delegation clauses in medical practice acts that allows for physicians' delegation of nursing acts is inappropriate.

4. Pieces of care should not be provided in isolation by unlicensed persons functioning independently of the nurse if the health, safety and welfare of the public is to be assured.

5. Boards of nursing need to monitor guidelines and regulations of federal and state regulatory agencies with the understanding that the state's nursing practice act has the higher legal authority.

6. Boards of nursing need to work to assure evidence of adequate nurse involvement where nursing services are being provided.

7. Boards should promulgate clear rules on the utilization of unlicensed persons in all settings where nursing care is delivered.

8. Boards need to clearly define delegation in regulation.

9. A limited supply of nurses is not an excuse for the inappropriate utilization of unlicensed persons.

10. Boards must set standards based on the health, safety, and welfare of the public regardless of cost containment or arguments for lower standards.

11. Regulations regarding the delegation of nursing functions must be linked to the disciplinary process (for dealing with complaints against licensees).

12. Boards need to pursue criminal prosecution when there is clear evidence that unlicensed persons are performing nursing activities.

1987 that establishes federal requirements for training and evaluation of nurse aides. The provisions of this law (P.L. 100-203) require the state agency with jurisdiction over Medicaid to administer the nurse aid program or to contract with another agency in state government to monitor, register, and approve training programs for nurse aides employed in nursing home settings. Several states place the authority for the regulation of nurse aides under the jurisdiction of state boards of nursing, using the argument that if nurses are to delegate nursing tasks to nurse aides, then nursing should control that aspect of the nurse aide training and approval. Because the job description of nurse aides falls within nursing practice and licensed nurses are accountable for nursing care on a 24 hour per day basis in nursing homes, it is reasonable that boards of nursing would assume authority over the regulation of nurse aides. In addition, cohesiveness and consistency in regulation of nursing are facilitated by one state regulatory agency setting requirements for such practice and it would enable licensed nurses to exercise authority and the concomitant accountability in the provision of care by nurse aides.

FUTURE TRENDS IN REGULATION

The regulation of the health professions, including nursing, has and continues to be closely studied by state governmental regulatory groups, the federal government, independent and private organizations, and business groups. The focus of the study and concerns is cost containment and maintaining quality. Several other factors will influence future licensure trends; one of which is delivery of health care within corporate systems.

Corporate health care has grown rapidly in the past 15 years. Large hospital corporations with holdings extending to the international level are a way of life, as are corporations owning nursing homes on a national basis. Home health care is another area in which private industry is growing rapidly. This growth is not diminishing but is accelerating, due to emphasis on deinstitutionalizing care.

The vast complexities and array of differences in regulating health care workers, including the licensure of nurses, produce an environment that may encourage efforts to allow corporate credentialing mechanisms much akin to institutional licensure discussed in the past. It is not unreasonable to envision a corporation that operates nursing homes on a nationwide basis to lobby for control of credentialing of individuals who provide care. As a result of the current shortage of nurses, hospital corporations transfer nurses from one hospital to another, crossing state lines, which requires licensure of those nurses. "Mobile nurses" already exist within corporate health care systems. Cost alone for licensure of individual nurses may be an argument for looking at a different credentialing system for nurses in the future. Any change in credentialing nurses should be carefully evaluated to maintain the profession's autonomy, social significance, and identity.

The stress on cost containment and quality services may require stringent mechanisms for assuring competence of nurse licensees other than voluntary mechanisms to date. Periodic retesting for the generalist license currently issued to licensed practical/vocational nurses and registered nurses is under discussion, as is certification requirements for specialty practice. As the federal government exerts more control over health care through reimbursement programs such as Medicare and Medicaid, the idea of a national credentialing system for nurses may gain popularity. Although states likely will be reluctant to relinquish jurisdiction over such matters that relate directly to the public health, safety, and welfare, cost containment may be a single driving force that will eventually lead to the development of national credentialing.

Increased scrutiny by the FTC is anticipated particularly as it relates to the specialty practice of nursing. As indicated previously, the recognition to practice in the expanded role is dependent in many jurisdictions on certification by private bodies. Anticompetitive issues will surely arise. Pricing, advertising, monopolization or attempts to monopolize, practice arrangements that are exclusive, activities that restrain trade, and business practices of licensees are governed by such federal laws as the Sherman Antitrust Act, the Clayton Act, the Federal Trade Commission Act, and the Robinson-Patman Act. Careful scrutiny will be applied and nursing, like other health groups, will be monitored.

Whereas nursing is concerned about individuals who are not licensed and are practicing nursing, the medical profession may view nursing as infringing on medical practice in its efforts to gain prescription authority and treatment ability. Other groups that are seeking licensure will attempt to enter areas to practice that may in fact impinge on the scope of the practice of nursing. These include such groups as occupational therapists, physical therapists, counselors, nutritionists, paramedics, and emergency medical technicians. These groups will continue efforts to legitimize their practice by legal regulation, and such regulation will affect the scope of practice of nurses in the future.

•   •   •

In summary, the growth of regulation in this country is on a crash course with concerns for cost containment and quality care delivery systems. An expanded technology produces a myriad of health care workers, there are serious demographic and social issues, and an AIDS epidemic is projected. In the midst of the numerous controversies between federal and state government authorities, in and among health occupations, and the overriding concern of cost, states are obligated to protect their individual citizens by promulgation of requirements for the practice of all health care occupations within their borders. At the same time, they are influenced by powerful forces such as that of the federal government and corporate health care systems. As an integral part of health care, nursing has and continues to make a contribution, and that contribution is safeguarded by individual licensure of nurses. The question of individual licensure surviving cost containment measures, corporate control of health care, and federal influences for reimbursement of health care services is far from being answered in the context of essential health care being a right of all citizens.

STUDY ACTIVITIES

1. When did the first regulations of nursing begin?
2. Who, as US nurses, are credited with the earliest efforts to credential nurses?
3. What nation enacted the first licensing laws and when?

4. In what year did the state you reside in enact nurse licensure laws?
5. What do you think are some major challenges facing boards of nursing today?

REFERENCES

1. American Nurses' Association: The scope of nursing practice, Kansas City, MO, 1987, the American Nurses' Association.
2. Birnbach NS: Credentialing—chaos to accountability. In Fitzpatrick ML: Prologue to professionalism, Bowie, Maryland, 1983, Robert J Brady Co.
3. Cleveland VL: Professional/legal definitions: are there differences. Issues 1(1), 1980, Chicago, National Council of State Boards of Nursing.
4. Committee on Curriculum of the National League of Nursing: a curriculum guide for schools of nursing, New York, 1937, National League of Nursing Education.
5. Commonwealth of Virginia Policy review: The regulation of the health profession, Richmond, Virginia, 1983, Department of Health Regulatory Boards.
6. Council of State Governments: State government organization charts, Lexington, 1988, The Council of State Governments.
7. Flanagan L: One strong voice, Kansas City, 1976, American Nurses' Association.
8. Graddy EA and Nichol MB: Public members on occupational licensing boards: effects on legislative regulatory reforms, Los Angeles, 1988, University of Southern California.
9. Institute of Medicine: Allied health services: avoiding crises, Washington, DC, 1989, National Academy Press.
10. International Council of Nurses: Report on the regulation of nursing, Geneva, Switzerland, 1986, International Council of Nurses.
11. Massaro TM: Legal opinion on advanced practice, 1984, (Unpublished).
12. National Council of State Boards of Nursing: Position paper on advanced clinical nursing practice, Chicago, 1986, NCSBN.
13. National Council of State Boards of Nursing: Position paper on continued competence, Chicago, 1984, NCSBN.
14. National Council of State Boards of Nursing: Statement on the nursing activities of unlicensed persons, Chicago, 1988, NCSBN.
15. Professional Licensing Report: Washington, DC, October 1988, Paxton Associates.
16. *Sermchief v. Gonzales:* 660 S.W. 2d 683 (Missouri banc 1983).
17. U.S. Congress, Office of Technology Assessment: Nurse practitioners, physician assistants, and certified nurse-midwives: a policy analysis, (Health Technology Case Study 37), OTA-HCS-37, Washington, DC, December 1986, U.S. Government Printing Office.
18. U.S. Department of Health, Education and Welfare: Credentialing health manpower, Publication No. (OS) 77-50057, Washington, DC, 1977, U.S. Department of Health, Education and Welfare.

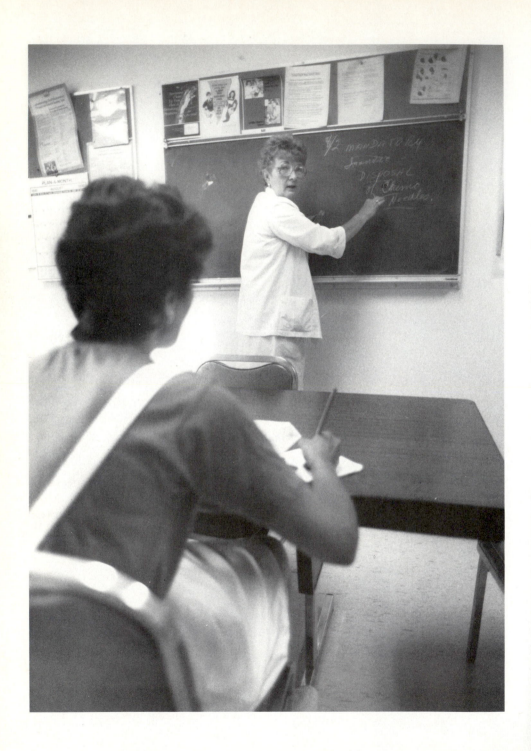

10

CONTINUING EDUCATION FOR RELICENSURE

Gloria Y. York

OBJECTIVES

After completing this chapter the reader should be able to:

- Discuss reasons why continuing education is necessary for nurses

- Identify who is credited with being the first nurse to recognize the need for continuing education

- Explain the history of continuing education for nurses since its beginnings in the early 1900s

- Explain the role of professional nursing organizations in the development of continuing education for nurses

- Explain the role of university schools of nursing in the development of continuing education for nurses

- Describe ways in which the federal government was supportive in the development of mandatory continuing education for nurses and other health professionals

- Discuss the challenges that face groups, organizations, and institutions offering continuing education for nurses

- Discuss some of the problems that must be addressed by boards of nursing as they relate to the multiplicity of continuing education providers, course offerings, and needs of nurses

DO NURSES NEED CONTINUING EDUCATION?

One of nursing's early founders, Florence Nightingale, identified the need for nurses of her day to continue learning after their training.[5] Today's need is even more acute, because nurses are challenged with keeping current in a field that is exploding with new information. Technical and scientific advances in medicine, and increasing consumer demand for high quality health care, increase the need for continued learning by nurses.[14] These advances are changing medical and nursing science so rapidly that nurses who graduated from nursing school five years ago are finding that some of their nursing education is already obsolete. New graduates can no longer feel confident because their nursing science and nursing theory courses are fresh in their memories. After graduation, they quickly discover they have tremendous amounts to learn in their first years out of school.

Today's nurses, like today's physicians, must contend with the information explosion. One way they are doing this is by becoming specialists in narrower fields of practice. Nursing specialization helps provide the overwhelming amount of information nurses need to know, but it does not extinguish the need for continued learning. The rapidity of advancement in medical science, even in specialized areas, must also be dealt with. This rapidity can be dealt with by nurses taking an active responsible role in their own continued growth and learning. Many nurses find this challenge exciting and seek out continuing education (CE) courses in their speciality area. These nurses are fulfilling the idea of CE as many of nursing's founders envisioned it.

CE TODAY

Nursing CE has seen many changes in the past 10 years. One of the most positive changes is a trend toward increased support. In California (the state that first mandated CE) the mandate stimulated more courses to be developed, and nurses report a greater quality and quantity of courses than in Michigan, a state that has not yet mandated CE.[16] The Florida State Board of Nursing has found the following information:

1. The mandate has been accepted by most nurses
2. Nurses have not failed to renew their licenses in increased numbers
3. CE costs are not escalating
4. The system is flexible
5. Administrative requirements are not prohibitive[15]

These studies indicate a growing satisfaction with mandated CE among nurses, and state board administrators who are using a mandated system. This does not mean that the states implementing the systems do not have problems. The task of setting up workable and equitable systems for providers, nurses, and consumers is tremendous. There are problems in any new regulatory system, and mandated CE is no exception. State nursing boards and accrediting agencies have problems setting up equitable regulations, setting up sufficient recording systems, and developing systems that make sure players in the CE scenarios conform to regulations. The most difficult tasks for the states have not been getting the nurses to conform, but assuring that providers of CE are conforming to standards that assure the development of quality courses.

A NEED FOR MORE SPECIFIC GUIDELINES

Since the first state passed mandatory CE for relicensure, there has been a growing number of CE providers, both profit and nonprofit organizations, with very few guidelines to help them develop CE courses. Today the American Nurses' Association (ANA) defines CE for nursing as "those planned educational activities intended to build upon the educational and experiential bases of the professional nurse for the enhancement of practice, education, administration, research, or theory development to the end of improving the health of the public."[1]

This statement is more of a goal for CE than a definition. Many courses could be said to fulfill the criteria of enhancing nurses' practice. For example, would a course in yoga enhance nursing skills in dealing with the stresses of caring for dying patients and allow nurses to be more responsive to patients and their families, thereby improving their practice of nursing and the health care they are delivering to the public?

With the lack of specific guidelines for providers, a wide disparity in the quality of nursing CE course content has developed. What the accrediting bodies wanted to create was a flexible definition of CE, to ensure that courses were developed to meet the educational needs of all nurses. This, in fact, is still a possibility.

However, there is a percentage of nurses who are not motivated to take CE courses addressing nursing topics, but seek out self-help courses (such as yoga) if they are accepted as appropriate content for CE. It is apparent to many providers that self-help courses are sometimes more popular and profitable than courses that deal with nursing practice. Because of this, many state boards and accrediting bodies are developing more specific nursing guidelines for CE in an effort to assure that courses provide high quality and appropriate content.

HISTORY OF CE IN NURSING

Most nursing CE literature identifies postgraduate courses as the earliest sources of CE for nurses. These courses were prevalent in the early 1900s and, for many years, were almost the only source of CE for nurses. Most of the postgraduate courses were offered by hospitals and provided training in selected clinical areas. Because there was no educational requirements for the courses, they often became a means for hospitals to obtain free help from course participants.[5]

In the 1920s, the ANA and the National League of Nursing Education sponsored institutes for nurses. Also, universities became involved. Lecture courses became more popular by the 1940s as nurses began to obtain college preparation for their profession. In-service education and refresher courses were available by the early 1930s, and the Social Security Act provided the first federal funds for CE in 1935.[3]

By 1941, New York developed the first statewide refresher program for inactive nurses. Federal legislation supporting refresher courses resulted in 1941 with Public Law 146 (77th Congress) and federal funds were allocated the following year. The Manpower Development and Training Act of 1962 makes provisions for many of the refresher courses offered today.[5]

In 1955, the University of Wisconsin department of nursing created an extension division to provide CE for nurses throughout the state. This started the trend for university schools of nursing to accept responsibility for nursing CE.[5]

The 1965 Title I of the Higher Education Assistance Act provided funds for some states to provide CE courses.[5] By 1970 the Carnegie Commission report on Higher Education and the Nation's Health stated that: "In view of the rapid rate of progress of medical and dental knowledge and the associated problem of educational obsolescence of practicing physicians and dentists, the Commission recommends the development of national requirements for periodic reexamination and recertification of physicians and dentists."[11]

In 1974 the Office of Prevention, Control, and Education of the National Heart, Lung, and Blood Institute initiated a review of continuing medical education. The report from this review states: "Conceivably, the issue of malpractice insurance may become linked to either recertification or relicensure as a means of reducing risk. Should that occur, effective continuing education would become essential to every physician as a means of ensuring his livelihood."[20]

These reports, and others with similar recommendations, have led many states to develop a system for monitoring and requiring CE for license renewal of physicians and nurses. In 1971, California became the first state to pass a law requiring CE for nursing relicensure.[6] By early 1988 there were 26 states that had mandated that nurses participate in CE as a requirement for relicensing.[23]

CHALLENGES FACING CE

CE for relicensure has not been welcomed by all. Some of the arguments against mandated CE are listed as follows[23]:

1. Participation in educational opportunities is no guarantee of learning
2. Education cannot be equated with competence and accountability
3. The mandate will result in programs designed for the median needs of all nurses, which will result in inferior learning opportunities for some nurses
4. It violates the principles of adult education to make education mandatory
5. There is no proof that what is taught in courses affects job performance

These arguments stimulate studies on motivational factors affecting attendance of CE offerings. Many studies conclude that most nurses attend CE opportunities by a desire for job improvement and advancement, and indicate that the more educated nurses are the most motivated to attend.[19] Studies in some midwestern states show 24% to 28% of nurses would not attend CE on a voluntary basis.[17,18] In one of these studies the typical profile of nonparticipants was documented as nurses who (1) worked part time in single nurse or chronic care settings, (2) had relatively low-level positions and (3) had no education beyond professional training. Apparently the nurses least likely to voluntarily attend CE offerings are the ones who might need them the most.[17]

These findings, as well as a lack of guidelines, present challenges for educators interested in developing high-quality courses for CE. How can accrediting agencies and providers meet the challenges? By determining appropriate audiences, subject matters, education levels, contact hours, medias, evaluation techniques, and costs for CE offerings.

What Nurses Need to Know

What do nurses need to know? Health care agencies, educational institutions, state boards, accrediting agencies, and independent providers all have difficulty finding the answer. Part of the difficulty in assessing learner needs is that nurses are a heterogeneous group. Some factors include the following:

1. Diversity of types of educational preparation
2. Diversity of speciality areas
3. Diversity of work settings
4. Diversity of types of job descriptions within each work setting

Programs frequently develop in health care settings because of needs identified by supervisors or by a few staff members. Often, after the development of programs, continuing educators discover there were only a few nurses who really needed to attend the offering. From a financial standpoint, no CE provider can afford to develop programs that only fill the needs of a handful of nurses. Part of the solution to this problem is for CE providers to conduct careful needs assessments of nurses' true professional learning needs.

Health care agencies have access to data that provides excellent opportunities to conduct valid needs assessments. In health care agencies, data can be collected in the following ways:

1. Interviews with supervisors and head nurses
2. Data from nursing care audits of patient records
3. Reports from quality assurance committees
4. Recommendations from JCAH*
5. Needs assessment surveys of staff[2]

Health care organizations have access to data about performance problems nurses have on the job. Nursing care audits and quality assurance reports, when used in conjunction with other needs assessment tools, can provide needs analyses that differentiate perceived learning needs from actual performance needs.

---

*The Joint Commission on Accreditation of Hospitals.

If assessment leads to the design and implementation of a CE course, this same data can be used to evaluate the success or failure of the program. Decreased incident reports, better patient care, and decreased nursing turnover are ways in which health care agencies can measure the success of CE.

Educational institutions and independent providers need to explore the demographics of the nurses in their target audiences before developing CE programs. If their courses are on site or seminar-type presentations the demographics of nurses in the close vicinities need to be researched, as well as how far nurses will travel for particular offerings. Reports from state boards, state nurses' associations, state affiliations of national professional specialty organizations, and data about nurses in local health care settings need to be collected so that nursing educators can decide to which audiences they can best provide CE programs.[2]

The point of mandating CE is to fulfill needs that exist for nurses to stay current. Astute nursing educators realize that needs assessments, and instruction designed according to those assessments, is where continuing education must be headed to be of value.

Appropriate Subject Matter

Many states adopt similar specifications for subject matter that is considered appropriate for CE. California's content statement is a good example:

The content of all courses of continuing education must be relevant to the practice of nursing and must: (a) be related to the scientific knowledge and/or technical skills required for the practice of nursing, or (b) be related to direct and/or indirect patient/client care. (c) Learning experiences are expected to enhance the knowledge of the Registered Nurse at a level above that required for licensure. Courses related to the scientific knowledge for the practice of nursing include basic and advanced courses in the physical, social, and behavioral sciences, as well as advanced nursing in general or specialty areas. Content which includes the application of scientific knowledge to patient care in addition to advanced nursing courses may include courses in related areas,...Courses in nursing administration, management, education, research, or other functional areas of nursing relating to indirect patient/client care would be acceptable. Courses which deal with self-improvement, changes in attitude, financial gain, and those courses designed for lay people are not acceptable for meeting requirements for license renewal.[12]

Although this statement is clear, abuses still exist. In the spring of 1988, a board member cited a California nursing school that offered a course in "Colors" for nurses! Because the nursing boards that approve the providers only ask for sample programs or outlines of sample programs, few courses that are offered for CE are actually reviewed. Additionally, reviewers, usually CE consultants to the boards, have extraordinarily large workloads.

This situation results in inappropriate CE courses. California Nursing Board members cite a lack of feedback from nurses as consumers as part of the problem. In light of this, the California Board may require that providers furnish a statement to nurses informing them that they should notify the board if the quality of the course is poor. As CE providers continue to increase in number and state boards are faced with the added workloads, feedback from nurses will become invaluable for boards trying to monitor providers.

Educational Level of Materials

At what entry level should CE courses be designed? The standard educational content is now left to the CE provider. Although many accrediting bodies would like to see the level of all CE courses rise above the baccalaureate course level, this would not fit the learning needs of all the groups involved. A system has not been developed for dividing nurses into more homogeneous target groups and monitoring each group to make sure they only take courses appropriate for their level of education. Until some type of standardized system is implemented, and providers required to use the system to place their programs in categories, a "shotgun" approach to content level will continue. The result is nurses, as consumers, have a difficult time ascertaining if courses will be at the appropriate educational level for them. However, even if state boards and accrediting bodies mandate that providers analyse their courses and rate them by such a system, they still would need to make courses on the lower levels available to nurses who are more highly educated. The rationale for this is, if it is an educational need, that need should be addressed.

Making lower-level courses available to all nurses is necessary, because there is a great demand by nurses for refresher courses in certain subject areas. This demand for review courses has caused an ideological dilemma among accrediting councils. For example, California's regulations state that "Learning experiences are expected to enhance the knowledge of the Registered Nurse at a level above that required for licensure.[12]" This statement, and ones like it in other states, has resulted in some courses that nurses are requesting to be deemed inappropriate for CE. However, courses such as Cardio-Pulmonary Resuscitation are considered acceptable in some states and can be used for relicensure in every renewal period. If the goal of CE is to provide nurses with knowledge and skills that will prevent obsolescence and enable them to provide safe patient care, how can educators ignore the issue of learner retention?

CE must include relearning in areas where nurses identify needs. If all courses must be above the participants' level of schooling to be appropriate for CE, the idea that every chapter and verse learned in school is permanently implanted in memory no matter how seldom called on to use, is unrealistic. The common quote "If you don't use it, you lose it" is appropriate here. In addition, no two humans leave any particular learning experience knowing the same thing. The whole concept of CE must be based on the realization that all individuals have different learning needs, no matter what their educational background. Continued learning must include learning new things, relearning old things, and revising new schemas to fit the pieces of information together.

CE Hours

In 1968 34 national organizations developed a standard measurement of educational activity other than collegiate credit. As a result the continuing education unit (CEU) was developed.[9] The CEU is defined as: "Ten contact hours of participation in an organized CE experience under responsible sponsorship, capable direction, and qualified instruction."[7]

A contact hour is 50 minutes long and equals 0.1 CEU. CEUs are awarded by providers of CE courses. If providers award CEUs to participants of the course programs, they are confirming that the programs meet the criteria set up by the Council on the Continuing Education Unit.[7] Fortunately, this system for measuring credit is accepted by all nursing boards as the standard for measuring CE. Each state sets its own standard for a number of CEUs needed for relicensure in a license renewal period. Most states fall somewhere in the 1.5 to 4.5 CEU range.

The problem with using contact hours as a measure of achievement is the acceptance of nontraditional learning modalities in CE. *Nontraditional* courses are not grouped or monitored meetings. For example, seminars are traditional classroom situations and contact hours are measured by the time participants are actually present at seminars "under responsible sponsorship, capable direction, and qualified instruction."[7] In home study, however, the amount of actual time spent depends on how long it takes individual learners to read materials, and if they simply look up answers to post-tests, or study materials until they can answer the questions closed book. (Participants may pass the post-test without following directions and spending time to study the course.)

In past nontraditional learning, the number of hours was assigned by providers estimating length of time participants would need to complete the programs. Before 1988, most state boards did not require that providers use a systematic approach to estimate the number of hours assigned to each course; nor did they require documentation that the courses actually took the amount of time assigned to them. Florida was the first state to address this problem by organizing a task force of continuing educators to develop specific guidelines for nontraditional learning modalities. Recommendations made in the fall of 1988 include suggestions that providers should retain documentation of summative evaluations that prove that average learner times are the same as the number of hours providers are assigning to courses.

Video, audio tapes, computer programs, and interactive video instruction (IVI) are also a part of nontraditional learning. Contact hours for linear video and audio tapes are considered easy to measure because tape playing times and average testing times will be only slightly variable among participants. In computer and interactive video programs, however, nurses may do several reviews, practice exercises, or select different submenus that contain expanded information on the subject. In other words, the content of the program and amount of detail presented to learners is learner controlled. With interactive video and computer programs, average participant completion times are not valid measurement tools for contact hours. If participants are not monitored, providers of these types of programs have to be able to justify learner self-reporting. Because self-reporting is not acceptable for written material, providers of written materials want to know why it should be acceptable for computer and interactive video programs. The solution to this problem is for providers of IVI and computer programs to offer these programs in a way that actual contact hours can be verified.

Home study providers maintain that seminar and group presentations frequently do not require participants to do anything but passively sit, and courses that are based on reading or responding (such as computer or interactive video programs) require much more participation. Participants may be learning more from home study programs and receiving less credit, because they are not monitored.

Predetermining credit based on averages of contact hours presents many problems for learners and providers alike. This system, which is basically the system used for all formal education, is here to stay. Many students probably feel that the four-credit chemistry course struggled through would have given eight credits if the college system could actually measure the work put into the course!

Appropriate Methods and Media

The first courses in CE for nurses were formal classroom programs and clinical practicums. Today, advanced technology not only influences how quickly fields of practice change, it influences the methods used to educate students about those changes. CE programs are offered via the medias of print, video tapes, computers, interactive videodisc systems, teleconferencing systems, and live presentations.

Nurses have the choice of obtaining CE credit offered in the following formats:

1. Seminars
2. Institutes
3. Conferences
4. Symposiums
5. Workshops
6. Home study
7. Teleconferences
8. Clinical practicums
9. Self-directed learning projects

Seminars, institutes, conferences, symposiums, workshops, and teleconferences are all popular group presentations that are frequently provided for large groups of nurses and marketed to large geographical areas. These large-group programs may be sponsored by health care organizations, professional nursing organizations, university schools of nursing, university departments of CE, national or state health care organizations, or private CE businesses. Home study courses are developed by these organizations in addition to nursing journal publishers and book publishers. Home study courses are marketed to large geographic cross sections of nurses. Courses prepared for nurses within the health care organizations use multiple formats and are provided for the employees of the organization and sometimes other nurses in the community. These courses may or may not be marketed to the nurses in the local or state community.

Self-directed learning is a process in which learners assume the initiative for identifying, developing, and evaluating their own learning activities. The ANA has published guidelines for nurses wishing to use this as an alternative to learning programs designed by others.[18] At present, not all states that have mandated CE allow nurses to use self-directed programs as an option for relicensure requirements. The criteria for approval in many states is basically the same as a provider has to develop for acquiring a provider number. The individual must submit a proposal before starting the learning experience. Although nurses using this alternative are increasing, the process is lengthy and may limit the growth of self-directed learning as a viable alternative for many nurses.[8]

Live presentations such as seminars, conferences, institutes, and symposiums may use two or three types of medias, e.g., oral presentations, written materials, and films or slides. Some home study courses combine video or audio tapes and written materials. Media selections make programs more interesting, and are designed for the convenience of the providers.

If instruction is systematically designed, the medias in which subjects are presented should be determined by the subject matters, and learner assessments. Ideally, analyses of the subjects, learners, and learning environments should be done before selection of the medias. Realistically, this is usually only done by professional instructional designers or companies who specialize in developing custom educational products. Most providers of CE programs provide subjects that will fit into their medias. Providers are involved in some of the following businesses:

1. Seminars
2. Journals
3. Home study courses
4. Computer programs
5. Interactive videos
6. Videos
7. Teleconferencing

Nursing educators, who are not restrained by having to produce programs in a particular media, can best develop CE programs that are appropriate for their learners and subjects. As the field of instructional design becomes more well known and health care organizations, nursing schools, specialty nursing organizations, and private providers become more aware of the increasing learning that takes place when media selection is a result of front-end analyses, professional help from this field will be used more often.

Educational Effectiveness of CE

Evaluation is gathering, analyzing, and interpreting indications of how well an instructional product or system performs.[10] The ANA states: "Evaluation is an integral, ongoing, and systematic quality assurance process of the continuing education provider unit and each program. Evaluation includes measuring the impact on the learner, and where possible, on the organization and on health care."[1]

Until 1988, evaluations were required by some regulatory agencies, e.g., the ANA, but not by many state boards. This lack of regulations led to variation in the number and quality of evaluation systems used by CE providers. It has also led to a gap in the amount of data on the effectiveness of the majority of CE programs and an inability of the nursing boards to more closely monitor the quality of CE offerings. In 1988, California and Florida enacted requirements for participant program evaluations as a part of the CE offerings.

Before these regulatory changes, most providers in these states developed only eval-

---

_____ TYPICAL QUESTIONS ON A HAPPINESS EVALUATION FORM _____

Did the offering meet your educational needs?
How would you rate the quality of the program?
Did the program meet the stated objectives?
Was the program well presented?
Will you use your new knowledge in your workplace?
What suggestions do you have for improvement of the program?
What other topics would you like to have offered?

---

uations to find out what topics nurses were interested in. Providers of traditional courses often only offer program evaluations or "happiness evaluations," which are question-naires presented at the end of courses asking participants to rate the offerings (see box).

Although these evaluations provide valuable information for providers about improving their programs, they do not measure what participants have learned or the effectiveness of programs. Unmonitored nontraditional programs develop post-tests to ascertain if participants have actually taken the course. The post-tests measure partici-pant satisfaction and learning as a result of the CE offerings.

Many state boards do not require that providers give post-tests, or that providers who do give post-tests require participants to achieve minimum passing scores. The lack of regulations for all providers to measure learning, and the lack of specifying standards for passing scores on post-tests, has been explained in the following way: There is no large scale documentation that CE has an effect on patient care. Nurses who take CE for reli-censure and have evidence of participation (i.e., monitored attendance or attempt at com-pleting a post-test) are entitled to CE credits. If the state boards specify that participants must show evidence of learning (i.e., an acceptable post-test score) and participants take courses and fail post-tests, these nurses could be denied renewal of their licenses and suspended from work until completion of their CE requirements. Some state boards feel they cannot defend the refusal of nurses' licenses on the basis of failed post-tests. They feel that nurses could challenge the assumption that the courses have a bearing on their ability to practice competently. Until more data exists to prove impact, some state boards are hesitant to require that participants pass post-tests.

Impact of CE

CE impact studies, conducted by some health care and educational institutions, result in cost-benefit analyses to health care agencies or research studies by universities. Nursing audits are used to determine effect of CE on patient care. Although some studies show a positive correlation between CE and impact on patient care, the results of most studies are mixed and portray a difficulty in establishing any CE correlation.[22] Nursing audits may measure the impact of CE courses on patient care, but other variables that cannot be controlled may be the reason for low impact scores. Some factors that influence patient care, and interfere with a positive correlation between education and increased job performance, include the following[13]:

1. Staffing patterns
2. Workload
3. Fluctuations in patient census
4. Variations in hospital and administrative support
5. Role modeling and motivational factors

Nurses in a study conducted at Marquette University, however, had an increased probability of practice change if the participants perceived the program as being applicable to their current nursing practice.[21]

The problem of low-impact correlations is caused by a general lack of thorough front-end analyses of performance problems. If, for example, IV medication errors are noted as a problem and tests reflect a lack of knowledge in this area, the solution might not be simply to develop an educational program. Nursing educators who understand the concept of front-end analyses know that although there might be educational needs, it may represent only a small portion of the reason for the performance discrepancy. A thorough analysis may reveal, in the case of the IV medication errors, some of the following examples:

1. The pharmacy packaged IV medications in a confusing way
2. The method established for staffing the floor is inadequate and nurses are making mistakes because their workload is too heavy
3. The system set up for doublechecking the medication may be ineffective
4. The unit may be very busy and kardexes not changed until many hours after orders are received

Cost Effectiveness of CE

The cost of assessments and developing, implementing, and evaluating CE often outweighs cost effectiveness. Independent providers and educational institutions must show a profit, or at least break even, to continue to provide CE courses. They cannot claim decreased incident reports, improved patient care, or less nursing turnover as an effect on their organizations' financial status.

Often, providers are more concerned with getting the most return for dollars spent on course development than on filling the learning needs of particular target groups. Many providers send mailers to all nurses in states in which they have provider numbers three to six months before the nurses' license renewal dates. Relying on the fact that many nurses procrastinate about obtaining their CEs, and often select courses out of interest, convenience, and price, rather than real learning needs, these providers get better responses than those who mail to groups targeted because of their learning needs. However, mail advertising response is about 1%.

The competition is strong between providers in states such as California and Florida, who have long offered mandatory CE. The competition, although helping to lower the cost of CE to nurse consumers, can also have negative effects. Cutting costs of program development and overestimating the number of hours assigned to a particular

CE offering is sometimes a method used by providers to stay in business. The problems caused by providers cutting quality and overestimating hours assigned to a course in order to compete caused California and Iowa State Nursing Boards, in the spring of 1988, to propose that all nurses taking home study courses be allowed only 1 hour of credit for every 2 hours of credit they received. This proposed change resulted in so much protest in both states that the proposal was dropped by state boards. But the problem of overestimating hours still exists, and California, Iowa, and Florida are developing stricter guidelines for providers in an effort to curtail this problem.

Providers must take the responsibility of careful and realistic program planning before beginning CE program development. Additionally, all accrediting agencies must develop stricter guidelines for providers, to prevent cutting quality, instead of using careful planning, to maintain cost effectiveness.

FUTURE RECOMMENDATIONS

With all the problems that exist, what is the future of CE in nursing? If the problems are analyzed, it appears that solutions to many of them will take time to resolve, but are never-the-less attainable. Although CE for relicensure has problems, it also has some positive effects. One educator found that because the large majority of nurses are women, the mandate helps to release the restrictions they place on themselves. The fact that CE is the law releases some nurses from feelings of guilt regarding spending additional time away from home and spending money on CE.[4] Another positive effect of increased availability and quality of courses in states where CE is mandatory might be contrasted with the problems caused by so many providers trying to compete for nurse participants. Although competition is keeping prices lower and increasing the availability of courses, it also causes problems for accrediting agencies, who must monitor providers who cut the quality of courses to offer their programs at competitive prices. Increasing provider regulations may help solve this problem. I suggest changes in regulations in the following areas:

1. Requirements that courses be categorized at specific education levels so that participants may choose courses appropriate for their education and learning needs
2. Requirements that providers furnish a statement to nurses informing them they should notify the board if the quality of the course is poor
3. Requirements that all courses develop post-tests to measure learning and course evaluations to collect data on quality of courses and actual time spent completing the courses; these should be kept as records for audits and studies by accrediting agencies
4. Requirements that providers use the expertise of credentialed educators, develop needs assessments for at least 25% of their offerings and providers that are of significant size, and measure and report at least one impact study per year
5. Requirements that providers help reduce board workloads by participating in peer review at least once a year

6. Requirements that all nurses take CE courses that have been identified by the state as being a large-scale learning need, (e.g., a study of AIDS) and requirements that nurses update their education in areas that have been added to nursing school curriculums (e.g., child abuse and substance abuse)
7. Revisions in the definition of CE to include review courses and courses that encompass all nursing learning needs

Besides these regulatory changes, state boards should conduct large-scale studies to help establish general needs assessments and the impact of CE on nursing practice. Because large-scale studies could be used to justify CE for all licensed professions, funds from all of the Departments of Consumer Affairs could be used for the studies. States with large nursing populations could pool resources and obtain funds from the Federal Department of Education. Biennium large-scale needs assessments could be conducted. Providers could be required to offer at least one of the topics that was identified in these studies.

•   •   •

These studies and regulations would increase the accountability of providers and nurses, and lead to improved CE systems. Nurses are a highly motivated and dynamic group of professionals. If states continue to mandate CE for relicensure, they must also mandate higher standards. Many nursing educators are eager to meet the challenges of nurses' learning needs. As professionals, they want to offer nurses the best possible CE system.

STUDY ACTIVITIES

1. What was the first state to require continuing education (CE) as mandatory for relicensure?
2. Describe the development of CE for nurses, beginning with the early 1900s to the present.
3. What are some of the pro and con arguments regarding the issue of mandatory CE for relicensure?
4. Does the state in which you reside or plan to practice nursing have mandatory CE for relicensure?

REFERENCES

1. American Nurses' Association: Standards for continuing education in nursing, Kansas City, 1984, American Nurses' Association.
2. Bell EA: Needs assessment in continuing education: designing a system that works, J Continu Educat Nurs 17(4):112, 1986.
3. Bowser MR: Selected factors related to participation in continuing education of dental hygienists, nurses, and physical therapists, Doctoral thesis, 1979, University of Pittsburgh.
4. Brooks CM: In defense of mandate, J Continu Educat Nurs 19(3):129, 1988.
5. Cooper SS and Hornback MS: Continuing nursing education, New York, 1973, McGraw-Hill.
6. Cooper SS and Neal MC, eds: Perspectives on continuing education in nursing, California, 1980, NURSCO.
7. Council on the Continuing Education Unit: criteria and guidelines for use of the continuing education unit, Silver Springs, 1979.
8. De Silets L: Self-directed learning in voluntary and mandatory continuing education programs, J Continu Educat Nurs 17(3):81, 1986.
9. Dolphin P and Holtzclaw BJ: Continuing education in nursing, Virginia, 1983, Reston Publishing Co, Inc.
10. Gagne RM and Briggs LJ: Principles of instructional design, New York, 1974, Holt, Rinehart and Winston, Inc.

11. Hennelly M et al., eds: Higher education and the nation's health: a digest of the Carnegie Commission on Higher Education, Berkeley, CA, 1974, McGraw-Hill.
12. Laws Relating to Nursing Education Licensure-Practice with Rules and Regulations, section 1456, pg. 84, Sacramento, 1985, California Board of Registered Nursing.
13. Meservy D and Monsond MA: Impact of continuing education on nursing practice and quality of patient care, J Continu Educat Nurs 18(6):214, 1987.
14. O'Conner AB: Nursing staff development and continuing education, Canada, 1986, Little, Brown and Co.
15. Penny JT: Mandatory continuing education for Florida nurses: a description of the second biennium (1981-1983), Jacksonville, 1985, Florida State Board of Nursing.
16. Pituch MJ: Perceptions of nurses toward mandatory CE (Doctoral dissertation, University of Michigan, 1979), Ann Arbor, Mich, 1979, University Microfilms International.
17. Puetz BE: Providing an empirical basis: legislating a CE requirement for licensure renewal, J Continu Educat Nurs 14(5):5, 1983.
18. Schoen DC: Continuing education and the professional orientation of nurses, Res Nurs Health 5:183, 1982.
19. Urbano M, et al.: What really motivates nurses to participate in mandatory professional continuing education? J Continu Educat Nurs 19(1):38, 1988.
20. US Department of Health, Education and Welfare: Competence in the medical professions: a strategy. Hyattsville, MD, 1974, US Department of Health, Education and Welfare.
21. Wake M: Effective instruction in continuing education, J Continu Educat Nurs 18(6):188, 1987.
22. Warmuth J: In search of impact of continuing education, J Continu Educat Nurs 18(1):4, 1987.
23. Weiss-Farnan P and Reynold W: Mandatory continuing education: the discussions a decade apart, J Continu Educat Nurs 19(2):73, 1988.

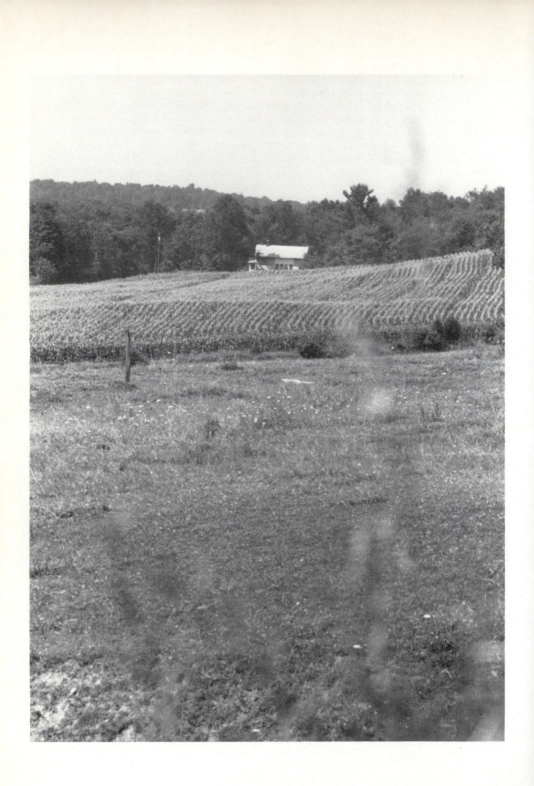

CHAPTER 11

RURAL NURSING

Heidi R. Sulis
Grace L. Deloughery

OBJECTIVES

After completing this chapter the reader should be able to:

*   Identify some features of rural areas that affect health of people residing there

*   Identify two major populations that reside in rural areas

*   Discuss some governmental interventions that were developed to improve health of underserved and vulnerable populations, especially those in rural areas

*   Describe development of the Frontier Nursing Service and its contribution to rural health

*   Discuss ways in which nurses can develop a professional practice and make a contribution to improve health of people in rural areas

The delivery of quality health care to Americans living in rural communities has become one of the most challenging and intransigent problems in our modern society.[14]

The delivery of health care in rural areas historically has been neglected, and presently continues to be inadequate and beset with problems. Although the American system of health care is highly acclaimed as one of the best in the world, there are areas in the United States where health care is less advanced. On the contrary, it is, at best, rudimentary and hardly sufficient for some populations. One group for whom this is true is the rural population.

In many rural areas of the United States the health care systems are characterized by blatant problems that influence health status and the overall delivery of health care. Basically these gross deficiencies encompass the following areas:

1. Limited accessibility
2. Limited affordability
3. Inequities in the reimbursement system (urban versus rural)
4. Inadequate attention of the national statistical system(s) to rural areas, resulting in a paucity of information and data
5. Insufficient political support and voice
6. Limited availability—there are disproportionately fewer numbers of practitioners and facilities in rural areas, resulting in fewer alternatives for the individual

Breindel et al.[6] claim that "people in rural areas have traditionally lacked knowledge of the choices that might be available to them regarding health care, and they have historically had to rely on acceptance of available health care irrespective of its quality or quantity."

In essence, these problems are demonstrated by higher infant mortality rates, higher incidence of certain chronic diseases, and higher incidence of accidents (especially related to mining and farming occupations). The status of health care in rural communities is profoundly affected, and negatively compounded by geographical, sociological and economic factors, including poor roads and other deficiencies of transportation, the sparsity of population in many rural areas, the disproportionate share of elderly people and low-income families with greater health needs than average, and, generally speaking, lower educational levels. [6,8]

DEFINITIONS

Any thorough examination and assessment of a problem requires some understanding of its past. Thus, to adequately describe and discuss the delivery of health and nursing care in rural areas, it is necessary to look at the definition of *rural* as a literal term and concept, as well as the relevant events and actions that take place, with or without impact, on the evolving process of rural health care. It is only with a historical perspective that one can understand and accurately evaluate the existing situation and its companion problems.

No single concept or definition of "rural" dominates in policy formulations, analytic work, or popular literature. While the lack of consistency is frustrating, most of the diversity is a legitimate reflection of the multidimensional character of rural life. But this diversity does not imply that the many definitions are arbitrary matters that can be approached casually. Indeed, the multidimensional nature of rural is precisely why its definition and the resulting implications for the rural data system must be approached thoughtfully and with special care.[9]

As defined by the US Census,* *rural* means "the population not classified as urban." (It is easy to understand why its meaning often becomes ambiguous and deceptively simple.) However, despite the difficulty in the definition of the idea of rural, the word carries some characteristic distinctions.

Rural is not a homogeneous classification. Geographically, the term includes areas that are remote and isolated, as well as communities that border major Standard Metropolitan Statistical Areas (SMSAs). Although rural inhabitants live in places of fewer than 2500 people, this in itself does not lend any uniform meaning to the concept of rurality. Population density, size of settlement, distance to services, resource base, and physical environment are characteristics that distinguish rural from urban areas.[9]

Furthermore, the people residing in rural areas are not homogeneous, on several levels: educational, income or occupational. Some occupations include farming, mining, fishing, small industry, and recreational enterprises. Yet despite the disparity that exists among rural residents, Reynolds insists there is an element of commonality between them. He claims that common features characterizing rural areas include the following:

1. Sparse populations
2. Low family income
3. Unemployment
4. Poor schools
5. Inadequate to almost nonexistent health care systems

All of the listed features exacerbate the problems accompanying the shortage of health care personnel in rural areas.[15]

Today, 26.3% of our entire population live in rural areas of the United States.[21] In the first half of this century, the US population increased from 90 to 150 million people. The rural population also increased at this time, but as a percentage of the total population, rural inhabitants decreased from 60% to 36%.[20]

Typically, the rural population is divided into two categories—farm and nonfarm. The rural nonfarm population consists of people living in the open country (2/3) or in small towns (1/3) and outnumbers the rural farm population by about 7:1.[10] Hassinger states that it is the farm portion of the rural population that has declined sharply since the 1920s. In 1920, the farm population represented 30% of the total US population.[10] Today, further decline of our farm population is even more threatened by the most acute agricultural crisis since the Great Depression. Not only is the present crisis rooted in decades of agricultural policy oriented to large-scale, technologically sophisticated, and heavily capitalized farming, but in a number of other variables that force thousands of families off the farm.

Since 1980, the growing strength of the dollar, high interest rates, low livestock and crop prices, declining land values, ever-mounting debt loads, government programs, and tax policies increasingly favor the larger producer, and unfavorable weather patterns have added to the stressful and severe economic conditions in rural agrarian America.

---

*The US Census is commonly used throughout the nursing literature.

In 1983, national net farm income dropped to its lowest level since 1971, and by 1984 farm debt in the United States climbed to over 216 billion dollars. This debt continues to grow and unfortunately is primarily concentrated among operators heading for insolvency. Nationally, farm families and community based businesses face land values declining at rates greater than 50% from pre-1980 appraisals. Correspondingly, real estate collateral for loans has diminished, creating stressed banking and loan situations, arbitrary loan terminations, and ultimately, foreclosures. If these trends continue, over 80% of currently existing farms will no longer exist by the year 2000 and almost all black-owned family farms will be gone by 1990.[1]

Rural communities have lost, in the past 10 to 20 years, financial security, farming families, businesses, vitality, and self-esteem. Ironically, these factors create perhaps the greatest need and demand for health care services in decades. The impact and net result of financial stress have often been severe. "Strained and broken marriages, spouse and child abuse, misuse of drugs and alcohol, frustration, anger, violence, grief, and depression and suicide are no longer uncommon.'"[1]

TRENDS IN EVOLUTION OF RURAL HEALTH CARE

Deficiencies unique to the rural population were recognized as far back as the Civil War, and since the late 1800s numerous attempts, originating at local, state, and national levels, have been implemented to provide or improve health services for these populations (see box). A summation of the relevant issues and events highlighting the continuum of trends in the evolution of rural health care will follow.

These programs have involved social actions in many spheres[16]:

1. The organized prevention of disease, communicable and other
2. Efforts to improve the distribution of physicians and allied health manpower emanating from several governmental levels and from voluntary efforts
3. The construction of health facilities with federal subsidies and special priorities for rural areas
4. Programs for particularly disadvantaged rural groups such as migratory farm workers or American Indians
5. Efforts to improve or maintain the quality of medical care in rural districts
6. Measures to increase the economic accessibility of care
7. The movement to strengthen overall health service planning

Health problems specific to rural areas were first formally introduced and addressed in 1862 in the First Report by the Commissioner of Agriculture to President Lincoln. In this report Dr. W.W. Hall claimed, "the high incidence of insanity and respiratory disease among farm people, the hazard of miasmas around farm houses, gastrointestinal problems associated with the use of outdoor privies, and the longevity of farmers to be 'not so great as we might suppose.'"[16]

In an attempt to establish the evolution of public health activity in the delivery of rural health care, one can look back to 1797 when Massachusetts established a system of local

_____ SIGNIFICANT EVENTS IN THE EVOLUTION OF RURAL HEALTH CARE _____

1797	Massachusetts established local boards of health
1862	First Report by the Commissioner of Agriculture to President Lincoln
1865	Development of the Rockefeller Sanitary Commission (later known as the International Health Board)
1921	The Sheppard-Towner Act
1935	Passage of the Social Security Act
1935	Launching of the Voluntary Prepaid Health Plan program
1946	Enactment of the Hospital Survey and Construction Act (also known as the Hill Burton Act)
1950s	United Mine Workers of America Welfare and Retirement Fund
1957	The Sears Roebuck Foundation introduced the Community Medical Assistance Program (CMAP)
1965	Medicaid and Medicare programs initiated
1960 to 1970s	Establishment of (1) Regional Medical Program (RMP), (2) National Health Services Corps (NHSC), (3) Health in Underserved Areas (HURA), and (4) Rural Health Initiative (RHI)
mid-1970s	Establishment of the Community Health Centers Program
1977	The Rural Health Clinic Services Act amended Titles XVIII and XIX of the Social Security Act
1978	Department of Health, Education and Welfare established agreement with the Farmer's Home Administration to allow low-interest loans

boards of health. Connecticut followed in 1805, but subsequent efforts continued slowly, until the Civil War, at which time only seven states had provided for local boards of health.

By 1865, at termination of the Civil War, progress toward improving health in rural areas renewed vigorously. Probably the two most influential institutions responsible for the early development of full-time rural health service were the Rockefeller Sanitary Commission (later known as the International Health Board), whose principal interest was in hookworm disease, and the US Public Health Service.[12] It was also at this time that the first health departments, for systemic protection of preventive service, were organized on a county basis, rather than on a city basis.

The Sheppard-Towner Act of 1921 helped strengthen rural county health departments by providing federal grants to states for supporting maternal and child health stations; however, by 1929, this support was terminated under the conservative administration of Herbert Hoover. 1929 marked the beginning of the Great Depression and this essentially halted all rural, as well as urban, health efforts.

By the early 1930s, one-fifth of the rural counties in the United States had a full-time public health service, though fewer than 50 of them were sufficiently staffed and budgeted. Thus, generally speaking, early public health efforts in rural areas were rudimentary. Local health departments, dependent on, but not satisfied by, external or outside financial support systems to provide efficient full-time health services, could only offer limit-

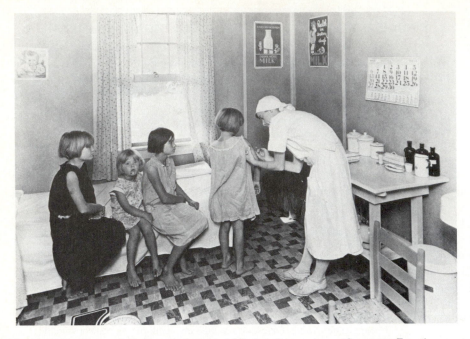

Innoculations were a vital aspect of early public health nursing. *(Courtesy Frontier Nursing Service.)*

ed services through the 1930s. Furthermore, there was a lack of competency, or at best, adequate training among the health offices in rural areas. This compounded or certainly contributed to the slow development of health care and services in these environments.

It was not until 1935, with the passage of the Social Security Act, that efforts to improve the public's health resumed in both rural and urban areas. The Social Security Act is noteworthy because its passage brought some rather dramatic changes in government's role in public policy and health care. It was the government's first attempt to share in the responsibility for the public's health. It was also the major federal program for the provision of maternal and child health, until the passage of Medicaid in 1965.

Included in the Social Security Act of 1935 were Titles V and VI. Title V benefited urban and rural areas by providing federal grant money to the states for both maternal and child health services and crippled children's services. Title VI (terminated in 1946) of the original Social Security Act gave grants to the state and local health departments for public health work.

Another program of the 1930s was the Voluntary Prepaid Health Plan, set up by the US Farm Security Administration in 1935. This was an example of a federal program that was specifically directed to low income farm families and implemented to deal with rural health problems. This program was designed to furnish and improve the delivery of medical services, including general practitioner care, dental services, and hospitalization and surgical services, to dependent farm families through the concept of voluntary group action.[17]

At its peak in 1942, over 600,000 people in 1100 rural counties were enrolled in the program, but by the mid-1940s the program began to decline because there were not enough enrollees to make it viable. To be successful, it should have been available to all rural farmers, not just those who were borrowers from the Farm Security Administration. This solution, or dilemma, highlights the problem of how to collectivize a geographically scattered population, which is so often characteristic of rural populations. Eventually, after World War II and subsequent withdrawal of federal funds, the program ceased.

By 1940, the shortage of rural health practitioners became acute with only 18.6% located in rural areas, a highly disproportionate amount given the fact that 43.5% of the total population lived in rural areas. World War II brought a lack of financial resources, which, combined with a lack of human resources, attributed to a period of decline in rural health care facilities and the delivery of services.[17]

It was hoped that the enactment of the Hospital Survey and Construction Act of 1946, better known as the Hill Burton Act, would address the problem of disproportionate physician/practitioner distribution, but it actually had little effect on enhancing physician recruitment to rural areas. Other attempts to solve this problem of distribution were of no avail; recruitment and retention were, and still remain, difficult problems.

One significant rural program of the 1950s was the United Mine Workers of America Welfare and Retirement Fund, which provided a full range of health services benefits for miners and their families, and is claimed to have had a significant impact on the medical care delivery system in Southern Appalachia. But when the bottom fell out of the coal industry in the early 1960s, financial difficulties plagued the Fund, and like so many other previous attempts to boost services and accessibility in rural areas, this one became unstable and ineffective.[4]

In 1957, the Sears Roebuck Foundation introduced its Community Medical Assistance Program (CMAP) to assist rural communities in building medical clinic facilities. As with the Hill Burton Act, this effort was based on the assumption that modern new facilities would enhance physician recruitment to rural areas.[4]

During the existence of this program, from 1958 to 1970, a total of 625 communities completed the survey, and 253 of them were accepted into the program by the Foundation. Within this 12-year span, the CMAP provided design, fund-raising, and planning assistance to 165 physicians' offices in rural areas. However, the turnover rate was high, with approximately 30% of the recruited physicians leaving after 1 year or less. Thus, while this attempt demonstrated that a new facility had some ability to lure a new physician into the area, it had a very short-term effect and failed to anticipate or deal with the problem of retention.

Many health care programs developed in the 1960s were also characterized by inequities with regard to rural populations. The Medicaid and Medicare programs were initiated in 1965 as amendments to the Social Security Act of 1935, with a major goal of improving access to health care for the disadvantaged. However, as Kathleen Murrin claims in *Management of Rural Primary Care—Concepts and Cases,* "the medically underserved rural population represented a significant gap in the programs' intent. Both Medicare and Medicaid discriminated against rural communities through lower reimbursement levels for the same kinds of services provided in urban areas with higher prevailing charges."[4]

There were numerous attempts, though sporadic and sometimes late, to implement, increase, and improve health care in rural areas. Unfortunately, none of these efforts was characterized by longevity; in fact, the effect was very short-term. The ultimate effect that these efforts had on the overall situation of health care in rural areas is debatable. What cannot be argued is that by the mid to late 1960s, there was substantial deterioration of rural health care resources, resulting in considerable national concern.

At this time the federal government became actively involved and began to sponsor direct programs to combat further erosion. Between 1970 and 1980, millions of dollars in grant funding were provided for the following efforts:

Regional Medical Programs (RMP)

National Health Service Corps (NHSC)

Health Underserved Rural Areas Program (HURA)

Rural Health Initiative (RHI)

Community Health Centers Program

Migrant Health Program

Rural Health Services Clinic Act

Farmers Home Administration Rural Health Facility Loan Program

One of the earliest Congressional attempts to improve access and availability of health care services to rural areas resulted in the development of the Regional Medical Programs, initiated in the mid-1960s and established throughout the United States. The inception of this program was largely in response to widespread concern, from public and professional parties, regarding the need to institute effective and efficient mechanisms for providing education, research opportunities, and health resources to rural areas, thereby improving the physical, mental, and social well-being of many underserved populations. This effort to stimulate initiative and innovation at the regional level through planning, coordinating, and sharing limited health care resources and facilities was thought to be the most effective way of providing and maximizing the quality and quantity of care and services available to populations of many rural regions.

The Regional Medical Programs became particularly instrumental in improving the care of patients with heart disease, cancer, and stroke, but also focused on the following issues:

1. Biochemical screening (Missouri)
2. Development of a comprehensive utilization and patient information statistical system (Connecticut)
3. Provision of optimum clinical lab services for 3 million people (Connecticut)
4. A multimedia approach to enhance the learning of health science personnel (Colorado and Wyoming)
5. A telephone network for continuing education (Central New York)
6. Continuing education for physicians (West Virginia and the District of Columbia)
7. Guest resident programs (Maine)
8. Studies to determine whether comprehensive, family-oriented health care in a neighborhood Health Center, coordinated with an automated multiphase screening

lab, could result in improved mortality, morbidity, health service use, and health attitudes (Tennessee-Mid-South)

By the end of 1967, 54 such programs were established throughout the United States and continued into the 1970s until dwindling federal funding and support led to their demise. As Milton Roemer said, "Except for the recent major cutbacks in federal Regional Medical Program funds, this program was helping to extend the qualitative influence of the urban medical center to rural locations."[16]

The National Health Service Corps was the first federal effort designed to directly place physicians and other health professionals in rural areas. As the NHSC increased in size, it shifted from the development of self-sufficient rural practices to become the staffing mechanism for other federal rural health projects.[17]

Health in Underserved Rural Areas (HURA) was established in 1974 to develop comprehensive health care systems for underserved populations in rural areas. These programs include primary care, radiology, dentistry, pharmacy services, and other specialized programs in an area-wide network of health services.[3] The Rural Health Initiative (RHI) was an administrative effort to improve the development of health care systems in rural areas by managing and integrating the activities and resources of all existing federal programs operating in rural areas.

All four of the preceding efforts—RMP, NHSC, HURA, and RHI—implemented in the 1960s and 1970s represented joint ventures between the federal government and local communities. Whereas HURA emphasized research and evaluation of existing models delivering health care, RHI was an effort to efficiently direct federal resources toward the development of comprehensive primary care delivery systems in rural areas.

The Community Health Centers Program, combining three independent programs—the Neighborhood Health Centers (NHC), Family Health Centers (FHC), and the Community Health Networks (CHN)—was established to support ambulatory health care projects in areas with scarce or nonexistent health services.

In 1977, the Rural Health Clinic Services Act amended Titles XVIII and XIX of the Social Security Act to permit cost-related Medicare reimbursement for nurse practitioner and physician assistant services provided by health care centers in rural, federally designated, medically underserved areas. Implementation of this law was gradual, with only a small proportion of the clinics participating, and many states unwilling to promote the program. This is largely attributed to inertia, strained state Medicaid budgets, complexities of the cost reimbursement formula, excessive paperwork, inadequate load to make certification worthwhile, and physician opposition.[17]

In 1978, the Department of Health, Education and Welfare embarked on an agreement with the Farmer's Home Administration (Department of Agriculture) under which rural health centers, supported by RHI funding, could acquire low-interest loans for facility construction.

Essentially, the extensive efforts of the 1970s resulted in the diffusion of federal monies through a wide variety of programs that too often duplicated and overlapped each other. It is not surprising then, that the 1970s received criticism for this and the fact that the delivery of health care in rural areas did not markedly improve during this time.

Unfortunately, the majority of efforts that occurred with regard to delivery of health care in rural areas were too often characterized by fragmentation, duplication, ineffectiveness, and finally, lack of longevity, thus perpetuating a critical situation in our country. In fact, Rosenblatt and Moscovice[17] refer to it as a *rural health care crisis,* claiming "the study of rural health care shows that the government tends to go from crisis to crisis, rather than coming to grips with the true, underlying problems of rural health care." They argue that rural programs have consistently been developed without sufficient thought regarding concurrent technological processes, and concern about the consequences on rural residents.

Breindel et al.[6] share similar concerns with Rosenblatt and Moscovice and claim that "too often, rural communities have been approached as if they were without talent and competence." Plans and models were superimposed on a community fabric that was misunderstood, mistrusted, and discounted.

Up to this point, primary emphasis was placed on government's attempts to improve the delivery of health care in rural areas. Although many of these met with failure, or at least not noteworthy success, other private efforts to improve the system of health care in rural areas are successful. The Frontier Nursing Service (FNS) is an example of successful planning in a rural area.

FRONTIER NURSING SERVICE

The FNS, located in Hyden, Kentucky, was founded in 1925 by a pioneering woman and nurse, Mary Breckinridge, a member of a prominent Kentucky family, who decided to devote her life to the health care of women and children after her own two children died in their early childhood.

Today, FNS provides preventive, primary, and acute secondary care to approximately 20,000 people, involving four counties and inhabiting a 700 square-mile mountainous area of the Appalachian region of southeastern Kentucky. FNS is a decentralized system of health care, providing its services through a hospital, four district clinics, and a home health care program via an extensive network of certified nurse-midwives and family nurse practitioners, and supported by a small number of physicians.

Nothing in Mary Breckinridge's origins or upbringing would have led one to guess that she would become one of the greatest nurses in history, to follow in the footsteps of Florence Nightingale and Clara Barton. Her great achievements lay in introducing into the United States the concept of the trained nurse-midwife, modeled on those of the British Isles, and in establishing a demonstration project of complete family health care in a remote rural area through the organization which she founded in 1925 and directed until her death in 1965—the Frontier Nursing Service.   (Marvin Breckinridge Patterson)[5]

Life of Mary Breckinridge

Much as I loved my people and much as I enjoyed the life I led, especially when it was in forests and on lakes and streams, I chafed at the complete lack of purpose in the things I was allowed to do. Several times I suggested to my mother that it would be nice to do something use-ful, but I never got anywhere with such an idea. I could range freely and read deeply. That was considered enough until I made up my mind whom I wanted to marry, and this I didn't do right away.[5]   (Mary Breckinridge)[5]

Mary Breckinridge, founder and director of FNS until her death in 1965, was mar-ried twice and had two children. Her first husband died; her second marriage ended in divorce. The death of her children, and especially of her son, Breckie, at the age of four, profoundly affected her and propelled her into a new career—nursing.

After graduating from St. Luke's Hospital School of Nursing in New York in 1910, Mary Breckinridge began to travel as a spokesperson for the Children's Bureau. She went to France during World War I to work with the American Committee for Devastated France. It was during this time that she met a British nurse and midwife—an event that led her to eventually study nurse-midwifery at the British Hospital for Mothers and Babies in London and that motivated her to think about alternative options for delivering quality care in America.

In France midwives were not nurses. In America nurses were not midwives. In England trained women were both nurses and midwives. After I had met British nurse-midwives, first in France and then on my visits to London, it grew upon me that nurse-midwifery was the logical response to the needs of the young child in rural America. But in America much had been done for city children, whereas remotely rural children had been neglected. My work would be for them.[5]

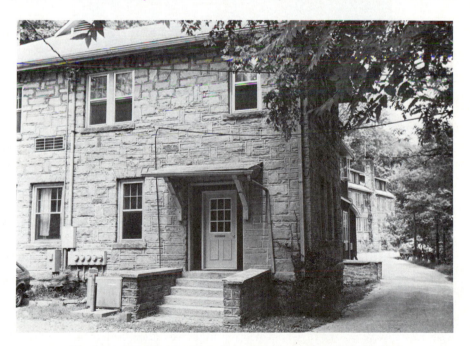

The Mary Breckinridge Hospital. *(Photo by Gabrielle Beasley.)*

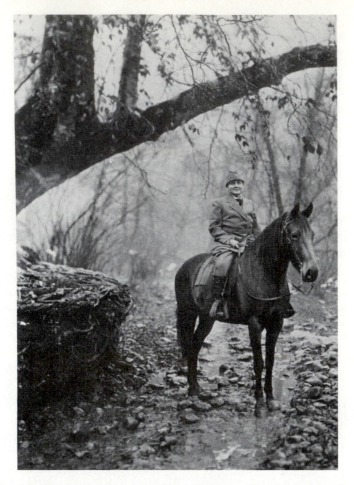

Mary Breckinridge on horseback in 1930. *(Courtesy Frontier Nursing Service.)*

After completing her work in France, Mary Breckinridge returned to the States to supplement her education by taking a year of courses in public health nursing at Teachers College, Columbia University; after which she began her work in the remote regions of Southeastern Kentucky.

A native of Kentucky, Mary Breckinridge set out during the summer of 1923, on her own initiative and with her own money, to survey Leslie, Knott, and Owsley Counties. Traveling alone and spending nights in mountaineer cabins, she covered nearly 700 miles on horseback before completing her survey. She learned from the people what their greatest needs were and how they might best be met. During this time, she interviewed 53 midwives, most of whom became midwives after their own families were grown, to help neighbor women who had no other means of support or help. She found many of them intelligent, and over $1/3$ were of greater than average ability. Nevertheless, at the end of her journey she concluded, "...the care given women in childbirth and their babies, thousands of them in thousands of square miles, was as medieval as the nursing care of the sick in the public hospitals in France."[5]

Because of the survey and her goal to help women and children in an area where infant and maternal mortality rates were high, Mrs. Breckinridge decided to focus her efforts, and ultimately devote her life, to the mountains of southeastern Kentucky. At the time, there were no roads within 60 miles, and not one licensed physician in the county. She felt that if her efforts and plans were successful in such an inaccessible area, they could be successful anywhere. "I felt that if the work I had in mind could be done there, it could be duplicated anywhere else in the United States with less effort."[5]

After her adventurous and enlightening summer, Mary Breckinridge returned to London where she studied nurse-midwifery at the British Hospital for Mothers and Babies. After completing this program, she thought it would be beneficial to gain additional exposure in an environment similar to that where she wished to ultimately settle—Leslie County, Kentucky. Therefore she went to Scotland where she observed the work of The Highlands and Island Medical and Nursing Service, which provided the kind of decentralized care that became the model for FNS.

She returned to the United States in 1925 and created the nucleus of the FNS at the first meeting of a "Kentucky Committee for Mothers and Babies," (renamed in 1928 as the Frontier Nursing Service.)

Early Development

The objectives of the FNS, as originally stated in the Articles of Incorporation, identify the nurse-midwife as the major provider of primary health services. The objectives, recently amended in June, 1984, read as follows:

To safeguard the lives and health of mothers and children by providing and preparing trained nurse-midwives for rural areas where there is inadequate medical service; to give skilled care to women in childbirth; to give nursing care to the sick of both sexes and all ages; to establish, own, maintain and operate hospitals, clinics, nursing centers and midwife training schools for graduate nurses; to carry out preventive public health measures; to educate the rural population in the laws of health, and parents in baby hygiene and child care; to provide expert social service; to obtain medical, dental and surgical services for those who need them, at a price they can afford to pay; to promote the general welfare of the elderly and handicapped; to ameliorate economic conditions inimical to health and growth, and to conduct research toward that end; to do any and all other things in any way incident to, or connected with, these objects, and, in pursuit of them, to cooperate with individuals and with organizations private, state or federal; and through the fulfillment of these aims to advance the cause of health, social welfare and economic independence in rural districts with the help of their own leading citizens.

The Articles of Incorporation of the Frontier Nursing Service, Article III

In 1925, with the first nurse-midwives recruited from England, Mary Breckinridge began the FNS, with headquarters in Wendover, located four miles from Hyden.

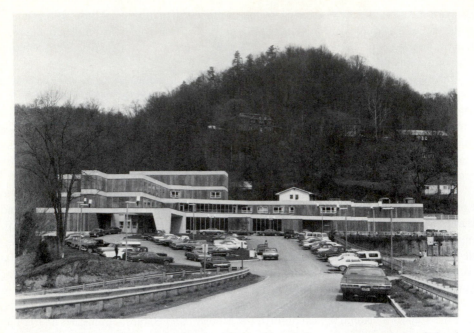

The Morton Gill Building, originally the Hyden Hospital, now home of the School of Midwifery and Family Nursing. *(Courtesy Frontier Nursing Service.)*

As she said in her book, *Wide Neighborhoods,* "First we must give a demonstration in a remotely rural area of the value of nurse-midwives and only then backed by statistical findings, would we be ready to awaken public interest in the development of the nurse as a midwife."[5]

One of the first organizational steps was the establishment of the Hyden Hospital and Health Center (1928) and six outpost nursing centers built between 1927 and 1930. The outpost clinics (now called district clinics) were built along two major rivers in the area, the Middle Fork of the Kentucky, and the Red Bird River, because the rivers provided transportation in those days. The outposts were located in Leslie and the adjoining counties of Clay and Perry, and were placed between 9 to 12 miles apart. Each clinic was staffed by a nurse-midwife and became a "district" of the FNS service region. By 1930, the FNS nurse-midwives provided bedside nursing, midwifery, and public health nursing and education to nearly 10,000 people in a 700 square mile area. Starting from Wendover or the Hyden Hospital and spending one night at each site, it took Mrs. Breckinridge 7 days to complete rounds of all the outpost clinics, because the terrain was rugged and travel was very rough at times. Transportation did not change substantially until the 1940s when roads were built in Leslie County, after which the organization began using jeeps.

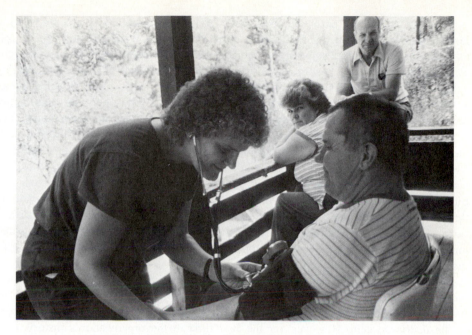

A family nurse practitioner (FNP) visiting patient at home.

FNS Today

The FNS Graduate School of Midwifery was established in 1939, and in 1970 the school was expanded to include a graduate program in family nursing. Also highlighting the 1970s was the opening of the Mary Breckinridge Hospital (MBH) in 1975. This 40-bed facility, which remains in operation today, replaced the original 25-bed Hyden Hospital. Today, the MBH features an outpatient clinic, emergency services, social services, surgery, x-ray, laboratory, physical and respiratory therapy, a labor and delivery suite, a birthing room, and a nursery.

In addition to the Frontier School of Midwifery and Family Nursing and the Mary Breckinridge Hospital, the FNS presently comprises eight other practices, including the following:

1. The Hyden Clinic, located within the hospital
2. The Hyden Medical Center, situated in a small shopping plaza two miles from the hospital
3. The Kate Ireland Women's Health Care Center, which is adjacent to the hospital
4. A home health agency
5. Four district nursing clinics, two of which are in the adjacent counties of Clay and Harlan

The four district clinics are between 8 to 40 miles from the hospital.

Staffing patterns for each site vary. The Hyden Clinic is staffed by a pediatrician, a family practice physician, 1.5 family nurse practitioners, and a support staff. The hospital additionally employs a surgeon, 1.5 family nurse practitioners for day-time emergency room coverage, and a host of ancillary staff. The Hyden Medical Center is staffed by a cardiologist, an internist, and a support staff; and the Women's Center is staffed by an obstetrician/gynecologist, five certified nurse-midwives (CNMs), one part-time family nurse practitioner (FNP), a licensed practical nurse (LPN), aide, and receptionist. The CNMs also work in the hospital and in a number of neighboring county health departments. The home health agency employs an RN coordinator and four additional full-time RNs, as well as five nursing assistants, a billing manager, and secretary. The district clinics are managed by FNPs and supported by very small ancillary staffs. Of the four district practices, the smallest has only one FNP and a receptionist, whereas the remaining three each consist of two FNPs, one secretary/receptionist, and one aide. The qualifications of the nurses and nurse practitioners vary from diploma and certificate-prepared nurses to Bachelor Degree (or dually prepared Bachelor Degrees) and Masters-prepared individuals.

Because the districts are licensed as rural health clinics, the state requires that a physician visit each site at least once a week. Due to periodic problems of short-staffing, this regulation has, at times, imposed difficult constraints on the delivery of health care in the district system. However, for the first time in the organization's history, FNS employs a family practice physician to work exclusively with the district nurses and home health agency. This is an exciting development and promises greater stability and continuity of care. Already results can be seen of the tremendous advantages of consistent physician presence and collaborative practice through significant increases in patient encounters when compared to the preceding year's statistics. With 3 months remaining in the current fiscal year, three of the five rural health clinics have already attained 90% to 97% of last year's visits; the other two clinics have attained 72% and 82%, giving clear indication of continuous growth.

Average numbers of clinic visits vary from site to site, ranging between 330 to 420 per month (18-day month) at four of the sites, and at 165 per month at the smallest and most isolated clinic. The FNPs average between 11 and 15 visits per day. FNP and physician fees are listed in the box.

FNP AND PHYSICIAN FEES

Patient Diagnosis	Fee ($)	
	FNP	Physician
Single uncomplicated problem	22	27
Multiple uncomplicated problem	30	35
New major problem	40	45

FNS Finances

For more than 40 years, the budget of the FNS was dependent on charitable contributions from donors throughout the United States. Today, contributions in total dollars are at the highest level in the organization's 64-year history—but these dollars only represent 10% of total annual revenue.

The significant rise in health care costs and the introduction of Medicare and Medicaid in 1966 changed the complexion of health care financing in the United States, and the complexion of the FNS.

Today, 80% of FNS revenue is derived from patient services, 10% comes from charitable contributions, and 10% from income on the organization's investment funds. Regarding expenses, more than 40% are related to personnel costs—not unlike most health care organizations, which tend to be labor-intensive. From 1980 to 1988, the annual operating budget of the FNS grew from $4.5 million to $9.6 million.

ARNP Practice

Working in collaborative practice with the district and staff physicians, Advanced Registered Nurse Practitioners (ARNPs) follow written protocols, known as the *Medical Directives of the Frontier Nursing Service*, that are mutually developed by FNS physicians and ARNPs. It is this type of joint practice that characterizes the current model of the FNS. Although FNPs still perform some of the functions more directly associated with nursing, they also assume many functions that traditionally were performed by physicians. Particularly with regard to the family nurse practitioner, Isaacs points out:

The primary care nurse helps to combine preventive measures with the management of common health problems. Heavy emphasis is placed on helping family to cope with their own health problem. The aim is to lessen the need for costly hospitalization and nursing home care. If the health care system is organized in a manner whereby primary care is readily accessible with good specialty care linkages, much can be done to lessen chronic disability and perhaps maintain and revive the community spirit that used to be so vital in the development of this county.[7]

Indeed, ARNPs perform routine health care and immediate urgent care, treat most common medical problems, and provide patient education and counseling. The latter elements often characterize the unique and special elements of their practice.

Browne and Isaacs report the following common disorders in this area[7] (in order of decreasing incidence):
1. Upper respiratory infections
2. Otitis media
3. Hypertension
4. Arteriosclerotic heart disease
5. Influenza and bronchitis
6. Kidney and urinary tract infection
7. Diabetes mellitus
8. Chronic obstructive pulmonary disease

They further claim that the majority of illnesses (75%) can be diagnosed and managed by the FNP. "She also screens patients and directs them to appropriate health and social services. She is a port of entry to the health care system for many."[11]

Undoubtedly, FNPs and nurse-midwives, serving as primary health care providers since the establishment of the FNS in 1925, play a vital, and crucial, role in improving health care in their area. Beasley reports the following statistics: With regard to FNS's first 10,000 births, most of which were delivered in the home (approximately 75%), nurse-midwives achieved a maternal mortality rate of 11 per 10,000 live births, at a time when the nation, as well as the state of Kentucky, carried a rate of 34 per 10,000 live births.

Today, FNS boasts a maternal mortality rate of zero. Furthermore, during the mid-1950s, the FNS delivered more than 500 babies each year in an area that hosted the highest birth rate in the nation. But between 1960 and 1970, the birth rate decreased by 60% and the annual number of births decreased by 30%, while at the same time the population increased by 7% and the proportion of childbearing women increased by 2%. This improvement can be largely attributed to pracitutioners' active involvement in intensive family planning efforts.[2] Today Leslie County has a birth rate of 15.2 and an infant mortality rate of 12.9.[19]

In the Mountains and Beyond

Clearly, FNS evolved to meet the changing needs of its immediate target population, and those of the state and federal health care systems as well. Sometimes these changes came about with great energy and enthusiasm; but at other junctures they occurred through a more painful and arduous struggle.

As discussed earlier in the chapter, the problems associated with and often so characteristic of rural health care have at times certainly confronted the FNS—and all too often with relentless persistence. Chief among these are the lack of prescriptive privileges for ARNPs in the state of Kentucky, compounded by the recruitment and retention of professional staff and an unsteady financial system made further vulnerable by the national health care environment that has become increasingly precarious itself, especially in rural areas. These problems continually challenge the organization's longstanding mission, and adversely affect the practitioners' full potential and ability to provide for their patients.

Despite the fact that regulations of the state nursing board support and advocate prescriptive privileges for the ARNPs the lack thereof, made evident through the lack of supporting state legislation, definitely impedes the current practice of FNS practitioners and all of their colleagues throughout the state. Compounding this problem are gradual but profound changes within other state professional boards, i.e., the Medical Association and Pharmacy Board, which have resulted in a number of imposed restrictions and constraints on the ARNP practice.

A small group of ARNPs from Kentucky, known as the *Kentucky Coalition of Nurse Practitioners and Midwives,* collectivized in September of 1987 to combat this critical issue. One of their first tasks was to determine how many nurse practitioners (NPs), nurse-midwives (NMs), nurse anesthetists, and clinical specialists (517) were practicing in the state. After reviewing state records, they learned that approximately 215 NPs and NMs are currently practicing in Kentucky.

The Coalition's priority was to obtain prescriptive privilege legislation for the ARNPs in Kentucky. Several meetings of interested ARNPs, the Kentucky State Nurses' Association, and a political action lobbyist led to many discussions as to how to proceed toward this goal and what language to use in creating such a bill. Unfortunately, the Coalition's efforts occurred well into the legislative session, resulting in a handicap of time.

When the Coalition and newly-formed bill met resistance from the Medical Association, the executive director of the Kentucky Nurses' Association (KNA) began to support the Coalition's activities and cause... with this reasoning:

In Kentucky 33% of the patients who are seen in NPs and NMs earn less than $15,000 per year, most of these people have little or no health insurance benefits; there are only two clinics in the state for the homeless, both are run by NPs; 50% of Kentucky NPs and NMs work in rural, under-served areas; and finally, NPs are the bulk of prenatal and indigent care providers in the state.[18]

Through letters and, later, testimony, many physicians joined the effort to persuade the legislators of the need to provide nurse practitioners with prescriptive privileges. Consumers/patients were also asked to write letters of support and call their individual legislators.

Ultimately, the Chairman of the House Health and Welfare Committee sponsored the bill, which precipitated rounds of hearings, testimony, and distribution of data to educate the legislature about this important issue. Although the bill never passed committee, the Coalition's efforts hadn't gone unnoticed, and certainly with regard to harnessing statewide resources, and through exposure and initial steps at educating both public sectors, significant gains were made. Further impetus was given to work even harder, and the Coalition is currently doing just that. As Michael Sheets optimistically ended his article, "we are prepared to win our case next time around".[18]

Thus earlier obstacles to smooth running of the FNS—no roads, no transportation, no electricity, no means of obtaining any kind of health care—have been either rectified or resolved, but there are plenty of new obstacles today and it is ironic to think that they are potentially even more threatening to the delivery of health care than the obstacles of 40 to 60 years ago.

However, as reported by the National Rural Health Association (NRHA) in their most recent newsletter, "there is a strong base of support for rural health issues in the Congress as is evidenced by the membership of the House Rural Health Care Coalition and the Senate Rural Health Caucus."[13] The House Coalition, founded in February, 1987, is a bipartisan group of 100 members of the House. It has set the following three main goals:

1. Medicare reimbursement equity
2. Reduction of rural health manpower shortages
3. Increased support for rural health services in general

Similarly, the NRHA has a full legislative agenda for 1989, including the following focal points:

1. Equity in Medicare payments
2. Federal coordination of rural health policy
3. State rural health access plans
4. Rural health clinics
5. Funding for rural health programs

The NRHA supports legislation to eliminate the urban-rural differential (up to 50%) in Diagnosis Related Group (DRG) standardized amounts, and, as the sole plaintiff, has filed a lawsuit against the federal government Health Care Finance Administration (HCFA), challenging the inequity of DRG payments to rural hospitals. The Association also supports a refinement of the area wage index to accurately reflect the cost of labor for rural hospitals, and legislation to eliminate the geographic differentials in payments to physicians.

Because access to primary care services is inhibited by acute shortages of health professionals and hospital closures and because rural areas have a higher percentage of uninsured and higher rates of infant mortality, chronic illness, accidents and disability, the NRHA supports expanded Medicaid coverage of prenatal, obstetrical, and perinatal care. It also supports and seeks expanded Medicaid and Medicare coverage for preventive and primary care.

The Rural Health Clinic Services Act of 1977 envisioned 2000 clinics by 1990, but there are only 450 such clinics in existence today. The NRHA recommends amending the Rural Health Clinic Services Act to promote the creation of more clinics to increase access to primary care services in rural areas. NRHA suggests that federally funded community and migrant health centers should automatically be eligible for Medicare and Medicaid reimbursement under the Rural Health Clinic Services Act. It is also their belief that states should be given greater flexibility in designating underserved areas to qualify for reimbursement under this act.

Finally, the NRHA advocates continued support of many rural health programs, including Community and Migrant Health Centers, the National Health Services Corps, the Area Health Education Centers, the Maternal and Child Health Block Grant Program, Primary Care Health Professions Education (including nursing and allied health), the Rural Hospital Transition Grants Program, and Rural Health Research.

In addition to the political challenges on state and national levels, the culture and physical environment specific to this region of the country are also challenging. The FNS is based in Leslie County, an area partially defined by the Daniel Boone National Forest, the rugged Appalachian mountains, and paved and unpaved roads alike. Hyden is a small town, with a population of approximately 600 people, and offers coal mining as its primary industry. It is a relatively immobile society with perhaps the greatest transient activity centering around the FNS. As one might expect, family fabric is tightly knit and the extended family plays a specific and important role in this culture.

Working for the FNS provides many individuals with their first experience in a new region of the country; in an isolated rural area; in a new and different culture and lifestyle, characterized by a different language or speech pattern, set of values, etc; in an area where the county literacy rate is over 30%, the number of inhabitants below the federal poverty level is 34.1%,* and a fluctuating unemployment rate hovers around 15%; and finally in an area that has been scrutinized, studied, and at times ravaged by good and bad intentions alike, which has left this population leery and cautious of outsiders.

Continual success of providing health care in this area requires an understanding of the educational, political, and economic values specific to this culture, the ramifications they have on health care and finally, the necessary creativity and commitment required to deliver care that is acceptable, accessible, and affordable. Finding ways to educate those who cannot read, realizing the blunt reality that when a mine closes in a depressed economy it so often means the immediate loss of all health insurance for its employees, and trying to arouse financial support in an area deplete of resources are just a few examples of what factors influence health care in this area. The challenge is obviously multifaceted and requires a willingness to cross cultural barriers to truly implement change.

However, characteristic of most challenges, the resulting rewards—gradual but progressive success in meeting need by providing services otherwise unobtainable, lowering maternal and infant mortality rates, influencing positive change in diet and nutrition, learning about and becoming educated by a new culture, and forming lasting and genuine relationships with mountain folk—can be infinitely satisfying and worthwhile elements of a rural practice.

Indeed, the FNS family nurse practitioners and certified nurse-midwives have played, and continue to play, an integral role in the delivery of health care in southeastern Kentucky. Without a doubt, Mary Breckinridge was a true innovator for developing a system of health care with a nucleus formed by nurse-midwives and family nurse practitioners. She met her initial goals with success. She demonstrated the value of the nurse-midwife, and was instrumental in awakening public interest regarding the development of the nurse as a midwife and family nurse practitioner. However, the viability of her successes are being challenged, and felt especially hard in rural areas where ironically there is such tremendous need for cost-effective, quality health care. A renewed effort to explore and establish systems to prepare and use nurses more effectively is appropriate and essential to the improvement of rural health care.

Rosenblatt and Moscovice[17] claim that extensive literature concerning the use of ARNPs in rural areas supports evidence that ARNPs provide acceptable quality of care, yield high patient satisfaction, and are cost-effective. Certainly this is characteristic of FNS experience, in which nurses play a vital role in improving the population's health care, make great strides in raising the population's consciousness, and teach people to become more responsible for their own health.

• • •

Especially regarding delivery of rural health care, every avenue that will empower and strengthen the nursing profession must be vigorously pursued. As

---

*Health Resources Developmnet Branch, Kentucky cabinet of Human Resources.

Mary Breckinridge summarized at the conclusion of a chapter in *Wide Neighbor-hoods*[5]:

"At the beginning of this long chapter I explained why a program which combined bedside and public health with midwifery was peculiarly suited to remotely rural nursing. After more than a quarter-century of experience, it is my conviction that bedside nursing and public health will always yield better results, each in its own field, when they are carried on together. I think now, as I did in 1926, when I wrote the following words to Miss Morgan and Mrs. Dike, in answer to an inquiry from them about my old nursing service in France: 'Adaptations are more administrative than anything else. The basic principle of nursing the sick in their homes, and through that human touch creating a spirit of public health to prevent sickness, is peculiar to the people of no one nation. The nurse who tends the sick only, and teaches nothing and prevents nothing, is abortive in her work. On the other hand the nurse who attempts instruction and prevention without combining with them an appreciation of the sickbed, and without meeting its appeal, has failed in the one element which differentiates her profession from all others and out of which it was created.'"

STUDY QUESTIONS

1. What are some of the critical health problems in rural America today?
2. Describe possible practice/career opportunities for nurses in rural areas.
3. Name at least one well-known example of nurses who have developed nursing practice into a system that provides health care to people to rural areas.

REFERENCES

1. Advisory Council on Church and Society and the Presbyterian Hunger Program: Rural community in crisis: a report from rural America to the Presbyterian church (USA), New York, May 1986.
2. Beasley RWB: After office hours: coping with family planning in a rural area, Obstet Gynecol 41(1):155, 1973.
3. Bernstein JD, Hege FP, and Farran CC: Rural health centers in the United States. Rural Health Center Development Series, no. 1. Cambridge, Mass, 1979, Ballinger Publishing Co.
4. Bisbee GE Jr, ed: Management of rural primary care—concepts and cases, Chicago, Ill, 1982, The Hospital Research and Education Trust.
5. Breckinridge M: Wide neighborhoods: the story of the frontier nursing service, Lexington, Ky, 1952, The University Press of Kentucky.
6. Breindel CL et al.: Marketing strategies in rural areas, J Ambulat Care Manage 4:15, Nov 1981.
7. Browne HE and Isaacs G: The frontier nursing service: the primary care nurse in the community hospital, American J Obstet Gynecol 124(1):14, 1976.
8. Ford TR, ed: Rural USA Persistence and Change, Ames, Iowa, 1978, Iowa State University Press.
9. Gilford DM, Nelson GL, and Ingram L, eds: 101 Rural American in Passage: statistics for policy, Washington, DC: 1981, National Academy Press.
10. Hassinger EW: Rural health organization: social networks and regionalization, Ames, Iowa, 1982, Iowa State University Press.
11. Isaacs G: The frontier nursing service: family nursing in rural areas, Clinical Obstet Gynecol 15(2):394, 1972.
12. Mustard HS: Rural health practice, New York, 1983, The Commonwealth Fund.
13. National Rural Health Association: NRHA/NACHC Joint task force on rural health report reveals inadequate funding for the nation's community health centers, Rural Health Care, 11:1, Jan-Feb, 1989.
14. Nolan RL and Schwartz JL, eds: Rural and appalachian health, Ill, 1973, Charles C. Thomas, Pub.
15. Reynolds RC et al.: The health of a rural country: perspectives and problems, Gainesville, Fla, 1976, The University Presses of Florida.

16. Roemer MI: Rural health care, St. Louis, Missouri, 1976, C.V. Mosby Co.
17. Rosenblatt RA and Moscovice IS: Rural health care, New York, 1982, John Wiley and Sons, Inc.
18. Sheets MA: NPs and nurse midwives organize in Kentucky, Council of Primary Health Care Nurse Practitioners Newsletter II:3, 1988.
19. State Center for Health Statistics: 1984 Vital Statistics Report, Department for Health Services, Division of State Health Planning, Health Information Branch, Frankfort, Kentucky, 1986.
20. US Bureau of the Census: Historical statistics of the United States: colonial times to 1970, Part 1, Washington, DC, GPO.
21. US Bureau of the Census: Statistical abstract of the United States: 1984, 104th ed, Washington, DC, 1983.
22. US Department of Health, Education and Welfare: Proceedings: conference-Workshop on RMPs (Vols. I and II), January 1968, National Institute of Health, Public Health Service.

ADDITIONAL READINGS

Banahan BF et al.: Evaluation of the use of rural health clinics: knowledge, attitudes, and behaviors of consumers, Public Health Reports, 97(3):261, 1982.

Ford TR: The Southern Appalachian region: a survey, Lexington, Kentucky, 1962, University Press of Kentucky.

Goldsmith SB: Management of health manpower in rural ambulatory care programs: responding to the trends, J Ambulat Care Manage 5:77, Feb 1982.

Goldsmith SB: Rural health personnel: management issues in availability, recruitment, and hospital relationships, J Ambulat Care Manage 5(4):49, Nov 1982.

Hassinger EW and Whiting LR: Rural health services: organization, delivery and use, Ames, Iowa, 1976, Iowa State University Press.

McCleary E: Delivery of health care in rural America, Chicago, Ill, 1977, American Hospital Association.

Moscovice IS et al.: Rural health care delivery amidst federal retrenchment: lessons from the Robert Wood Johnson Foundation's Rural Practice Project, American J Public Health 72(12):1380, Dec 1982.

Mott FD and Roemer M: Rural health and medical care, New York, 1948, McGraw Hill Book Co.

Rosenblatt RA: Planning ensures local referral care for remote rural areas, Hospitals 53:83, Nov 1979.

Sharpe TR et al.: Evaluation of the use of rural health clinics: attitudes and behaviors of primary care physicians in service areas of nurse practitioner clinics, Public Health Reports 97(6):566, Nov-Dec 1982.

Tripp-Reimer T: Barriers to health care: variations in interpretation of Appalachian client behavior by Appalachian and non-Appalachian health professionals, West J Nurs Res 4:179, 1982.

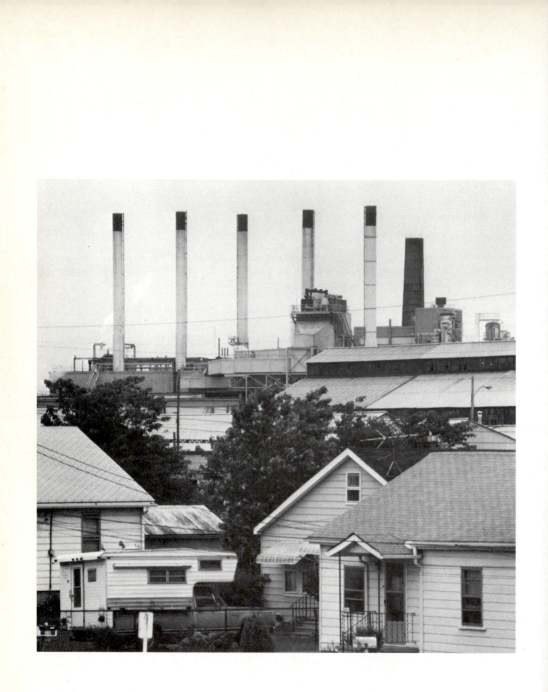

URBAN
NURSING

Iris R. Shannon

OBJECTIVES

After completing this chapter the reader should be able to:

- Describe various aspects of what is meant by an urban community

- Define environmental health and discuss social, psychological, and physical problems related to urban living

- List diseases that are urban related

- Assess characteristics of the inner city and poverty and health care related to them

- Discuss dynamics involved in public access to health resources (including nurses and other health care professionals) in urban communities

- Discuss the nurse's role as patient/client advocate in urban areas

The focus of this chapter* is on inner-city populations because (1) these populations are frequently at higher risk of illness, disability, and premature death, (2) resources in inner-city communities are frequently inadequate to meet the multiple social and health problems of the populations living there, and (3) inner-city settings, with their cultural and organizational diversity, provide opportunities for nurses to participate in problem-solving with multiple types of clients, caregivers, and organizations. Although urban

---

*Appreciation is expressed to Dr. Carolyn Eastwood for her assistance in researching the materials in this chapter.

areas represent many communities, nurses who understand and apply the theories of cultural diversity in their practice can function more effectively in delivering nursing services.

The World Health Organization (WHO) defines health as a "state of complete well-being, physical, social, and mental, and not merely the absence of disease or infirmity." As expressed in the Institute of Medicine, National Academy of Sciences' report (1988) on *The Future of Public Health,* this definition implies that the definition focuses on "...commitment to extend community efforts beyond the narrow concerns of special interests and the boundaries of any one professional discipline."[31] A general discussion of urban health is followed by discussion of three aspects of health that greatly influence urban residents: environment, society, and the organization and delivery of health care. The issues are complex and the chapter makes no attempt to exhaustively represent the subjects. Readers are encouraged to consult other references to increase their knowledge and understanding of these subjects.

Urban health

The terms *urban* and *community,* in their modern embodiment, remain vague and ill-defined, with a shifting focus that depends on the emphasis of the author. Conceptual models for urban and community abound with formulations from classical times. Associated with these terms are different schools of thought regarding how urban communities are defined, their characteristics, and their evaluation. In considering urban health issues an attempt is made to explore the salient features of the concepts of urban and community.

According to Shamansky and Peznecker,[57] before the health status of the community can be assessed, the community health nurse must develop a clear and appropriate conception of the community being considered. In the case of urban health this is doubly complicated because of the confusing terminology. Spradley[59] notes, "The concept of community for community health nursing includes two important variables. One is people. The other is having something in common." In a study of definitions by Hillery, Shamansky and Peznecker[57] found that the area emphasized in many definitions of community includes "...the possession of common ends, norms, and means." In the Hillery study of 97 definitions, the influence of many different academic viewpoints was obvious, but Shamansky and Peznecker[57] found that for the concept to be meaningful in terms of community health issues, an operational definition was needed.

Adapting Moe's[43] definition, Shamansky and Peznecker devised an operational scheme that includes the following three major areas[51]:

1. Who or people factors
2. Where and when, or space and time factors
3. Why and how, or for-what-purpose factors

A professional nurse working within a particular community would fill in the details of this broad outline. In general terms, some sets of communities (as in a particular region of a country or those involved in certain economic activities) may share certain characteristics, but at the same time, each individual community has its own unique combination of features. Familiarity with generalizations about the "type" of community has value, but what is most important is a knowledge of that particular community; this would include the roles of individuals within the community and the role of the community within the general regional and national scheme. This kind of knowledge can promote a positive and constructive approach to work within the community.

Because the discussion is about particular genre of community (sometimes called *neighborhood*), the community is placed in an urban setting. The concept of *urban* produces numerous generalizations and approaches. but basically, the Western view of urban society is that it is morally corrupt. According to Durkheim, rural societies were self-sufficient, but the division of labor and interdependence characterizing city societies was more likely to break down the complex urban society.[49,67]

Sociologists of the "Chicago School," among them Louis Wirth, Robert Park, and E.W. Burgess, saw the city as an ecological system with "natural" interacting ecological areas. This model was based on Chicago in the 1920s and depicted the city as a set of concentric zones. According to Wirth,[70] a city may be defined as "a relatively large, dense, and permanent settlement of socially heterogeneous individuals." For some, an assumption that resulted from these characteristics is that city life produces pathologies.*

Although frequently used measures of urban are demographic (e.g., trait lists based on size, density, and heterogeneity), the overall philosophical emphasis is usually an assumed social illness in city life. Crime statistics are easier to obtain than positive measures of urban areas such as cultural institutions or community organizations. Official definitions of urban vary from country to country and often include a measure of density.

In the next section, selected environmental problems that affect the health of urban dwellers are explored. Attention is given to common problems that affect air, water, and soil and affect communities, individuals, and families.

ENVIRONMENTAL PROBLEMS

If the city is a hostile environment, then the city presents numerous barriers to social and physical good health for its citizens. The nurse working in urban areas encounters a host of environmental, medical, and social problems that may be more concentrated and intense in urban communities. Other than intervene after symptoms occur, nurses working with urban populations must recognize indicators of unhealthy environments that may be causing present health problems or lead to future ones.

In discussing the role of environmental health, Blumenthal[9] writes: "If the 1960s were the decade of access to health care and the 1970s the decade of primary care, then

---

*The definition of urban in the United States is simply, "Places of 2500 inhabitants or more incorporated as cities" (US Demographic Yearbook, 1975).

ENVIRONMENTAL HAZARDS

Air pollution	Food contamination	Water disposal
Dust	Bacterial	Household
Pollen	Chemical	Industrial
Chemical	Viral	Vector control
Nuclear	Noise pollution	Household pets
Water pollution	Industrial	Mosquitoes
Chemical	Traffic	Flies
Bacterial	Other	Rodents
Viral	Toxic chemical hazards	Other
Soil pollution	Household	Accidents
Sewage	Industrial	Motor vehicles
Chemical		Home
Other		Other

---

it might be said that the 1980s are the decade of environmental health." Blumenthal defines environmental health as the "study of disease-causing agents that are introduced into the environment *by humans,* as well as the diseases that are caused by these agents." Some of these agents affect air, water, and soil of the entire community and require large-scale solutions. Others cause problems on the individual and family level such as improperly designed heaters or toxic chemicals used in the home, and family education can help alleviate the problem.

The makeup and density of inner-city populations result in disease-causing agents that are likely to affect large numbers of people. Ford[22] writes that some illnesses that are concentrated in cities can be "...clearly explained as consequences of physical environments." For others, she states that the urban environment "...contributes either to the origin or to the severity of the disease."

It is not always possible to assign a specific cause when poor health, or death, is attributed to environmental causes or associated with a specific place of residence. Even mortality rates "...are marred by errors of completeness and accuracy."[22] In spite of this, an increasing number of studies show that environmental hazards (see box) in the air, water, and soil of cities are detrimental to good health. For example, it is believed that approximately 80% of newly reported cases of cancer (incidence rates) are environmentally induced.[62]

Part of the nurse's role in urban settings is to know the environment in relation to trends, incidence, and prevalence of environmentally associated disease and disability. It is also necessary for the nurse to understand which populations are at risk based on age, location, occupation, and other socioeconomic determinants.[23]

Sources and Types of Pollution

Community air pollution generally implies the presence of "substances put there by the activities of man in concentrations sufficient to interfere directly or indirectly with

---

_____ COMMON AIR POLLUTANTS _____

Ozone	Lead
Nitrogen dioxide	Carbon disulfide
Sulfur dioxide	Suspended particles (e.g., dust)
Carbon monoxide	Asbestos

---

one's comfort, safety, or health."[6] The Clean Air Act of 1970 empowered the Environmental Protection Agency (EPA) to achieve the following:

Establish and enforce national ambient air quality standards

Set emission standards for stationary pollution sources and for mobile sources

Approve state implementation plans specifying how the national standards will be achieved and maintained*

The relationship between health states and environmental states is repeatedly established. For example, Ford[22] in a study of mortality rates reported the following: "The average person living in a central city/county of the United States faces a 9 percent greater chance of dying in a given year than his fellow citizens who live in adjacent suburban counties and a 1.5 percent higher chance than residents of non-metropolitan counties."

There are many types of air pollutants in the atmosphere (see box). Many of these pollutants are identified in the Clean Air Act and are based on studies performed in a number of cities in the United States. Ambient standards are set for the pollutants, including ozone, nitrogen dioxide, sulfur dioxide, total suspended particles, carbon monoxide and lead.[24] Local television and newspapers report air pollution indexes to alert the public to daily conditions (Figure 12-1). Because these pollutants affect the respiratory tract and are associated with acute and chronic pulmonary disease, efforts are made to control their levels.[22] Ford notes that the smog of Los Angeles is particularly well studied. She states, "The effects of air pollution on human health in Los Angeles and other similar cities include death from pulmonary disease, impaired breathing, aggravation of heart disease, sensory irritation, the storage of potentially harmful pollutants in the body, and interference with well being." One report about this problem claimed that ozone levels, ("a major component of urban smog" formed when pollutants from automobiles, factories, and other sources react with sunlight) are three times higher than the federal standard in Los Angeles.†

Most pollutants result from the burning of fossil fuels in industries and homes. Power plants are frequently implicated as sources of pollution. Large disasters such as the London smog that resulted in almost 3000 deaths in the 1950s[24] are associated with air pollution.

---

*General Accounting Office, 1982.

†From Stevenson W: *The New York Times*, 8/7/88, 3:1 +

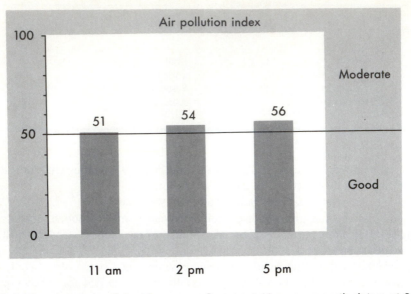

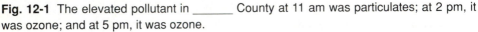

Fig. 12-1 The elevated pollutant in _____ County at 11 am was particulates; at 2 pm, it was ozone; and at 5 pm, it was ozone.

Other pollutants concentrated in urban air are not named as primary air pollutants in the Clean Air Act. For example, "long-term exposure to carbon disulfide has been associated with heart disease."[24]

The liver is also a target organ according to Gallo et al.[24] because foreign compounds concentrate in the liver and this vulnerability "... is enhanced in individuals who possess certain risk factors, such as poor nutrition ...." The inner-city resident may suffer from any combination of these factors to a greater degree than residents of outlying districts. Indisputably, the quality of nutrition is less likely to be satisfactory for many inner-city residents.

The long-term effects on young children of the inner city who breathe pollutants on a daily basis may be more obvious to the school nurse or public health nurse who sees the children on a long-term basis.

There is a higher incidence of respiratory diseases in cities, and the distribution of cancer deaths within cities is also related to urbanization and industry.[22]

EXAMPLE: Mortality rates for all malignancies show a direct correlation with air pollution in Cleveland, Ohio. In Los Angeles, California, rates of lung cancer were higher among residents of certain highly industrialized areas where elevated levels of known carcinogens were present. Asbestos is an air contaminant. It is associated with obstructive lung disease and mesothelioma (a form of cancer). Workers in asbestos plants and residents and school children in buildings where asbestos was used for insulation are particularly vulnerable.[20] Removing the asbestos insulation from older homes, schools, and buildings in inner-city communities is a costly operation. Hence, many residents, particularly children, remain at risk of asbestos-related health problems.

Lead Poisoning

Lead is a toxic heavy metal. It primarily affects the hematopoietic, renal, and central nervous systems.[10] Lead poisoning is frequently associated with urban living. Cited among the causes of this problem are the following:

1. Increased amounts of air-borne lead emitted by cars and trucks
2. Chipped or peeling paint in old inner-city housing
3. High levels in the soil because of heavy auto traffic

The main source of airborne lead is gasoline. "Blood levels have been shown to increase with proximity to major urban highways or exposure to heavy traffic density."[22] However, there is a steady reduction in lead pollution from gasoline because of EPA regulations. Other factors contributing to the reduction in average blood lead for all Americans "…may have included a simultaneous reduction in the lead content of foodstuffs, the impact of targeted screening programs in high-risk areas and an increase in public awareness of the hazards of lead."[2]

The most devastating form of lead poisoning is in inner cities where old dilapidated housing, containing chipped and peeling paint, is responsible for poisoning thousands of children. Peeling paint with a lead base forms colorful sweet-tasting chips that may be attractive to children. In the early 1970s, the average lead level in the blood of urban children and adults was twice as high as the average lead level of suburban and rural residents.[22] A National Health and Nutrition Examination Survey (NHANESII) was conducted from 1976 to 1980, and prevalence rates for elevated lead blood levels were found highest among families in densely populated urban areas and among those with incomes of less than $15,000 per year.

One source of lead poisoning for urban children may be in the soil where they play. Because of the additional traffic and exhaust fumes in urban areas, and the possibility of paint chips in homes, young children are particularly at risk. Among children, inhalation is the second major route of lead absorption.[2] Lead poisoning may also result when an older home is renovated and lead-based paint is removed.

Community nurses are in an excellent position to observe and educate the public about the dangers of peeling paint in older houses and to recognize the symptoms of lead poisoning, which may begin with signs of lassitude and "slowness."

In 1988, the Agency for Toxic Substances and Disease Registry said that lead in the environment is still a potential threat for 3 to 4 million children in metropolitan areas.[5] Legislation passed by Congress in 1988 provided for the following:

1. Screening children for blood lead levels
2. Assuring referrals for treatment and intervention
3. Providing education about this problem

US Representative Sikorski (Dem, Minnesota) who authored House Bill 4939 said, "This crippler of young minds and bodies rivals the proliferation of mind-numbing drugs in our schools, but there is no local pusher to blame: just water fountains and plumbing."

Other sources of urban soil pollution in addition to lead are the long-term health dangers of toxic waste dumps. Two pieces of legislation are designed to deal with the management of hazardous chemical waste: the Resource Conservation and Recovery Act of 1976 to control waste that is being presently produced and the Comprehensive Environmental Response, Compensation and Liability Act of 1980, which assists in the cleanup of hazardous waste sites.[14] Surface and ground water present ways in which most hazardous wastes pose a threat to the health of residents of a community. However, the effects sometime take years to (1) manifest and (2) establish a correlation between waste that is dumped and morbidity and mortality. A nurse can assist in the education of the community and public officials about these hazards.

A hazard of urban living is the accumulation of waste, which breeds rats and other pests harboring pathogens. Most metropolitan governments have some form of rodent control programs. Occasionally, a newpaper reports that a child is bitten by rats, but the ongoing problem of the spread of disease from rat droppings and mice is rarely reported. Measures to educate the public on the control and elimination of rodents are necessary and should include[6]: (1) keeping all food inaccessible to rats and mice and (2) using all possible safety measures in the application of rat killing rodenticides and fumigants.

Occupational Health Issues

Issues of occupational health and safety must be included in any discussion of environment. After the Industrial Revolution, the development of cities and factories were closely related. Factories were associated with harsh working conditions for men, women, and children.

Although government, professional groups, and organizations were active in occupational health issues for many years, higher standards for occupational health were established only with the passage of the Occupational Safety and Health Act of 1970. Today, considerable improvement in occupational health and safety for workers exists; hours are shorter, children are no longer allowed to work in factories, and machines are, on the whole, safer. Occupational health nursing is one of the many health specialties that has emerged and that has made tremendous contributions to making the work environment safer and healthier. According to Ford,[22] "Accident mortality and work-related injuries are less common today among city dwellers than among individuals who live outside metropolitan areas." Nevertheless, occupation-related injuries and illnesses that affect city workers have far-reaching effects in terms of the health and wellbeing of the family. Melius and Landrigan[41] state that each year, approximately one of every 11 workers suffers an illness or injury as a result of hazardous exposure, and approximately 4500 job-related deaths and 578 million job-related injuries occur in workplaces with 11 or more employees.

Today, concern for the health of workers includes toxic chemicals in the workplace. Many of the hazards of these chemicals were previously unknown and are beginning to surface, but frequently, because of costs involved, there is often a marked reluctance on the part of manufacturers to remedy a dangerous situation. Melius and Landrigan[41] note: "New and growing industries such as synthetic fiber products, electronics, and biotechnological production involve possibly unrecognized hazards from these new work environments." Neurotoxic disorders (diseases of the nervous system) are on the National Institute of Occupational Safety and Health (NIOSH) list of 10 leading work-related diseases and injuries because of their potential severity.*

The National Safety Council estimates an annual toll of work-related injuries to be as high as 11,500 workers and that an additional 50,000 to 70,000 Americans die each year as a result of work-related exposure to toxic substances.[19]

Another health hazard to workers compounded by general urban conditions is noise. "The pervasiveness and magnitude of this noise (industrial and community) has been increasing for at least 30 years and has reached a level in many places where it is believed to constitute a public health hazard."[60] However, at the same time that noise-induced hearing loss as an occupational health problem is recognized, higher noise levels are accepted by the public as a way of life. Health promotion activites are needed to promote preserving hearing functions. Nurses can assist in screening workers exposed to noise and in suggesting means of reducing noise exposure.

In 1984 and 1986, the American Public Health Association (APHA) issued policy statements (8416 and 8607) addressing the question of worker notification of adverse health findings. Not only are workers still at risk in many industries, but often when information is available about health risks, the information is withheld. The APHA' states (8607) the following: "Noting that between 200,000 and 250,000 workers, who are surviving members of occupational cohorts studied by the National Institute for Occupational Health and Safety and identified as being at increased risk of contracting cancer and other occupational illnesses, have not been notified individually of the risk information about themselves."

The APHA also recognizes that coalitions for occupational safety and health (COSH) have an important role in providing training and education so that workers understand the health risks. A policy statement (8606) notes: "COSH groups have provided a vehicle for occupational health professionals to be involved in assisting workers and unions to deal effectively with a growing number of occupational health and safety problems."

The above discussion includes disease-causing agents that are introduced into the environment and their effect on residents living in the inner-city setting. Other health problems have special relevancy when people are poor and living in overcrowded conditions and when people are unemployed and malnourished. These social and health problems will be addressed in the following section.

SOCIAL PROBLEMS

To assess health risks of some urban residents, it is necessary to appreciate the complex characteristics of the inner-city ghetto. The mix of residents is not the same as it

---

*From Mortality and Morbidity Weekly Report: leading work-related diseases and injuries—United States, JAMA, 255(12):1552-1559, 1986.

_____ SOCIAL PROBLEMS AFFECTING URBAN POPULATIONS _____

Poverty	Hunger and malnutrition
Unemployment	Homelessness
Lack of education	Racial differences
Social isolation	Lack of medical care
Crime and violence	

---

was 25 years ago, although the present situation rests on historic underpinnings. This section will discuss some of the major problems of inner-city residents (see box).

Poverty

The overriding characteristic of the inner city is poverty. Poverty in the inner city today is not necessarily the same as it was in times past. In a study cited by Ford,[22] when 19 large cities of the United States were examined, it was found that low income areas within these large cities experienced higher rates of low birth-weight infants, infant mortality, inadequate prenatal care, unplanned pregnancies, tuberculosis, and violence that were generally from one to three times higher than in high income areas.

William Julius Wilson[69] maintains that communities of the underclass are "plagued by massive joblessness, flagrant and open lawlessness, and low-achieving schools." A study (1987) involving 26 cities by the US Conference of Mayors' Task Force on Hunger, Homelessness and Poverty found that although unemployment in general is down, hunger, homelessness, and poverty continue to increase in urban America. For example, the number of people needing emergency food increased by 18% from the year before and the number of people seeking emergency shelter rose by 21%.

A report on the changing faces of poverty in the United States[64] asks the question, "Who are the Poor?". This study[27] found that the working poor are a significant and increasing proportion of the poor. In 1986, 41.5% of all poor people over the age of 14 worked; this is equal to the highest percentage of poor who worked since 1968. This is an important finding because of the frequent argument that poor people are all on welfare.

The report also found that children constituted the poorest age group in the United States when, in 1986, one fifth of all children lived below poverty levels. Hence, "children of the poor bear a disproportionate share of the poverty burden." The poverty rate for black children under 18 years of age in 1986 was 43.1%; more than three times the rate for all Americans (13.6%). The poverty rate for Hispanic children was 37.7% in 1986.

Education

Harrington found that growing up poor is likely to increase the number of school dropouts. In 1983, the dropout rate for nonpoor whites was 8.6%, and 9.3% for nonpoor blacks. The demonstrated dropout rates for the poor were much higher: 17.1% for whites and 24.6% for blacks. Harrington noted that the data indicates a relationship between educational attainment and poverty. In 1986, 34.5% of the poor over 25 years of age had no schooling. Twenty-five percent of the poor had less than 8 years of schooling; 15.5% had only 8 years of education; and 18.5% had 1 to 3 years of high school.

In his studies of the total effects of poverty on inner-city populations, Wilson[69] states "A vicious cycle is perpetuated through the family, through the community, and through the schools." Using the example of schools in Chicago, he notes that of the 39,500 students who enrolled in ninth grade in the public schools in 1980, only 18,500, or 47% of those who enrolled, graduated from high school 4 years later. However, of those who graduated only 6000 had reading levels at or above the twelfth grade. This situation is compounded by the fact that of the 25,500 ninth-grade black and hispanic students originally enrolled in high school, 16,000 did not graduate. The Census Bureau states that nationally the dropout rate among black high school students is 57%.

Social Isolation

Wilson[69] uses the term *ghetto underclass* to describe a "heterogeneous group of families and individuals who inhabit the cores of the nation's central cities." He maintains that the groups represented by this term are different from the more socially isolated who lived in these communities in earlier years. The social isolation in inner-city areas described by Wilson is attributed to two factors. First, because middle class professionals, as well as working-class blacks, move out of the inner cities, the role models for achieving a more hopeful future are no longer there. The professionals are upwardly mobile. Industry moves out of the inner city neighborhoods, resulting in a lack of working-class jobs. The few remaining jobs for unskilled workers usually pay less than subsistence wages, so that even if there are numbers of "working poor" within the neighborhood, the operative part of the phase for health and well-being is "poor."

The second aspect of isolation is that as the moderate-income blacks move out of the neighborhoods, institutions become more and more difficult to maintain, thus increasing the distance between poor ghetto residents from the main stream of society. This was discussed previously in access to health care. Unlike the turn-of-the-century immigrant neighborhoods and the later black neighborhoods that now characterize inner-city residents, few residents "move up the ladder" and out of the neighborhood. The present inner-city residents are restricted by lack of low-income affordable housing and other income constraints.

Public Attitude. The hardening of public attitudes toward those less successful is another contributing factor to social isolation experienced by many inner-city residents.[38] During the sixties, the public had concern for ghetto residents and there was a strong will to conquer the problems presented by inner-city life. Wilson[69] has posited that it is not the residents of the inner city who are to blame but the macroforces of the nation's economy that create the problems. Not only did heavy industry such as steel and automobile manufacturing leave the northern cities for the south and other countries, but many forms of industry (particularly light industry) left the inner cities for the suburbs. At the same time, freeways were being built that cut through neighborhoods to form direct pathways to the suburbs from the central city.

The number of poor people in metropolitan areas increased steadily, from 8 million in 1969 to 12.7 million in 1982 (or by 59%), whereas the proportion in poverty increased by 57%. Therefore, Wilson states, "To say that poverty has become increasingly urbanized is to note a remarkable change in the concentration of poor people in the United States in only slightly more than a decade."

Crime and Violence

The frustration of joblessness is hard to measure, but there are far-reaching health and psychological effects that disturb the fabric of the community. Although direct linkages are sometimes hard to prove, studies show that there is a rise in crime during periods of severe unemployment, families are under greater psychological stress, and individuals show a greater frequency of illness. The associations between unemployment and crime are complex, but a fundamental relationship can be seen in the fact that violent crimes are associated not only with times of severe recession, but also that the rates of violent crimes vary according to the economic status of a community.

EXAMPLE: Wilson[69] indicates that during the severe recession of 1974, Chicago experienced a record number of 970 murders. However, Chicago's murder rate was lower than the rates in Detroit, Cleveland, Washington, DC, and Baltimore. In another recession year, 1981, Chicago experienced its second highest number of murders: 877. This number placed Chicago fifth in a ranking of the 10 largest urban areas of the nation. Wilson also demonstrated that the highest rates of crime were associated with the communities of the underclass. He states, "More than half of the city's 1983 murders and aggravated assaults occurred in seven of the 24 police districts, the areas with a heavy concentration of low-income black and Latino residents."[69]

Ford[22] cites studies in Birmingham, Houston, Philadelphia, and Cleveland, noting that these studies also show that higher rates of homicide occur in poor sections of the city and are associated with crowding, bad housing, and unemployment. Ford states, homicide may be considered an index of powerful cultural and interpersonal stress in our society. Obviously, the social cost of homicide is significant. Violence is usually committed against a family member or at least a member of the community.

A second point is that although homicide is the most extreme form of violence, there are other indices such as forcible rape, robbery, and aggravated assault. One barometer of violence in a community may be reflected in the way children are abused. Children are often caught in the crossfire of gang warfare, even when they are not the intended victims, but increasing numbers of children are abused within their own homes. McNulty and Gratteau[39] cite a study done between 1974 and 1984 of children at a single inner-city hospital. This study was confined to violence to children under the age of 15 and included 300 children. More than half of this number were shot by one of their parents or by their mother's companions. Sixteen percent were victims of random gunfire or indiscriminate drive-by shootings. Many of the remainder were believed to have been caught in crossfire or other gang-related shootings.

Child Neglect

It is increasingly important for health professionals to recognize the signs of the violence component of family life, to advocate for and protect children, and to intervene effectively as helping persons. These postures are necessary as society addresses its ambivalence about abuse and other values such as gun control.

The important point is that the average case is not outright child abuse but child neglect. This occurs when children are not fed, left alone, or the parent does not follow up on health matters. Gangs are common occurrences in cities. The negative outcomes of gang participation do not nullify the feelings of belonging that young people apparently do not get in other groups.

Hunger

When a disaster occurs such as an earthquake or flood, the health effects are immediate and obvious, but the long-term results of malnutrition and homelessness on urban populations is less dramatic and is ignored to a great extent. As the Physician Task Force on Hunger (1985) points out, when hunger reaches epidemic proportions as in Ethiopia, the outcome is not in question; for large numbers of people, the deprivation proves fatal.[48] In the United States, the Task Force[48] states, "Instead of a single clear cut outcome—starvation leading to death—we have to look for the multiplicity of outcomes that may result from mild or moderate nutrition."

The American Dietetic Association[3] warns that if the problems resulting from hunger are not confronted, the resulting costs will be high. These costs include the following:

1. Infant prematurity and retardation
2. Inadequate growth and development
3. Poor school performance
4. Decreased output
5. Chronic disease morbidity

The Physician Task Force on Hunger (1985) states that about 20 million people in the United States, including 12 million children, were hungry at some time in the month. In other words, children make up 60% of hungry Americans and their present as well as their future health is at risk because of the long-term effects of malnutrition.

The *Scientific American* used a definition of hunger that is generally accepted in the medical community; "...a hungry person is chronically short of the nutrients necessary for growth and good health."[13] The crisis of the middle 1980s documented by a number of reports,[3,13,48,64] is that by this definition, hunger has reappeared as a serious national problem.

Les Blumenthal, Associated Press, reports in *The Seattle Times* (12/25/89, D3) that a 1989 survey completed by the US Conference of Mayors representing 27 cities and examining hunger and homelessness indicates that the demand for emergency food assistance was up an average of 19% for all surveyed cities. It concludes that hunger and homelessness continue to grow and the outlook for 1990 is "grim." An indication of the interdependence of social and medical issues can be supported from the fact that physicians in some parts of the country saw correlations between patients' malnutrition and illnesses such as anemia and tuberculosis. Brown[13] notes that pregnant women, infants, children, and elderly people are likely to suffer the most harm when food is inadequate. Malnutrition is also likely to make a person more susceptible to infectious diseases.

The Elderly. Problems for the elderly living in inner cities are compounded by several factors. There may be many obstacles to obtaining and consuming an adequate diet. They are more likely to be living on fixed incomes and below poverty level and may be unable to buy the foods they need to maintain a good health state. Food suppliers may not be within reasonable distances. Many inner-city elderly are afraid to shop because of the risk of robbery and mugging even when a grocery is relatively close. This situation is compounded by the fact that many elderly live alone or with an elderly spouse and are without extended family support.

Brown[13] lists three factors in the "disease" of hunger. One is the condition of the nation's safety net or the system of support for people who live in or close to poverty. A second factor is the rise in poverty resulting from economic recession. Structural causes of urban poverty, particularly in midwestern cities in Illinois, Ohio, and Michigan, and eastern cities in New York, New Jersey, Pennsylvania, result from an exodus of industry and employment from these areas.

In a study of needs and social services in three low-income Chicago communities,[28] the researchers found that in 1983, 42% of the households had fallen behind in rent and gone hungry at some time because they lacked money to buy food. The number of households experiencing multiple hardships increased from 10% in 1983 to 16% in 1985 "suggesting that a number of people are becoming worse off." Those who had experienced an improvement in the 2 years attributed the improvement to their economic situation to increased employment rather than income assistance.

The third factor in hunger in America is due to public policy, particularly in cutbacks in federal programs relating specifically to nutrition. In 1981, the Reagan Administration began cutting back on programs such as school lunch and breakfast programs and supplemental feeding programs for pregnant women. For example, Brown[13] indicates that "Nearly half of the Americans in poverty receive no food stamps. Those who do get stamps receive an average benefit of 49¢ per meal."

The Homeless

Hunger and homelessness are twin specters of poverty: poor health is often the end result. In 1987, the report of the US Conference of Mayors showed that in 26 cities, 20% more people were seeking emergency shelter and that nearly two thirds of the cities had to turn people away because their shelters were full. Even the conservative National Bureau of Economic Research states that the population group with the greatest increases in homelessness are families with children. In some cities such as New York City, where 76% of the homeless are families with children, the figures are higher. These populations offer special challenges to health agencies because they are mobile and are at high risk of disease, disability, and premature death. Nurses are among the many providers of health care in the variety of private and public community-based programs providing care to the homeless.

The National Coalition for the Homeless indicates that 30% of the homeless are veterans. Unlike the post-World War II days when large amounts of affordable housing was available for veterans, affordable housing for all types of low-income families is disappearing. Harrington[27] notes that federally-assisted housing funds designed to provide low-income housing have been cut by 75% since 1981.

Tax reform of 1986 encouraged the construction of low cost rental housing for the following reasons:

1. To address the problem of homelessness caused by high costs of rentals
2. To provide tax deductions to owners who would build low cost multiunit rental properties
3. To provide financial support for the hiring of the unemployed in the construction of low cost housing

How much this actually helped to alleviate homelessness in America is difficult to measure, but it serves as an initial effort.

The figures for homeless families imply that although the families have no permanent home, at least they are united. Homeless youths present another picture. In Illinois, a governor's task force on homeless youth defined this population as "those who are aged 20 and under, who cannot be reunited with their parents and lack housing and the skills to legitimately support themselves." This group estimates that there are as many as 21,500 homeless youth in Illinois, and the Chicago Coalition for the Homeless estimate that 10,000 of these young people are in Chicago.

In the early 1980s, a Los Angeles police commissioners' study reported that "if a kid is not resolved in a homeless situation within 12 months, their life expectancy from that point on averages to about five to seven years." Using statistics supplied by the Federal Office of Juvenile Justice and Delinquency Prevention, the Chicago Coalition for the Homeless reported in 1985 that 75% of youth who are homeless for more than 2 weeks, without the resources of friends or relatives, become prostitutes. Added to the physical abuse that they may endure, these youths are also likely to endanger their health through the use of drugs, contraction of infectious diseases, particularly AIDS, and violence.

In testimony about the general mental health of the homeless before a US Senate Subcommittee, Dr William Mayer conservatively estimated that between 35% and 40% of the homeless have a primary alcohol, drug abuse, or mental health disorder.[21] One reason for this is that a proportion of patients have been deinstitutionalized and released from mental hospitals. Because many of these patients are without homes, they reside in the streets. Some receive continuing mental health care through systems of out-patient mental health clinics. However, in addition to those previously mentally ill, there are many people who become mentally stressed because of their experiences with homelessness and feelings of powerlessness.

The problem of finding the homeless is illuminated by a Census Bureau decision to hire thousands of people to search, with flashlights, for the homeless on March 20, 1990, to secure a more accurate tally. Berke[8] states: "With many homeless people now out of the shadows and on the streets their existence cannot be ignored. Yet no one knows their true number, and estimates vary from 250,000 to as high as 3 million, prompting vigorous debate over how much to spend to aid them."

Part of the problem in assessing health problems and needs of the homeless is to locate this population. By definition, these people have no permanent address; therefore a survey of medical status is difficult and follow up is almost impossible.

Brickner[12] writes a summary of the general situation of the homeless: "The medical disorders of the homeless are all the ills to which flesh is heir, magnified by disordered living conditions, exposure to extremes of heat and cold, lack of protection from rain and snow, bizarre sleeping accommodations, and overcrowding in shelters."

Nevertheless, Brickner states, "The information base about health problems of the homeless is rudimentary." A series of articles in *Health Care of Homeless People*[12] outlines some of these problems. Green[26] discusses studies of scabies and lice in the homeless population and concludes that the primary means of transmission is the act of sleeping next to one another. Crowded living conditions, the sharing of sleeping accommodations, and infrequent laundering of clothes favor the spread of scabies. The problem of treating the homeless for lice or scabies is that contacts cannot be found and there is no way of treating all infected people at the same time.

Thermoregulatory disorders are related to the way of life of the homeless.[25] Homeless people are at risk because they are unprotected much of the time from the cold and the sun. Even when they are admitted to a shelter at night, they usually must vacate the shelter early in the morning. Green points out that heat stroke is a major risk for the homeless. Those who are aged or debilitated and malnourished are at grave risk when the temperature/humidity index rises. Hypothermia and frostbite are two cold-related disorders for which homeless are at risk. One of the common environmental disorders found in the homeless according to Goldfrank is *trench boot*. This is ". . . directly related to prolonged exposure to cold and damp, typically in the moist environment of winter boots." For extreme weather conditions, many cities have heating and cooling centers for the homeless and persons living in unhealthy housing conditions.

Frequently cited diseases that afflict the homeless are leg ulcers, cellulitis, and venous insufficiency.[37] These authors estimate that, based on previous studies, 2600 to 3200 homeless persons in New York City suffer from some form of insufficiency.

The specific diseases previously mentioned do not address the usual illnesses that affect the population as a whole: hypertension, diabetes mellitus, pulmonary disease, and tuberculosis.[12] In data from a study by Ropers,[53] consisting of 269 homeless men and women in Los Angeles County, 39.8% reported chronic health problems. Of these, 38.6% reported high blood pressure. Other chronic problems were bronchitis or emphysema.[53]

Screening and access to medical care is a major problem for the homeless, and although some strategies have developed such as health care teams working with the homeless there are still great difficulties in maintaining care. When homeless people need treatment in a hospital there are problems with admission and payment for service. Sharer and Price[54] state, "It is a preconception that in urban settings one hospital is responsible for the care of the indigent. However, information received from 42 of the most populous cities in the United States shows that 55% indicate the presence of more than one hospital willing to take care of the homeless." Some hospitals have special outreach programs such as the Sisters of Providence Hospital in Springfield, Massachusetts[18] and Saint Vincent's Hospital in New York City.[17]

The social issues discussed in this section and their relationship to medical outcomes are part of the complex mix of problems affecting inner-city residents (Figure 12-2). Some are related to structural causes and must be dealt with primarily on governmental levels. Many are related to poverty and unemployment and, although employment rates have improved on a national level, poverty is severe in most large cities of the United States, particularly in the north and east. Health care professionals care for the homeless in community settings where the hungry, homeless, ill, and injured abide. Frequently, health professionals function as advocates for the homeless in attempts to increase

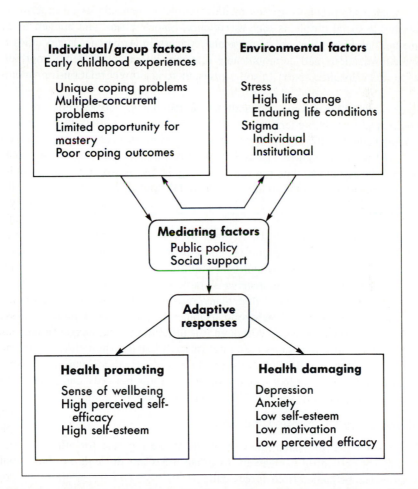

Fig. 12-2 Adaptational model of poverty. *(From Berne AS, Dato C, Mason DJ et al.: A nursing model for addressing the health needs of homeless families, Image (22)1:8, Spring 1990; modified from Pesznecker BL: The poor: a population at risk, Public Health Nurs 1(4):237-249, 1984.)*

needed resources. To provide health care to these people, nurses must be able to assess their problems comprehensively. Factors that affect homeless people and the potential interrelationships of these factors must be assessed. In the final section of this chapter, selected medical problems are discussed that have special significance to urban populations and that represent special challenges to nurses working in urban settings.

MEDICAL PROBLEMS

Throughout the previous section medical problems were discussed in terms of their relationship to social problems such as violence, homelessness, and hunger. In this section medical problems that are of particular concern in America's larger cities will be considered: infectious and communicable diseases, infant and maternal morbidity and mortality, and substance abuse. In some cases, there is a direct relationship among all of these.

Ford[22] notes, "Pneumonia, tuberculosis of the lungs, and syphilis are old urban plagues that persist in modern cities. All three continue to show higher mortality in metropolitan counties than elsewhere ..." In spite of the efficacy of antibiotics, tuberculosis has not been eliminated. The active case rate varies within central city counties, it continues to be associated with poverty, "and may be five or six times higher in the poor sections of the city than in the wealthy residential districts."

Tuberculosis

In an overview of tuberculosis, Iseman[33] uses the term *double jeopardy* to describe the situation of the homeless because: (1) they are at high risk of developing tuberculosis and (2) if they have tuberculosis their stressful life, crowded shelters, and poor nutrition make it unlikely that they will receive suitable treatment. A factor that concentrates tuberculosis victims in cities is that many members of minority groups come from regions where tuberculosis is epidemic. Another factor is that a pool of tuberculosis exists among substance abusers. Although it is difficult to obtain exact figures, Iseman[33] notes, "Estimates of tuberculosis case rates in unaffiliated or homeless urban alcoholics range as high as 500 per 100,000 per year." In a Public Health Report, Slutkin[58] concurs that treatment of urban indigents is a problem, and this not only endangers the patient but increases the danger of spread of infection throughout the community.

AIDS and Other Infectious Diseases

Ford[22] notes that the same kinds of problems are reported for other infectious diseases. Figures pertaining exclusively to urban areas are difficult to obtain, but some information can be gained from survey data.

EXAMPLE: Cases of syphilis were reported from 61 major cities of the United States at three times the rate reported from the rest of the country, and the gonorrhea rate was almost five times higher in cities than elsewhere. In the Institute of Medicine, National

Academy of Sciences report *Confronting AIDS, Update 1988,* in areas where high rates of HIV infections exist (e.g., New York City, Florida, and California) 30% increases in syphilis were reported for 1987. "The increases in syphilis cases suggest behavior that increases the probability of HIV infection among heterosexuals is not being effectively curtailed.

The most devastating and challenging of recent diseases for health care professionals is AIDS, or more correctly (by international agreement), human immunodeficiency virus or HIV. Clever and Omenn[15] state, "The (AIDS) epidemic is international, multigenerational, and one way or another, threatens the human race." Although much of the material published in America is based on studies in several major cities, the epidemic affects the whole country.

The first 5000 diagnosed cases were reported to the Center for Disease Control between July 1981 and June 1984.[5] Since the disease first entered medical awareness the number of cases has increased at a geometric rate. The US Public Health Service in 1986 projected that in the upcoming 5 years the number of US AIDS cases would increase at least tenfold.[47] Osborn states that these figures based on estimates of the disease expressivity and incubation period may be low in light of further evolution of experience since 1986.

After its initial acknowledgement, "...the speed of its recognition was quickly matched by an outpouring of research and clinical data."[47] In their preface, Cole and Lundberg[16] note that there are more than 10,000 medical and scientific citations on AIDS extant, and they are growing at the rate of 600 citations per month. Considering the volume of information and the evolving state of knowledge about HIV, we will discuss only some relevant aspects of the disease in relation to urban health. Osborn[47] states that even with the deluge of information, considerations of public policy and health care delivery lag behind epidemiological and virological information.

Research in two cities contributes to increased knowledge regarding aspects of the AIDS epidemic: first, New York City is the only city in the United States that maintains its own registry of vital statistics.[35] A report using these statistics examines how AIDS changed the patterns of premature mortality in New York City. In the 1980 to 1984 period, AIDS was one of the five leading causes of death for men between the ages of 24 and 54 and was the single leading cause of death for men aged 30 to 39 years. For women, AIDS was among the five leading causes of death for those between ages 25 and 29 years. Among males ages 15 to 64 years, AIDS mortality rates were significantly higher for blacks and Hispanics.[35] Many communities have serious drug-related AIDS problems, and in some areas such as New York/New Jersey, well over 60% of IV drug users are infected.[47]

The second city, San Francisco, responded to early stages of the epidemic by providing health care based on principles of multilevel response to patient needs, patient-centered medical care, and graded access to health care depending on level of need. This is known as the *San Francisco model.*[47] The impact of care of AIDS patients is most severe in cities, and health facilities are taxed severely. One study concludes that public hospitals bear a greater brunt of hospital care and cost than private hospitals, which means that the impact will be greatest on hospitals serving the poor.

Another aspect of the AIDS crisis is its effect on health care professionals. Brennan[11] states that as AIDS spreads, more and more nurses are ambivalent in terms of their own and their families' safety related to the work with AIDS patients, and also in terms of the dim prognoses for their patients. A survey of staff nurses caring for AIDS patients was conducted. Most are full-time nurses and 92% of them work in urban hospitals. They have been caring for AIDS patients an average of 3 years. Their responses indicate the following:

1. That "caring for people with AIDS consumes time and energy, but that the rewards are just as great"[11]
2. That three nurses are needed for every ten AIDS patients, and that ratio could change to one-to-one at any instant
3. Nurses want more information, about their own risks, about the disease, and about the patients they are treating

Brennan notes, "Our survey revealed a telling point, especially for hospitals and hospices with AIDS patients: the more informed the nurse is about these patients, the more likely she'll react positively to taking care of them."

The AIDS crisis is discussed here in terms of adults, but a report from Washington* indicates that AIDS is increasing as a child-death cause. It is now the ninth leading cause of death among children 1 to 4 years of age, and the seventh leading cause of death among young people 15 to 24 years of age. Dr. Antonia Novello states that the disease will soon be the Number Five killer of children from birth to age 24. Osborn[47] notes that predictions that the number of females with AIDS will increase at a relatively greater rate than males also affects pediatrics and AIDS. He also notes that there is a disproportion of minorities among AIDS cases in the United States. It is predicted that by 1991 over 90% of children with AIDS will be either black or Hispanic.

Infant Mortality and Morbidity

The discussion of pediatrics and AIDS leads directly to the more general problem of infant and maternal morbidity and mortality in the inner city. In one study, 16 low-income areas of New York City were compared with the rest of the city over a three-year period (1961 to 1963), and infant and maternal mortality ranged from 55% to 299% greater in the poor sections.[22] A more recent APHA position paper states that low birth weight in infants is the principal cause of high neonatal and infant mortality rates (IMRs) in the United States. It also causes numerous health and developmental problems and major economic burdens on the family and community. The paper states that the problem is especially serious in the black population because black women are twice as likely as white women to have a low birth-weight baby, and almost three times as likely to have a *very* low birth-weight baby.

Neresian[44] says it another way when he states that if mothers and infants of these

*Chicago Tribune, December 20, 1988.

"vulnerable populations" (i.e., those in poverty and certain minority groups) were as healthy as their "nonvulnerable" counterparts, as many as one third (approximately 12,000 deaths) of all infant deaths in the United States might be avoided each year. Neresian also notes, "Family income is probably the single best indicator of an infant's vulnerability."[44] This is why it should not be assumed that any one racial or ethnic group is homogeneous; for instance, Puerto Ricans have a high infant mortality rate (IMR) whereas Cubans and Mexican-Americans are close to the national norm. The "Hispanic" classification blurs this distinction. This is also why it is more satisfactory to look at IMRs for small neighborhood areas rather than for an entire city. For example, "...from 5.8 per thousand in New York's 'Silk Stocking District' to 25.6 per thousand live births in the impoverished community of Harlem."[12a]

Even though numerous authors consider income the best indicator of IMR, other risk factors include the following:

1. Lack of prenatal care
2. Unmarried mothers
3. Mothers with low educational levels
4. Medical complications during pregnancy or delivery

Medicaid has made a difference in infant mortality; from 1965 to 1980 the IMR fell by 49% and the death rate among black infants fell by more than 50%.[27] Yet these figures are hardly reassuring, because using international comparisons of IMRs, the United States ties for twentieth place. Countries that have better IMRs include Scandinavia, Western European nations (England, France and Germany), and Asian nations such as Japan, and Australia. Another international comparison shows that the black IMR in the United States is comparable to figures in Third World countries.

Substance Abuse

Medical and social ill-effects of substance abuse are extensively documented without effectively treating the cause. In urban communities close links are formed among sale and use of drugs, gangs, and the spread of AIDS and intravenous drug use; these combinations are having devastating effects on inner-city areas.

As a Chicago high school principal said, "They (gangs) have become better organized. It seems the gangs are now running the drug industry."[34] He states that 50 or 60 young people in the city were murdered last year because of gang-related activites. Irving Spirgel, a University of Chicago sociologist, estimates that the number of gang members existing in the city is about forty thousand.[34] These gang members prey on the elderly in the community and on single mothers and their children, often selling drugs in abandoned houses and empty apartments.

In New York City there was an all-time annual record in killings when, in August of 1988, there was a 74.8% increase in murders. The head of the Citizens Crime Commission, a nonprofit group that monitors crime of New York City said, "Everyone knows that drugs is the key problem." Officials and criminologists also blame the increase in killings on the continued effects of drugs and drug trafficking.

These problems are not exclusively inner-city problems, but as Ford[22] wrote,

"Though the abuse of alcohol is widespread, with definite urban concentrations, drug addiction is almost entirely an urban phenomenon." Freeman and Heinrich[23] note that substance abuse is a problem for members of health professions, as well as for educational, law enforcement, and welfare institutions. The widespread use of drugs in cities, suburbia, and other communities is well known and the basis of the Bush Administration's "War on Drugs."

Nurses in inner cities can play important roles in helping detect signs of substance abuse in individuals and its effects on the life and health of the family. Freeman and Henrich[23] note that nurses are in a position of knowing the community: where drug trafficking is occurring, working with community groups that are combatting the problem, and being familiar with drug treatment possibilities.

•   •   •

The environmental, social, and medical problems outlined in this section are not all of the problems encountered by inner-city residents, nor are they unique to urban areas. They occur in all parts of the country, but in the inner city they are more concentrated and inner-city residents are at higher risk and are more likely to experience the effects of these problems. They also are more likely to breathe unclean air, to be hungry or homeless, to be poor and living in dilapidated housing in high crime areas, and to have less opportunity for a proper education. Many of these conditions affect the health of the residents, who, if they are in need of medical solutions, may not have access to health care. Where do they go if they are ill or injured? Who looks after them and how do they pay for care? These issues will be addressed next.

Access to Health Care

If, as I look at the world around me, I see only what is there and don't see what is not there, I see scarcely anything at all.—Herbert Marcuse

Health care is widely recognized as a human right. In 1948 the United Nations General Assembly declared: "Everyone has a right to a standard of living adequate for the health and well-being of himself and of his family, including food, clothing, housing and medical care and necessary social services...."[52]

Although a greater proportion of America's income is spent on health care, some groups such as the poor of inner cities have problems gaining access to health care. Individual interpretations of the term *access* vary, but there is general agreement about the meaning of this concept and the indicators of adequate or inadequate access. Aday et al.[1] defined access to health care as "...those dimensions which describe the potential and actual entry of a given population group to the health care delivery system." If access to health care is a right, as stated in the UN declaration, then need is the important factor in determining the quality of access.[1]

A presidential commission appointed by President Carter published a report in 1983, in which it stated that equitable access requires that all citizens can secure an adequate

---

INDICATORS OF ACCESS TO HEALTH CARE

Structural indicators

Availability and organization of the health delivery system
Available supply of physicians and nurses
Accessibility of health care facilities
Sources of care providers
Sources of coverage for health care

Process indicators

Populations at risk
Age groups
Income levels
Race and ethnicity
Cultural factors

Outcome indicators

Measures of realized access to health care
Use of health care by defined populations
Perceptions about the services received
Level of compliance with the health advice received

---

level of health care without excessive burdens.[52] This norm of equity provides a standard to measure access of health care, but actual indicators are needed when looking at specific cases in individual communities (see box).

Indicators of Access to Health Care

Aday et al.[1] states that the structural indicators of access to care refer to the characteristics of the health delivery system such as the availability and organization of the system. These include the numbers of physicians and nurses in an area, whether transportation is available to health care facilities and how much time is involved in reaching the care, sources of care providers, and coverage for health care. Process indicators associated with access refer to characteristics of the population-at-risk and include demographic characteristics (age groups, income levels, race, and ethnicity) and cultural factors (health beliefs and general knowledge of health practices). Aday et al.[1] includes measures of perceived need (how individuals feel about their own symptoms and health status).

Outcome or use indicators of access to care are measures of realized access to health care. Thorpe and Brecher[61] note, "One common and critical outcome-based indicator is a measure of utilization by a defined population." Therefore the use of an inner-city prenatal care clinic by residents of the area might be assessed; such clinics probably keep records on the patients they serve, and these may be used for comparative purposes. Is the clinic available to women in the area, how do they feel about it, do they use it regularly, and is it equally accessible to anyone regardless of race, education, or ability to pay? For the women who use the clinic, some of the subjective indicators of accessibility would include feelings about the service received and the level of compliance with health and medical advice from clinic doctors or nurses. Studies show that usage varies from individual to individual and from group to group. Health education is an important component of accessibility.

A 1986 Robert Wood Johnson Foundation[51] survey found that, "...those whose access to health care is already constrained for financial reasons are likely to face even greater problems." This study looked at certain subgroups organized on the basis of age, gender, residence, ethnicity, income, insurance status, health status, and chronic illness. Included in the findings was that 16% of those surveyed (or the equivalent of 38.8 million Americans) reported needing health care but had difficulty obtaining it. From the findings it was estimated that one million people tried to obtain care but could not afford it. More important, especially for inner-city health populations, is the fact that 12% of the poor who reported a chronic or serious illness did not have health insurance, compared to the 4% of the nonpoor chronically ill who lack insurance.

These figures relate to the question of access and the principle of equality of "life chances" discussed by Wilson.[69] The latter concept recognizes that disadvantaged individuals may have less-than-equal opportunities compared to those from another social strata. Society must find some way to give a poor inner-city baby access to the same start in life afforded the nonpoor.

Poverty. Poverty is generally regarded as a condition where people are badly housed, undernourished, frequently ill, and poorly clothed. It also has a technical meaning in the United States that is based on the following measurement: the poverty line is determined by food expenditure data that is over 30 years old, and those below that line are officially poor.[42] Miller suggests that using this formula, the poor are probably worse off today than they were in 1960.

Racial Differences and Unemployment. Inner-city areas have wide racial differences in poverty and unemployment. The 1987 census figures show a sharp increase in the poverty rate among blacks and a drop in the rate among whties.[32] For example, 45.6% of black children were living in households with incomes below the poverty line in 1986 compared to 17.7% of white children.[42] Miller also states, "The black unemployment rate is twice that of whites and has remained at that multiple for 30 years." Therefore many residents, particularly of inner cities, cannot afford health care and because they are unemployed, do not have insurance coverage through their place of work. This results in dependency on public means for gaining access to health care. These problems will be discussed in more detail later, but first we will look at the distribution of medical and health resources: the distribution of physicians; the short supply of nurses; and the availability of hospitals and clinics for the inner city poor.

Bayer asserts, "Good health cannot be assured to everyone. But good health *care* can and should be guaranteed."[7] This means, "...that all Americans must have access to the full range of necessary health services." However, as Ford[22] notes, "the urban health care system is full of inequities such that complex technology may be available for some while at the same time immunization of children is neglected, or poor people live within walking distance of renowned hospitals but cannot afford their services." As an American Nurses' Association (ANA) Executive Director Judith Ryan, RN, states, "We need to figure out the most cost effective way to provide universal access to the basic level of services."[29]

Supply of Physicians. The supply of active physicians has increased in recent years; from 141 per 100,000 population in 1950 to 218 per 100,000 in 1985.[52] However, these are broadbased figures—they tell us nothing about where the physicians are practicing and what their specialties are. Although some specialties are in oversupply, areas of undersupply include general and child psychiatry, preventative medicine, and emergency medicine. In spite of attempts to encourage physicians to enter the primary care disciplines (general internal medicine, family practice, and general pediatrics) the trend continues toward specialty training.[40] Although most physicians receive payment through fees, many more are receiving third-party reimbursement. Medicare fees are important to physicians because 26% of office visits and almost 31% of hospital visits are reimbursed by Medicare. Changes in Medicare funding affect patient accessibility, and also physicians' incomes.

Accessibility of Hospitals. In addition to payment for service, another question is whether physicians and hospitals are accessible. A study shows that "...for those who live close to the central business district the average time required to reach the dentist or the physician is greater than it is for those who live elsewhere." Other studies of individual cities show that within a metropolitan county the distribution of physicians varies widely.[22] Many physicians do not practice in the poorer sections of the cities (except for work in medical centers) but practice in the suburbs where there are affluent clients. The result is that black communities have a limited number of health care providers. In 1985 one third of the 750 American counties with the highest proportion of black residents were designated by the federal government as "critical shortage areas" for primary care physicians.[55]

Increasing the numbers of trained black physicians would help the ghetto areas, but Wilson[69] maintains that the "...ultimate determinant of black access to medical care is not the supply of black physicians, even if an overwhelming majority choose to practice in the black community, but the availability of programs such as Medicaid, Medicare, and National Health Insurance." A Robert Wood Johnson Foundation[51] report notes that the poor fare worse than the more affluent when one of the most important access measures is used, ambulatory visits. This is true despite the poor's generally worse health and the greater likelihood of chronic or serious illness.

Supply of Nurses. Although there may be an oversupply of physicians in some areas and in certain specialties, there is no question that there is a shortage of nurses. Even though 68% of nurses work in hospitals, employment of registered professional nurses in public and community health has grown rapidly. One third of local health department staffs are registered nurses and most state agencies employ large numbers of nurses. The American Hospital Association (AHA) states that the most serious shortage of baccalaureate-prepared professional nurses will surface in nursing homes and community health settings, but there are shortages in all areas. Both rural and urban areas experience the nursing shortage, but as always, needs in medically underserved locations are likely to be neglected.

A report prepared by the US Department of Health and Human Services estimates that there will be a 50% shortage of baccalaureate-prepared nurses by 1990. These estimates were contained in the Fifth Report to the President and Congress on the Status of Health Personnel in the United States, March 1986. Estimates reflect anticipated nursing staffing needed in the organization and delivery of community health services, and role expectations of community and public health nurses. A baccalaureate degree is a prerequisite for public health nursing practice because of its focus on health promotion, disease prevention, and health education and on management, coordination, and continuity of care within the community, which are content areas in baccalaureate education.[66]

An AHA survey found that 54.3% of hospitals experienced a "moderate" or "severe" nursing shortage, and that the shortage is more pronounced in public hospitals.[4] This aspect of the shortage particularly affects inner-city populations. The report states that the shortage was responsible for temporary bed closure in more than 18% of the nation's large urban hospitals surveyed by the AHA in 1987. Another effect on urban residents is temporary closure of emergency departments in 14% of the hospitals in major urban areas. Because there is a pattern by inner-city residents of using emergency departments, rather than maintaining a long-term physician relationship, the closing of these departments may represent a real hardship.

Even though 78.7% of licensed RNs were working as nurses in 1984,[65] a relatively high participation rate, one reason for the shortage today is that hospitals have increased the nurse/patient ratio; health agencies are also hiring more nurses in relation to other personnel. At the same time, there are increasing demands on nurses because of older patients and patients who are more ill, more complex technology, and special problems associated with care for patients with infectious diseases such as AIDS and hepatitis. Nurses who work in community areas are increasingly concerned about their personal safety, even though they are also aware of the great need for their service.

The House Select Committee on Aging (September 20, 1988), notes that the present nursing shortage is the fourth documented crisis since 1965, but this one is different because "statistics are catching up with us." Their summary of the statistics includes the following:

1. An aging population
2. Increaisng numbers of uninsured
3. Increasing prevalence of chronic diseases
4. The AIDS epidemic
5. A decline in student enrollment in nurse education programs
6. The trivialization of a nursing career, secondary to low wages and low prestige

The effects of an inability to solve these crises are likely to be severe and continuing for inner-city residents as public hospitals, emergency departments, and home health and community nursing are cut back.

Sources of Care Providers and Coverage for Health Care. Changes have occurred in the hospital system in the 1980s; with the rest of the health care system, it has become more competitive and there have been sharp declines in hospital use. Schleisinger[55] notes that the decline in occupancy rates, from 76% in 1981 to 65% in 1985, results in increased pressures for hospitals to find patients. At the same time there is a steady growth in for-profit hospitals and ambulatory care facilities since 1975.[52] Many claim that the effect of profit-oriented hospitals is to "cream" the most profitable patients and illnesses while leaving high-risk and indigent patients entirely to the public sector.[40] With cost containment an issue, hospitals are no longer willing or able to follow a pattern of cross-subsidies, whereby charges are increased by those covered by insurance to fund care for those unable to pay.[7] There is a serious question whether for-profit hospitals can provide access to care[52] in the way that is provided by voluntary not-for-profit groups such as community groups, religious orders, unions, and cooperatives.

A study by Thorpe and Brecher[61] was undertaken to determine whether public hospitals in cities increased access to health care for the uninsured poor. They looked at the following aspects of the health policy problems:

1. Twenty-five million Americans lack health insurance and these individuals may not receive needed medical care because they cannot pay for it
2. If hospitals provide uncompensated care, they may undermine their financial condition
3. "The operation of a public hospital in a city significantly affects access to care for that city's uninsured poor"[61]
4. Where a public hospital does not exist or was closed, the community's private hospitals do not typically "pick up the slack"
5. Access to care "...is most enhanced in cities where there is a public hospital and a large number of teaching programs"[61]

There is no question that access to health care by inner-city residents is threatened by hospital closures, health worker shortages, and federal cuts in spending for health care programs.

Medicaid and Medicare

EXAMPLE: A home care nurse describes the situation of a 50-year-old home health aide who is married to a man with a heart condition. Their medicines cost $400 per month. Although she often works 40 hours a week, she is considered a part-time employee and therefore has no health insurance.[29] In another case described by Huey, an elderly woman needs oxygen for a pulmonary disease. Her private insurance pays for only 3 months. After that, she is told to apply to Medicaid. She said, "If I apply for Medicaid they will take a lien on my house, which is all I have to leave to my children. I would rather die." Huey[29] concludes, "Two months later, she did die."

These cases illustrate some of the problems of the uninsured and the underinsured, and the problems inherent in the two main government programs, Medicare and Medicaid, that deal with health care. In the Robert Wood Johnson Foundation report on access to health care,[51] the "uninsured" were those who did not have coverage under a health maintenance organization, Medicare, Medicaid, other government health insurance, self-paid health insurance, or employer-paid health insurance. This definition does not address the problems faced by those who have some coverage, but not enough to pay all the health costs or to maintain good preventative health care. Roemer[52] states "...some 15% or more than 37 million people are economically unprotected against the cost of even hospital care, let alone all the other elements of health service. Moreover, the health service benefits of the 'protected' population are extremely inadequate."

Huey[29] notes, the government pays for health care "in fragments." For a premium, Medicare, part B, pays partial medical cost, and although part A requires no premium, it also pays only partial medical costs for the elderly and disabled. Medicaid varies from state to state because, although the federal government matches state funds, the decision of funding care for the indigent and the management of benefits is left to the individual states. In 1984, Medicaid extended coverage to less than 50% of persons below the federal poverty level.[52]

Another aspect of Medicaid that severely affects inner-city residents, particularly children, is that Medicaid is tied to qualifications for other federal programs. If the allowable income for Aid to Families with Dependent Children is lowered, this affects eligibility for Medicaid. Also there are cases in which the law forbids out-of-pocket payment, so when the coverage is exhausted "...the consequence has been a refusal to treat those covered by the program by some hospitals and many physicians."[7]

These aspects of Medicaid can be related to inner-city residents because a substantial proportion of these residents are black. On the National Health Interview Survey (1987) it was found that blacks are 50% more likely than whites to have no health insurance and 40% of all Medicaid enrollees are black. Thus changes in Medicaid allowances can disproportionately affect this population.

Another group affected by changes in coverage in recent years is the elderly. An example of this is the adoption of diagnosis-related groups (DRGs) for determining payments for Medicare patients. Bayer[7] states, "...empirical studies have already begun to reveal that elderly patients are being discharged from hospitals before optimal, effective and necessary care has been provided, in order to stay within the DRG limits."

Even when health care is financially accessible, minorities may face discrimination and, for this reason, find it difficult to seek or acquire the care that they need. Also lack of information may prevent minorities from being aware of the health care that is available to them. Schleisinger[55] notes, "Surveys have shown that minority Americans are less informed than are whites about both the services available in their communities and the provisions of their health insurance policies." However, Miller[42] notes that when poor individuals are provided services that are accessible and appear to them to be useful, they will use them.

Access to health care is limited by cuts in other areas besides Medicare and Medicaid. The 1981 federal budget reform also affected programs such as maternal and child health, alcohol and drug abuse, and mental health services, as well as nutrition programs such as food stamps and school lunches. As Huey[29] stated, "What we save by limiting access to health care, we spend to treat other complications." In Illinois, 500,000 children have neither Medicaid nor medical insurance and therefore have no access to medical care.[46] In Chicago, more than 100,000 women and children who are eligible to receive food through the federal Women, Infants and Children (WIC) program are not getting it because of lack of funding.

Thus inner-city poor, particularly minority elderly and children, are suffering from hunger, homelessness, environmental hazards, and illness. Often they have no place to turn because they have no access to the food, housing, and medical care declared as their right by the UN General Assembly.

•   •   •

Urban health issues are multidimensional and complex. Nurses working with inner-city populations must consider an array of social, health, and environmental factors in their assessments of health problems and nursing needs. Many of the societal issues that negatively affect health such as poverty, racism, lack of a universal health program, unemployment, violence, and drugs can only be corrected if there is a political will to do so. Nurses and other health workers have responsibility to advocate for programs and environments in which citizens can maximize their full potential. The concentration of populations in urban areas who are at risk for disease, disability, and premature death make the cities special places for focusing on the promotion of health and the prevention of disease. Opportunities for nursing practice abound in cities: the current shortage of nurses is more intense because of the multiple health agencies and institutions employing nurses. Hospital and community health settings offer challenges to nurses prepared to work with diverse cultural groups. The contributions that can be made by nurses are unlimited.

STUDY ACTIVITIES

1. Suggest some incentives that would help recruit nurses to work with the urban poor, inner-city populations.
2. What experiences might be provided to nurses, as students, to create more interest and knowledge in urban practice?
3. How can nurses become active advocates to alleviate problems through policy making in relation to urban health issues?

REFERENCES

1. Aday L, Andersen R, and Fleming GV: Health care in the U.S.: equitable for whom?, Beverly Hills, 1980, Sage.
2. American Academy of Pediatrics Committee on Environmental Hazards and Committee on Accident and Poison Prevention: statement on childhood lead poisoning, Pediatr 79(3):457-465, 1987.
3. American Dietetic Association: Hunger in America: an American Dietetic Association perspective, J Am Dietet Assoc 87(11):1571-2, November 1987.
4. American Nurses Association: The nursing shortage: situations and solutions, Kansas City, 1988, The American Nurses Association.
5. American Public Health Association: The Nation's Health, December, 1988.
6. Anderson CL, Morton RF, and Green LW: Community health, Saint Louis, 1978, The CV Mosby Co.
7. Bayer R et al.: Toward justice in health care, Am J Public Health 78(5):583-588, 1988.
8. Berke RL: Girding for bid to count homeless, The New York Times, B6, December 16, 1988.

9. Blumenthal DS, ed.: Introduction to environmental health, New York, 1985, Springer Publishing Co., Inc.

10. Blumenthal DS and Greene M: Air pollution, In Blumenthal DS, ed.: Introduction to environmental health, New York, 1985, Springer Publishing Co., Inc.

11. Brennan L: The battle against AIDS, Nursing 60-64, April 1988.

12. Brickner PW et al., eds.: Health care of homeless people, New York, 1985, Springer Publishing Co., Inc.

12a. Brown JL and Allen D: Annual review of public health, J Annu Rev Pub Health 9:503, 1988.

13. Brown JL: Hunger in the US, Scientific American 256(2):37-41, February 1987.

14. Carden JL: Hazardous waste management. In Blumenthal DS, ed.: Introduction to environmental health, New York, 1985, Springer Publishing Co., Inc.

15. Clever LH and Omenn G: Hazards for health care workers, Annu Rev Public Health 9:273-303, 1988.

16. Cole HM and Lundberg GD: AIDS from the beginning, Chicago, 1986, American Medical Association.

17. Conanan B and O'Brien NJ: New York City: The Saint Vincent's Hospital SRO and shelter programs. In Brickner et al., eds.: Health care of homeless people, New York, 1985, Springer Publishing Co., Inc.

18. Crane J: Springfield, Massachusetts: the Sisters of Providence health care for the homeless program. In Brickner et al., eds.: Health care of homeless people, New York, 1985, Springer Publishing Co., Inc.

19. Drew C: OSHA policies undercut bed to protect workers, Chicago Tribune 1:25, December 16, 1988.

20. Drotman DP: Chemicals, health and the environment. In Blumenthal DS, ed.: Introduction to environmental health, New York, 1985, Springer Publishing Co., Inc.

21. Flynn K: The toll of deinstitutionalization. In Brickner et al., eds.: Health care of homeless people, New York, 1985, Springer Publishing Co., Inc.

22. Ford AB: Urban health in America, New York, 1976, Oxford University Press.

23. Freeman RB and Heinrich J: Community health nursing, Philadelphia, 1981, WB Saunders Co.

24. Gallo M, Gochfeld M, and Goldstein BD: Biomedical aspects of environmental toxology. In Lave LB and Upton AC, eds.: Toxic chemicals, health and environment, Baltimore, 1987, Johns Hopkins University Press.

25. Goldfrank L: Exposure: thermoregulatory disorders in the homeless patient. In Brickner et al., eds.: Health care of homeless people, New York, 1985, Springer Publishing Co., Inc.

26. Green RW: Infestations: scabies and lice. In Brickner et al., eds.: Health care of homeless people, New York, 1985, Springer Publishing Co., Inc.

27. Harrington, M: Who are the poor?, Washington, DC, 1987, Justice for All National Office.

28. Hemmens G, et al.: Changing needs and social services in three Chicago communities, Chicago, 1986, University of Illinois at Chicago.

29. Huey FL: To the President and Congress: nurses know that U.S. citizens can get better access to better health care at affordable costs. Are you ready to change the system? Am J Nurs 1483-1493, November 1988.

30. Institute of Medicine: Confronting AIDS: directions for public health, health care, and research, Washington, DC, 1986, National Academy Press.

31. Institute of Medicine: The future of public health, Washington, DC, 1988, National Academy Press.

32. Irwin V: U.S. poverty standard comes under attack, Christian Science Monitor, January 11, 1989.

33. Iseman M: tuberculosis: an overivew. In Brickner et al., eds.: Health care of homeless people, New York, 1985, Springer Publishing Co., Inc.

34. Kotlowitz A: Bad boys, Chicago Times, 40-46, January/February, 1989.

35. Kristal AR: The impact of the acquired immunodeficiency syndrome on patterns of premature death in New York City. In Cole HM and Lundberg GD, eds.: aids from the beginning, Chicago, 1986, American Medical Association.

36. Lave LB and Upton AC, eds.:Toxic chemicals, health and environment, Baltimore, 1987, Johns Hopkins University Press.

37. McBride K and Mulcare RF: Perpheral vascular disease in the homeless. In Brickner et al., eds.: Health care of homeless people, New York, 1985, Springer Publishing Co., Inc.

38. McNulty TJ: Lost society infects cities, Chicago Tribune, 1:20, September 15, 1985.

39. McNulty TJ and Gratteau H: The American milestone, Chicago Tribune, 2:1, December 1, 1985.

40. Mechanic D: A brief anatomy of the American health care system. In Schwartz HD: Dominant issues in medical sociology, New York, 1987, Random House.
41. Melius JM and Landrigan PJ: Occupational health. In Blumenthal DS, ed.: Introduction to environmental health, New York, 1985, Springer Publishing Co., Inc.
42. Miller SM: Race in the health of America, The Milbank Quarterly 65:500-531, supple 2, 1987.
43. Moe EO: Nature of today's community. In Reinhardt AM and Quinn MD, eds.: Current practice in family-centered community nursing, vol 1, St. Louis, 1977, The CV Mosby Co.
44. Neresian WS: Infant mortality in socially vulnerable populations, Annual Review Public Health 9:361-77, 1988.
45. Nursing education crisis heightens shortage: need for standardization, Chart 84(2)2-5, 1987.
45. Ogintz E: Children's health needs grow in the U.S. also, UNICEF says, Chicago Tribune 2:8, December 21, 1988.
47. Osborn JE: The AIDS epidemic: six years, Annu Rev Public Health 9:551-83, 1988
48. Physician Task Force on Hunger: hunger in America, Middletown, Connecticut, 1985, Wesleyan University Press.
49. Press I and Smith ME, eds.: Urban place and process, New York, 1980, Macmillan Publishing Co.
50. Reinhardt AM and Quinn D, eds.: Current practice in family-centered nursing, vol 1, St. Louis, 1977, The CV Mosby Co.
51. Robert Wood Johnson Foundation: Access to health care in the United States: results of a 1986 survey, Special Report Number Two, Princeton, New Jersey, Johnson Foundation, 1987.
52. Roemer R: The right to health care—gains and gaps, Am J Public Health 78(3):241-247.
53. Ropers RH: The invisible homeless: a new urban ecology, New York, 1988, Human Sciences Press.
54. Scharer LK and Price B: Working with hospitals. In Brickner et al.: Health care of homeless people, New York, 1985, Springer Publishing Co., Inc.
55. Schlesinger M: Paying the price: medical care, minorities, and the newly competitive health care system, The Milbank Quarterly 65:270-297, supple 2, 1987.
56. Schwartz HD: Dominant issues in medical sociology, New York, 1987, Random House.
57. Shamansky SL and Peznecker BL: A community is .... In Spradley B, ed.: Readings in community health nursing, Boston, 1982, Little, Brown and Company.
58. Slutkin G: Management of tuberculosis in urban homeless indigents, Public Health Report 101(5):481-5, 1986.
59. Spradley B, ed: Community assessment and health planning. In Spradley B, ed.: Readings in community nursing, Boston, 1982, Little, Brown and Company.
60. Stream R: Effects of industrial and community noise on health. In Trieff NM, ed.: Environment and health, Ann Arbor, 1980, Ann Arbor Science.
61. Thorpe KE and Brecher C: Improved access to care for the uninsured poor in large cities: do public hospitals make a difference? J Health Polit Policy Law 12(2):313-324, Summer 1987.
62. Trieff NM, ed.: Environment and health, Ann Arbor, 1980, Ann Arbor Science.
63. U.N. Demographic Yearbook 1975, 27th issue, New York, 1976.
64. U.S. Conference of Mayors' Task Force on Hunger and Homeless: The continuing growth of hunger, homelessness and poverty in America's cities, Washington, DC, 1987.
65. U.S. Department of Health and Human Services, Office of the Secretary, Secretary's Commission on Nursing, vol III, July 1988.
66. U.S. Department of Health & Human Services, Fifth Report to the President and Congress on the Status of Health Personnel in the United States, March 1986. Washington, DC, U.S. Department of Commerce.
67. Uzzell JD and Provencher R: Urban anthropology, Dubuque, Iowa, 1976, Wm C Brown Company.
68. Voices of Illinois Children: voices 2(1):1, Fall 1988.
69. Wilson WJ: The truly disadvantaged: the inner city, the underclass, and public policy, Chicago, 1987, University of Chicago Press.
70. Wirth, L: Urbanism as a way of life. In Press I and Smith ME, eds.: Urban place and process, New York, 1980, Macmillan.

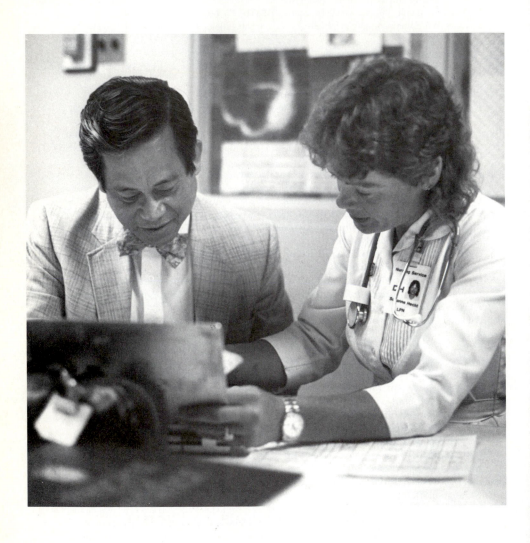

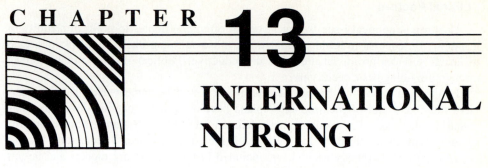

13

INTERNATIONAL NURSING

Sandra L. Jamison

OBJECTIVES

After completing this chapter the reader should be able to:

- List at least six forces that affect nursing internationally

- Define primary health care

- Discuss international trends in nursing education and research

- Name at least four international nursing organizations

- Describe the goals and functions of the World Health Organization (WHO)

- Describe how interested nurses might learn about job opportunities abroad

FORCES AFFECTING NURSING INTERNATIONALLY

Nurses from many nations report similar accounts of the social, economic, political, demographic, and environmental forces influencing nursing in their countries. The changing role of women, too, has a significant affect on the profession. Because nursing systems are part of larger health care systems, all forces affecting the latter have consequences for nursing.

Political Factors

Health is a political issue. As such, health often contributes to political stability or instability. In contrast to healthy populations, those suffering illness and lacking access to health services are dissatisfied and unproductive. Political support can be gained through providing basic health care.

Health care is political because it is an integral to development. Health-related services must be a part of socioeconomic plans developed at the national level. In many countries they are. For example, in Thailand, the Sixth National Socioeconomic Development Plan (NESDP) for 1986-1991 includes significant allocations for the implementation of primary health care. Included in the NESDP are monies and targets for the retraining of nurses to practice primary health care.

The interplay of health and politics is evident in matters such as national health insurance, drug control, long-term care for the chronically ill and elderly, and public funding for AIDS research. Nurses are directly influenced by these matters. Recruitment, retention, education, and practice of nurses are affected by the demand for services, reimbursement systems, prevalent health care problems, and research findings.

Political forces also influence the demands for health care.

EXAMPLE: In Africa and Asia, particularly in areas of major political unrest and open conflict, the needs of mushrooming refugee populations are increasing the demand for nursing services. Further, the nurses caring for the refugee populations must have specialized knowledge in the problems unique to these groups. Nurses working where imprisonment for political and religious reasons is not uncommon, are concerned with the requirement to participate in the torture of prisoners.[49]

Political factors influence legislated regulations about who may practice nursing.

EXAMPLE: In Europe, because of the political and economic arrangements among the Common Market countries, nursing licensure is reciprocal, and nurses can practice in any of the member countries without having to pass a licensure exam. In Brazil, nurses do not take an exam; rather they are licensed by the Regional Council of Nursing if they graduate from an accredited Brazilian school of nursing.[10] In Thailand, because nursing education is under two ministries, nurses studying in 4-year programs do not receive the equivalent degrees. Those in programs under the Ministry of University Affairs receive a baccalaureate degree, whereas those in colleges under the Ministry of Public Health receive only a diploma. Although both BS and diploma nurses are licensed by passing the national examination, there are strong feelings about the politics leading to two degrees for 4 years of education.

Political systems influence the working conditions and education of nurses.

EXAMPLE: Where socialism prevails, nurses are government employees who practice in institutions owned by the government. The administration of nursing services and nursing education is centralized; i.e., a few officials at the national level determine what will be taught in nursing education, how many nurses will be educated and hired, where these nurses will work, and nursing salaries. In democracies such as Canada where a national health insurance plan is in effect, nurses are less influenced by the government. Nursing education is decentralized and nurses practice in privately owned agencies. In the United States every nursing school has its own unique curriculum and the majority of nurses practice in nongovernmental institutions.

Indeed, political forces are affecting nursing worldwide.

Economic Factors

Closely associated with political forces are economic forces that influence nursing. Indirectly, the health status of people is positively correlated with economic status. When the economic picture is favorable, there is an improvement in health, as measured by indicators such as infant mortality and life expectancy. Countries in which the annual income averages $200 to $300, individuals have considerably less to spend on health.

More directly, the resources available and allocated for health care services, including nursing, depend on the economic status of the country. Poorer countries, although expending a larger percentage of the gross national product (GNP), may still be spending relatively small amounts for health. Wealthier countries may spend more on health while expending a lesser portion of the GNP. For example, in 1976 Honduras spent $10 per person, or 14.7% of its GNP on health, whereas the United States spent $259 per person, or 9.7% of its GNP.[52] In recent years, with an increasing percentage of many governments' budgets used for defense and debt reduction, the financial resources for health have diminished worldwide.

The economic forces influencing nursing extend beyond the availability of resources to include the distribution of these resources. The widening gap between the rich and the poor is a global concern. Those who can afford health care receive it. Those who cannot are left without health services. Further, they do not have the resources to obtain nutritious food, safe water, and education. Certainly, economic forces influence the health needs of people and how nurses meet these needs.

Demographic Factors

Demographic characteristics of populations affect nursing and the larger health care system. In developing countries in which 50% of the population are under the age of 21 years, nursing care must be directed more toward maternal-child care than toward the care of persons with chronic diseases. In Europe and North America, where an ever increasing proportion of the population is elderly, care of the aging is being incorporated in nursing cucrricula. Geriatric nursing has become a specialty. With increased industrialization, occupational health concerns and illnesses related to lifestyle are of more concern than infectious diseases.

The demographic shift from rural to urban areas has implications for nursing. Problems resulting from inadequate housing, poor sanitation, unsafe water, crowding, and unemployment are common in the rapidly growing cities of the world such as Mexico City, Cairo, Bangkok, and New Delhi. The existing health care facilities and the number of nurses prepared to deal with the massive public health problems are inadequate to meet the need.

Environmental Factors

Environmental forces affect nursing worldwide. For example, the increase in nuclear wastes and other hazardous materials influence the health of the world's population. Changes in the ozone layer and increases in air and water pollution are affecting health. Poisonings from pesticides and industrial injuries are not uncommon. Such problems are particularly serious in developing countries where the rate of industrialization has exceeded the implementation of safety measures.

Natural disasters such as the drought in East Africa and typhoons in Bangladesh provide nursing challenges. In Africa, nurses face the multifaceted heath care problems that result from severe malnutrition. Nurses in Bangladesh must provide care to large groups of persons with cholera, typhoid, or hepatitis.

Changes in Knowledge and Technology

Advancements in scientific knowledge and medical technology necessitate changes in the basic education of nurses, particularly for those who will work in acute care settings. Such advances raise ethical issues and questions about standards of practice in nursing. Applying technology appropriate to developing areas is extremely influential in improving the health status of millions, e.g., the use of oral rehydration solution—a solution of glucose, salts, and water taken orally—is estimated to prevent more than 600,000 deaths a year.[51]

Advances in communication technology make it possible for nurses to upgrade their educational preparation through televised extension programs. Public media also extend the possibilities for nurses in health education; e.g., nutrition lessons, information about immunizations, and methods for obtaining safe water can be taught over television to villagers who watch the village TV every evening for entertainment.

Role of Women

The role of women in various cultures influences nursing in two ways. First, the health needs of women are a reflection of the role of women in a society. Women suffer severe health problems from anemia and malnutrition in cultures where they must both work and bear numerous children. Second, the role and status of women influences the recruitment and education of nurses, the image of nursing, and the position of nurses in the health care system. In cultures where nursing activities are perceived as those of servants, it is difficult to recruit educated women into nursing. Further, in many countries women have fewer years of schooling than men. Because of their feelings of inferiority related to less education, as well as cultural attitudes toward women, nurses do not assert themselves and are not invited to take leadership positions on the health team. Recognizing the importance of women as health care providers and the problems for women because of their culturally appointed roles, the World Health Organization (WHO) is studying the problem and making recommendations. Two reports have been published on Consultation on Women as Providers of Health Care.[57,59]

The economic, political, demographic, technological, and environmental forces influencing health indicate the need for innovations in health care delivery systems. Recognizing the need for improvements, the WHO identified Primary Health Care as a strategy to cope with the expanding health care needs.

PRIMARY HEALTH CARE

In 1977, the Thirtieth World Health Assembly passed a resolution (WHA 30.43) stating that "the main social target of governments and WHO in the coming decades should be the attainment by all the citizens of the world by the year 2000 of a level of health that will permit them to lead a socially and economically productive life." The universal target was accepted as Health For All (HFA) by 2000. In 1978, the Declaration of Alma Ata, signed by the member states of WHO, recognized primary health care (PHC) as the means to attain HFA. PHC is defined as follows:

Essential health care based on practical, scientifically sound and socially acceptable methods and technology made universally accessible to individuals and families in the community through their full participation and at a cost that the community and country can afford to maintain at every stage of their development in the spirit of self-reliance and self-determination.

The above definition of PHC is based on five principles[53] (see box).

The Declaration of Alma Ata defined eight elements as essential to a primary health care service[53] (see box).

PHC is not endorsed as a substitute for current health care systems, but rather as a reorientation of health care. PHC "forms an integral part both of the country's health system, of which it is the central function and main focus, and of the overall social and economic development of the community. It is the first level of contact of individuals, the family, and the community with the national health system, bringing health care as close as possible to where people live and work, and constitutes the first element of a continuing health care process."[53]

PRINCIPLES OF PRIMARY HEALTH CARE

1. Equitable distribution—health care services should be equally accessible to all people
2. Community participation—individuals and communities should be actively involved in the planning and operation of health care services
3. Focus on prevention—priority should be given to prevention and promotion over cure
4. Appropriate technology—appropriate technology should be used, i.e., methods, procedures, techniques and equipment should be scientifically valid, adapted to local needs, and acceptable to uses and to those for whom they are used
5. Multisectoral approach—health care is only a part of total health development; health care providers must work with individuals in the other sectors such as education, nutrition, agriculture, and housing to achieve well being for all

---

_____ ESSENTIAL ELEMENTS OF PRIMARY HEALTH CARE SERVICE _____

1. Education concerning prevailing health problems and methods
   of preventing and controlling them
2. Promotion of food supply and proper nutrition
3. The provision of safe water and basic sanitation
4. Maternal and child health care, including family planning
5. Immunization against the major infectious diseases
6. Prevention and control of locally endemic diseases
7. Appropriate treatment of common diseases and injuries
8. Provision of essential drugs

How do nurses relate to PHC? In 1978 Dr. Halfdan Mahler, Director of WHO, addressed nurses with the following challenge:

If the needs of communities are to be met the ranks of health workers, including nursing and medical personnel, will need to consist predominantly of people who genuinely care about the health and welfare of impoverished communities, who want to help such communities, who are willing to learn what has to be done, and who cannot only do it, but do it without dependence on sophisticated and costly technology. (The world's population) needs nurses who can diagnose community health problems and institute measures to protect, advance, and monitor the health of populations as a whole, nurses who can care for the sick or the disabled, nurses who can teach people to care for themselves.[28]

Mahler also recognized the potential of nurses in PHC. After noting that there were at least 4 million professional nurses worldwide, Mahler said:

If the millions of nurses in a thousand different places articulate the same ideas and convictions about primary health care, and come together as one force, then they could act as a powerhouse for change...In order to realize the full potential of this powerhouse, nurses will need to be organized and equipped to break down resistance to change, to sustain the initial effort, and then to develop strategies and action plans. What is very clear is that the nursing profession is more than ready to respond to this challenge.[28]

In 1984 a WHO Expert Committee on the Education and Training of Nurse Teachers and Managers with Special Regard to PHC identified the critical importance of nurses being educated beyond the acute care hospital setting. The committee recommended that nurses be taught in community oriented, competency based, and learner-centered programs. Two years later another international committee with representation from 81 countries submitted a report on *the regulatory mechanisms for nursing training and practice: meeting primary health care needs.*[56] The report notes both legal constraints and recent advances in PHC-oriented nursing activities. In countries such as Indonesia, France, Luxembourg, Korea, Israel, and Spain, legislation regarding nursing activities was changed to incorporate the expanded role of nurses in PHC.

In 1986, two important events contributed to the momentum of nursing involvement in PHC. The first event was the Tokyo, Japan, meeting—Leadership in Nursing for Health for All: A Challenge and Strategy for Action.[54] Nursing leaders, senior health administrators, and politicians from 20 countries met to (1) identify roles of nursing leadership in the HFA, (2) define strategies to facilitate leadership roles, and (3) formulate recommendations relating to the development and performance of the nursing leadership role within the framework of individual countries. Many of the final recommendations relate to formal training within reoriented educational programs and informal training at each service level of health care systems.

The second event was the naming of two institutions as WHO Collaborating Centers for Nursing in PHC. One is the University of Illinois, which has a long-term commitment to international nursing. The purpose of the collaborating centers, now 13 in number, is to foster the exchange of experiences in PHC practice, to promote research related to PHC, and to share strategies for change in education and practice. Collaborating centers are located in Thailand, Denmark, Yugoslavia, Australia, France, India, Korea, Brazil, Columbia, Botswana, Kenya, the Philippines, and the United States.

Nursing in PHC includes the following roles[58]:
1. Assessing the health status of individuals and communities
2. Mobilizing community involvement in PHC
3. Providing integrated health care, including the treatment of emergencies and making referrals
4. Maintaining epidemiological surveillance
5. Training and supervising health workers
6. Collaborating with other development sectors
7. Monitoring progress in PHC

Nurses in Brazil are teaching and supervising village health workers.[31] In Kenya others are traveling with mobile clinics to teach health, give immunizations, and diagnose and treat illnesses. Nurses in Israel[47] are performing epidemiological surveys in kibutzes, and nurse midwives in Botswana are handling maternal-child care in a primarily rural population.[4] In Thailand professional nurses are working within health centers where the focus is definitely health promotion and disease prevention.[21] Canadian nurses have implemented PHC in self-help groups for parents who have lost a child or who have children with chronic diseases.[7]

Nurse educators are responding to the need of nurses for knowledge and practice relevant to PHC. Examples of curriculum changes are reported for India,[18] the United States,[13] Kenya,[34] Botswana,[4] Nepal,[11] the Philippines,[37] and Israel.[25] Changes in basic nursing education include integration of community health principles in all years of the curriculum and provision for clinical experiences beyond acute care hospitals. Attention is given to teaching prevention and health promotion, preparation to treat locally endemic diseases, and population-based care. Continuing education programs help nurses learn physical assessment skills, methods of health teaching, and epidemiological principles. The rate of change is slow because of a lack of faculty with experience in PHC, a scarcity of appropriate learning materials, and attitudes toward PHC within the health care system.

INTERNATIONAL NURSING ORGANIZATIONS

International nursing organizations provide collaboration of nurses, to improve the health of the public by exchanging knowledge and innovative approaches to health care. They also provide mechanisms for nurses to develop standards of care and codes of ethics, to cooperate in improving the socioeconomic and working conditions for nurses worldwide, to stimulate research and theory development, and to develop creative solutions to common concerns. Such organizations include the International Council of Nurses, WHO, Pan American Health Organization, Sigma Theta Tau International, and Nurses Christian Fellowship International.

International Council of Nurses

The International Council of Nurses (ICN), founded in 1899, is the oldest international professional organization in the health care field. For nearly a century this organization served as the worldwide voice of the nursing profession. In structure it is a nongovernmental federation of national nurses' associations from 98 countries, representing nurses who are members of constituent organizations. The purpose of the organization is to provide a medium through which the interests, needs, and concerns of member nurses' associations can be addressed, to the advantage of the public and nurses alike. Individual nurses belong indirectly through their national nurses' associations such as the American Nurses Association. The ICN, centrally located in Geneva, Switzerland, the traditional home of many humanitarian organizations, fosters global communication and networking.

The ICN, run by nurses for nurses, enables nurses from diverse backgrounds to exchange information of clinical and general interest and to explore nursing issues. Sharing is accomplished through seminars, publications, and meetings. Quadrennial congresses are conducted in various countries and provide unique and stimulating experiences. All nurses worldwide are invited to attend, although only those belonging to national nurses' associations may present papers.

Publications of the ICN provide news and useful knowledge about nursing. The *International Nursing Review,* published bimonthly, is the official journal. Other publications such as *Guidelines for Public Policy Development Related to Health, Guidelines for Nursing Research Development,* and *Guidelines for Nurses Applying for Senior Positions* provide directions for advancing the nursing profession. The *Caring for the Carers* series was developed to help nurses deal with a variety of work situations.

Three major contributions to nursing made by the ICN are as follows:
1. An internationally accepted definition of nursing
2. A code of ethics
3. The document on Conditions of work and life of nursing personnel, which was adopted by the International Labor Organization

In addition the ICN advances the profession by supporting education through the Florence Nightingale International Foundation and the ICN/3M Nursing Fellowship program, which awards three fellowships annually for advanced studies.

World Health Organization

Since its initiation in 1984, the WHO has had a profound impact on world health. The purpose of the WHO is to coordinate global efforts to prevent disease and promote health. In the WHO, nurses communicate with many other health and health-related personnel to identify health problems and strategies for coping with them. An international approach is needed to deal with many health problems because health and disease are not confined to national boundaries. The WHO collaborates with worldwide public and private institutions to implement its goals.

The WHO promotes education and research through a variety of programs, provides technical cooperation among nations, and develops guidelines for national policies on various health concerns. Publications such as *World Health Forum* and *World Health* communicate a sample of the global activities in health care. Major accomplishments of the WHO in the past 40 years include the following:

Smallpox disease has been eradicated worldwide, with no case reported since 1977

Half the world's children have been immunized against life-threatening diseases such as diphtheria, whooping cough, measles, tetanus, polio, and tuberculosis

Safe water and sanitation have been brought to 300 million Africans during the first 7 years of WHO's International Water Supply and Sanitation Decade

A massive oral rehydration program cosponsored by WHO and UNICEF is expected to save the lives of $1^1/_2$ million children suffering from diarrheal diseases

Recently WHO mobilized many of its resources to confront the global threat of AIDS

The WHO and ICN, both committed to HFA, have differences that influence their association and activities. The WHO is much larger (166 member countries) compared to ICN (98). The WHO is a part of the United Nations system and thus relates to governments. ICN is nongovernmental and nonpolitical. Both are divided into the same 7 regions of the world, but only WHO has offices in each of the regions.

Despite differences in size, structure, and political affiliation, there is remarkable and productive collaboration between ICN and WHO. Because of their relationship, the nursing profession and the health of the world's population have been advanced (see box).

Pan American Health Organization

The Pan American Health Organization (PAHO), although closely affiliated with the WHO, is an autonomous organization composed of 35 member governments in the Americas and three European governments with Western Hemisphere interests. It serves member countries in meeting the health needs of their populations. US nurses benefit from collaborating with nurses in other countries in North, Central, and South America through PAHO. One of the PAHO programs of interest to nurses is the Women in Health and Development Program, which focuses on women's special health needs and enhances women's role in providing health services.

Sigma Theta Tau International

Sigma Theta Tau, from its founding in 1922 until 1985, was confined to recognizing superior scholarship and leadership of nurses in the United States. In 1985 the honor

---

COLLABORATIVE ACTIVITIES OF INTERNATIONAL COUNCIL OF NURSING
_____ AND WORLD HEALTH ORGANIZATION _____

1948 ICN granted "official relationship" with WHO
1951 WHO supported studies of nursing education programs
1965 WHO and ICN published "World Directory of Post-Basic Nursing Schools"
1974 ICN participated in WHO Expert Committee on Community Health Nursing
1977 ICN supported WHO suggestions to develop community health nursing services
1978 At Alma Ata ICN presented "Contribution of Nursing to Primary Health Care"
1979 ICN-WHO conference in Nairobi "The Role of Nursing in Primary Health Care"
1982 ICN participated in WHO Expert Committee on "Nursing in Support of the Goal of Health for all by the year 2000"
1984 ICN-WHO worldwide survey of "Nurses and Physicians of Tomorrow"
1985 ICN/WHO panel on "Aging: Implications for Nursing" at ICN 18th Congress
1986 ICN participated in WHO and Japanese conference "Leadership in Nursing for Health for All"
1987 ICN-WHO cooperated in drafting Guidelines for Nursing Management of AIDS

---

society for nursing expanded its constitution to become the International Honor Society of Nursing. As evidence of the organization's commitment to excellence in nursing globally, three international chapters were chartered in 1989. The chapters are in Taiwan, Korea, and Canada. International nurses who become members of Sigma Theta Tau while studying in the United States will have local chapters.

The commitment of Sigma Theta Tau to excellence in nursing worldwide extends beyond membership. Such commitment was implemented in the establishment of the International Nursing Library, the publication of articles from nurses from several countries in *IMAGE: Journal of Nursing Scholarship,* and the promotion of research internationally. The International Research Congress cohosted by Sigma Theta Tau in Edinburgh, Scotland, July 1987, marked an advance in unifying global nursing scholarship.

Nurses Christian Fellowship International

Nurses are drawn together around the globe by religious organizations. Nurses Christian Fellowship International (NCFI) is an example. NCFI is an interdenominational organization for nurses that holds essential Christian beliefs. Its purposes include the development and maintenance of Christian beliefs among nurses worldwide and the promotion of Christian principles in professional life. The journal of NCFI, *Christian Nurse International,* includes discussions of issues of concern to nurses such as ethics, cross cultural communication and practices, standards of practice, and management problems.

• • •

All of the international organizations are involved in some way with initiating or perpetuating trends in practice, nursing education, and research. The major trend in practice is toward primary health care. Conference participants share details about education and research trends in their countries.

INTERNATIONAL TRENDS IN NURSING EDUCATION AND RESEARCH
Nursing Education

Historically there are three models for nursing education: The British, the French, and the American. Colonization of countries by Britain or France led to the perpetuation of their model of nursing education. Briefly, the British system involves a three-year training program within a hospital. Graduates qualify for nursing in general, sick children, or mental fields. After basic education, a nurse can continue in specialty certificate programs. In the French model, the curriculum is shorter but otherwise similar to the British in that it is an apprenticeship-based education within hospitals and focuses on the medical model. The American model began as the British model but quickly moved from hospitals to institutions of higher education.

The differences in models of nursing education are shrinking with the trend to move the educational preparation of nurses into institutions of higher learning. This shift is slow but consistent. Forces propelling the efforts to upgrade nursing education by academization include the desire for an improved image for nursing, the need to recruit more nurses, and the desire of nurses to affect the public's health by participating in policy making. Although desired by many, incorporation of nursing into university settings is a complex process necessitating the opening of new programs, the affiliation of existing programs with educational institutions, and the development of patterns for career mobility. Internationally, major obstacles to the academization of nursing include the lack of faculty with advanced preparation, lack of relevant learning resources, and a lack of influence in the bodies controlling advanced education within the country. The theory and clinical practice aspects of nursing curricula are under critical scrutiny, with significant revisions expected.

The trend for nurses to have advanced eduction preparation extends to the expansion of opportunites for obtaining master and doctoral degrees.

EXAMPLE: In Brazil the first masters program was established in 1972.[31] Nine years later there was a doctoral program. The Kellogg Foundation continues work with several Central and South American countries to extend the possibilities for advanced nursing education to their nurses. In other parts of the world—South Korea, Egypt, Norway, and The United Arab Emirates, doctoral studies for nurses are now a reality. In Taiwan, plans are developing to open a doctoral program at National Defense Medical Center in association with Yang Ming University.

Improvement in educational opportunities for nurses results in efforts to reorganize a multiplicity of programs offered in many countries and to develop a plan for career mobility. Generally the types of programs fall into the following three general categories:

1. Basic preparation—qualifies a nurse to apply for registration
2. Postbasic education—leads to certification in a specialty such as public health or midwifery
3. University nursing studies—most of which are postbasic, lead to either baccalaureate or masters degrees, and are primarily for the preparation of faculty

A Thailand representative illustrated the trend toward consolidation and upgrading of the nursing programs, a plan for career mobility in her country.[45] She described a multiplicity of programs as follows:

A 1-year program, which was phased-out as its graduates were given the chance for a second year program, leading to a certificate as a technical nurse

A 2-year technical program, which would be phased-out when there were no more 1-year graduates and there were enough 4-year programs available

A 2-year continuing program for graduates of a technical program to continue toward a diploma

A 4-year diploma program (comparable to a baccalaureate program, but in a nursing college rather than in a university)

A 4-year baccalaureate program in a university

A 2-year baccalaureate program in a university for graduates from 4-year diploma programs

She said that eventually there would be only 4-year programs, but it would take many years to achieve that goal.

Nursing research

Trends in international research were summarized by Meleis (1987) after an extensive review of nursing publications. Emerging trends, which will be discussed in subsequent chapters, are listed in the box.

There is growing recognition of the value of research and a concomitant desire among nurses to be involved in systematic investigation of nursing phenomena.

EMERGING TRENDS IN INTERNATIONAL NURSING

1. Professional concerns—image, status, role of nursing and nurses, immigration of nurses, and roles if indigenous workers in health care of nations
2. Educational concerns—types of programs effective in preparing nurses from other nations; recruitment and retention of students and graduates
3. Women's health—determinants and responses of women to universal events such as birthing, mothering, menstruating, and lactating
4. Family concerns—roles of family in support, care, and development of its members
5. Culture and country of origin as they influence responses of nurses and patients to health and illness events
6. Clinical therapeutics as practiced in other nations of cultures

---

From Meleis, A: International Nursing Research, Annu Rev Nurs Res 5:205-227, 1987 and International nursing research for knowledge development, West J Nurs Res 9(3): 285-287, 1987.

Research is needed to test the theories being developed in different countries such as those of Wanda De Augiar Horta in Brazil[2] and Usui in Japan.[23]

A great deal of information is available from contact with international nurses. Global forces and trends in nursing affect the profession. In addition, detailed information about nursing in individual countries provides information about nursing in specific areas of the world.

NURSING SYSTEMS IN SELECT AREAS
Brazil

A nurse from Brazil, the largest country in South America with a population of 130 million, described nursing quite different from nursing in other countries, with a national health insurance program for the majority of the people. One of the differences is in the ratio of nurses to other health professionals. Physicians outnumber nurses in a ratio of 6.7 to 1.[44] Professional nurses with a university degree constitute only 8.5% of the total nursing work force.[10] Auxiliary nurses with one to two years of training and attendants with no formal training provide most of the nursing care.

Ninety-seven percent of RNs provide curative care in hospitals or clinics.[10] The primary care system consisting of health centers and posts is staffed almost entirely by auxiliaries and attendants. On the average, there is one nurse for 11 health centers or 30,000 people, but this number varies considerably by regions of the country. Public health nursing and school nursing, are practiced very little.[44]

Nursing education and practice are centrally regulated by the Federal Council of Nursing (COFEN) and by Regional Councils (COREN), which are organs of the Ministry of Labor. By law all RNs must have a degree from a COREN-accredited university nursing program. The degree, rather than a licensing exam, qualifies a nurse to be registered. All RNs are required to pay dues to their COREN and to vote in their elections.

Nurses are also encouraged to belong to a labor union and to a variety of nursing associations. Because all nurses must pay a government union tax, it is to their advantage to receive the benefits of union membership. In 1983, 55% of Brazilian nurses were union members and 82% belonged to one or more nursing associations.[10] It is plausible that, with the current degree of organizations, nurses might improve the status of health care services, and the profession.

At present, nurses have little professional autonomy while they have heavy responsibilities for supervising and coordinating the activities of numerous minimally educated attendants. Working conditions and salaries, which have been deteriorating steadily,[46] discourage potential nurses. Germano[17] traces the series of professional difficulties in Brazilian nursing to a combination of long hours and low salaries compounded by the ideal of a nurse. Historically the image of a nurse is one of an obedient, disciplined person who consoles and assists society's victims, and does not exercise social criticism. Financial incentives and the upgrading of nursing education could influence the nurse image and thus increase the desirability of the profession.

The government has taken steps to increase nursing manpower but the results have not yet equalled the need. In 1982, the government funded a comprehensive study of nursing education and practice conducted by the Brazilian Nurses Association. The conclusion of the two-volume report was that nursing in Brazil was intricately associated with the economic, social, and health policies of the country. Recognizing the marked devaluation of all health professions in regard to career and income opportunities, the report stated that improvements in the quantity and quality of nurses could be made only with changes in national policy.[10] The future could be much brighter for Brazilian nurses, if the government could entice more potential nurses via support of advanced education, provision of desirable working conditions, and encouragement of autonomy in practice.

Russia

A feldsher, or Russian nurse, reported that in her country nursing is not considered an independent profession.[14] Rather, nurses are classified as *middle medical personnel* with physicians' assistants, sanitarians, and pharmacists. Their status as government employees is similar to that of schoolteachers and mechanics. All aspects of nursing education and practice are centrally planned and administered by the Ministry of Health.

Basic nursing education consists of a strictly standardized 1-year, 10-month program for women who are less than 30 years old and who have had 10 years of general education.[14] Physicians provide all the classroom teaching in the first year. In the second year, head nurses in hospitals teach basic nursing skills. Students are required to attend all classes and receive a small stipend for their efforts. After completing the program, they take a national examination that entitles them to one of two diplomas. Those achieving high scores receive an honors diploma that allows them to study medicine. Those with lower scores receive regular diplomas. Both diplomas certify them as licensed nurses. To continue in practice, nurses must take a reexamination every 2 years. There are no advanced certificate or university programs for nurses.

All nurses practice under direct physician supervision. Their duties vary according to their place of work. A number of nurses work in polyclinics, which are facilities delivering primary and ambulatory care. Their focus is on preventative health services, especially to children. As members of a health care team, nurses in the polyclinics are involved in health education, screening, and immunization. Unlike nurses in many other countries, Russian nurses are not involved in midwifery. Normal obstetrical care is the responsibility of trained midwives.

Any changes in nursing education and practice in Russia will evolve from changes in the national government, rather than from actions taken by nursing organizations or educational programs. The image of nursing will continue to reflect the value placed on nursing by those in power at the ministry level.

Nigeria

A nurse from Nigeria stated that nurses in her country face many of the same situations and concerns as nurses from other parts of Africa. She cited commonalities such as history of colonial influence; a predominantly rural population characterized by tribal group dominance, diversity of culture and religions; and health problems typical of developing areas.[12] The problems are all public health concerns: malnutrition, malaria, diarrhea and dysentery, parasitic diseases, and measles. Childhood diseases are the primary health concern because the mortality rate for children under the age of five is 182 per 1000.[51] Traditional and Western health care practices are used.

Health care services are regulated by the Ministry of Health (MOH). That is, health planning, preventive health services; administration of hospitals, education, and registration of health care practitioners; and regulation of pharmaceuticals are all responsibilities of the MOH.[41] A large proportion of the health care budget is allocated to a few hospital-based systems that are located in urban areas where only 23% of the population lives.[15] In its general economic development plan, the Nigerian government committed itself to establishing HFA by 2000 through primary health care. However, a primary health care system is still in the developmental stages.

The number and uneven distribution of health care professionals relate to some of the problems facing Nigerian nurses. For every 100,000 persons there are 31 nurses (the United States has 380 per 100,000) and nurses outnumber physicians 10 to 1.[41] A majority of physicians and nurses work in urban settings within hospitals. However, the number of nurses functioning in community settings is growing.[1]

Nursing education in Nigeria is rooted in the British system. Three types of basic programs not affiliated with universities qualify nurses for licensure in one of these specialties.[31] The 3 1/2-year programs require a high school diploma for entry and prepare nurses for midwifery and public health, psychiatry, or general nursing.[1] Nurses are registered by the Nursing and Midwifery Council of Nigeria on successful completion of a three-part exam. The exam consists of writing two theory papers, a 30 minute demonstration of nursing skills, and a 10 minute oral test.

Students entering a postbasic university program must have 1 year of practice as a registered nurse. At the end of their 3 1/2-year program they receive a BSc. A concern facing all educational programs is relevancy of education to the health care practices and needs of the population. Revisions are needed to prepare nurses for work in primary health care, and to work in an expanded role for health promotion and disease prevention in community settings.

The National Association of Nigerian nurses and Midwives, inaugurated in 1978, is a professional organization and seeks to advance nursing—the image, socioeconomic status, and educational preparation of nurses. Two professional journals are published: *Nigerian Nurse* and the *New Era of Nursing Image International.*[50] Nigerian nurses contribute to the body of research literature through these journals and through professional journals published abroad.[8,22] Unquestionably, Nigerian nurses provide an example for nurses in many of the African countries who experience similar situations and health concerns.

Japan

The nurse from Japan said that although there were advanced health care facilities in her country there were problems in providing quality health care for all people.[16] One of the problems is the shortage of nurses with the educational preparation to work in such facilities. Another problem relates to the lack of a plan for comprehensive and continuous health care rather than episodic acute care. There is an increasing need for rehabilitative and geriatric nursing services.

The role of the family in Japanese society adds a unique dimension to nursing practice. Patients are not seen as individuals but rather as members of a family. The extremely close relationships within the family should not be interrupted by anything, including hospitalization.[20] The family is considered more important to the patient psychologically than a good nurse. Thus families must be included in the patient's care, often to the point of staying with the patient and giving "attendance care" during hospitalization.

The educational preparation of nurses in Japan is specified in the Public Health Nurse, Midwife, and Nurse Law (the PMN Law), which was established in 1948. This law stipulates the education, qualifications, licensing and registration procedures and areas of practice for general nurses, public health nurses, midwives, nurses, and assistant nurses.[24] Nurses may take the national licensure examination after completing a minimum of 3 years of nursing education. After they are licensed, they may take courses in public health nursing or midwifery offered in junior colleges and universities. Presently the predominant educational model is the 3-year diploma program but there are a growing number of 4-year baccalaureate programs. Eleven universities offer a BS in nursing and two of these also have masters programs.

Although Japanese nurses are obtaining advanced education and contributing to nursing research and nursing theory, the gap between theory and practice in nursing is widening.[24] The steps taken to close this gap will serve as a model for nurses in many other countries, who also are seeking to advance the profession academically, although many unanswered problems remain in practice.

Europe

European nursing practices and education are similar to those in other countries previously discussed. The majority of nurses work for a public health care system, i.e., they are paid by the government. Most attend a 3-year basic program associated with some health care institution other than a university. Those who specialize continue for 6 to 12 months in a postbasic specialty course. Many of the nurses belong to the national nurses association, which is often affiliated with a recognized trade union and thus has bargaining power. In fact, the percentage of nurses belonging to the national nurses association in Denmark is 98%,[5] in Finland, 79.2%,[36] and in the United Kingdom, 65%.[38]

The Europeans relate that in their countries nurses practice in hospitals delivering curative care and in community settings. In the hospitals they work in a dependent role with physicians, whereas in the community they have much more autonomy,[26] particularly those with specialty training in midwifery, home health (health visitor), and public health.

EXAMPLE: The nurse midwife from Sweden related how she provided prenatal care, including education; performed uncomplicated deliveries; and provided family planning, including the distribution of contraceptives. Nurses from Denmark and Great Britain working as health visitors (similar to home health nurses) describe how they made home visits to expectant families before delivery to assess the home situation and then followed-up the children, performing physical examinations, developmental assessments, and immunizations. They said that other health visitors work in the schools. Norwegian nurses, working in public health, related their work coordinating services for the elderly.

Norway and the United Kingdom

Nursing in Norway and the United Kingdom demonstrate the commonalities and differences of nursing in different parts of Europe. In Norway, nurses are educated in 3-year programs.[48] Until 1980, the government specified every detail of the curriculum. Now, the 32 schools of nursing develop their own curricula. However, all schools are under the jurisdiction of the Department of Culture and Sciences of the Ministry of Education. An appointed national board of professionals approves each program. Students must pass a national state board examination to be licensed.

In Norway, there is a trend away from the medical model of nursing toward health organization, the Norwegian Association of Nursing. Current areas of emphasis are preventative health care, geriatric and home nursing, and midwifery. Specialty certification is possible in each of these areas, as well as the more traditional areas of pediatrics, anesthesiology, and intensive care. Nurses can pursue masters and doctoral degrees in the Institute of Advanced Nursing Education at the University of Oslow.

Nursing in The United Kingdom shares many features with nursing in Norway.[39] A high percentage of nurses belong to their national nursing association. Membership in the Royal College of Nursing represents approximately 65% of all qualified nurses and students. Education remains largely in non-university settings under the control of health authorities. As in Norway, nursing leaders of the United Kingdom advocate that nursing be placed within higher education. Nurses are licensed by a national board. Because of the diversity in the United Kingdom, each country has its own national board. A current debate in licensing is whether or not there should be periodic licensure rather than lifetime licensure.

In the United Kingdom as in Norway, most nurses work within hospitals and are paid by the government. Health visitors and midwives implement most of the nursing service beyond the hospital. Nurses in all places of work are concerned about reimbursement for their services. Salaries are determined at the national level for all civil servants, such as nurses who work in the National Health Care System.

While sharing commonalities, nurses in Europe also experience political and socioeconomic conditions, culture, and historical heritage of nursing unique to that nation. However, a landmark action in 1977 may bridge some of the differences among European nurses and thus achieve a more unified voice for nurses on the continent. In July 1977, the nine members of the European Economic Community (EEC)—Belgium, Denmark, France, Holland, Ireland, Italy, Luxembourg, West Germany, and the United Kingdom—signed the Nursing Directives.[9] The first directive said that "general nurses," born in and licensed in any of the nine EEC member countries, could practice nursing in any of the other countries without being licensed in that country. The second directive related to the coordination of legal and administrative outcomes of the first directive. A Permanent Nursing Committee was established to set minimum acceptable standards for entry into the profession and for nursing practice. Attaining comparable educational programs through growth production is frustrating and tedious for nurse educators throughout Europe.[38] European nurses are establishing a prototype for unifying standards of practice and education throughout the world.

European nurses identify the following as major challenges to their profession[55]:

1. Participating in setting policy nationally and locally
2. Establishing standards of practice with regard to quality of care and competence of professional nurses
3. Achieving a desirable socioeconomic status for nurses
4. Increasing contributions of nurses to the knowledge of nursing and health care delivery through research
5. Providing educational programs that prepare nurses to function effectively as multipurpose workers in nursing
6. Identifying the unique role and responsibilities of the nurse on the health team

With regard to the last challenge, participants in a WHO symposium on European nursing[55] agreed that "the nurse is the only professional in a position to plan and control the immediate environment of the patient." The potential for European nurses to meet the challenges facing them is promising, because of the increasing cooperation of nurses across the continent. Nurses in the United States are faced with challenges similar to those of the European nurses and will benefit from sharing solutions with their colleagues across the seas.

Opportunities for Nurses in International Settings

Rowe[43] estimates that the number of American nurses working in international settings is approximatley 22,000. Some nurses work for private multinational corporations. Others work for the US government or for national governments abroad. In fact, advertisements for working in Kuwait and Saudi Arabia appeared in a recent issue of the *American Journal of Nursing*. Universities through faculty exchange programs, nongovernmental volunteer agencies such as CARE and Project HOPE, and organizations with religious affiliations also hire nurses for employment abroad. Organizations such as the National Council on International Health post openings for nurses in many countries.

Most American nurses abroad are, according to Masson,[29] working in teaching, supervisory, or consultant roles. A relatively small number are giving direct patient care as clinicians. Information about the work of nurses abroad comes from personal experiences shared through presentation or recorded as anecdotes in nursing literature. Two research studies give an organized overview of nurses working internationally.[6,19] Andrews[6] surveyed 91 American nurses, working as international nursing consultants, regarding their educational preparation, country of work, employment arrangements, areas of consultation, adequacy of preparation, and demographic characteristics. Ninety-six percent of the consultants were women with a mean age of 41 to 50. Eighty-nine percent were masters-prepared and 55% doctorally prepared. One third of them had certification in a specialty area. The geographical areas in which the majority were practicing are as follows:

Middle East	30%
Latin America	30%
East Africa	30%
West Africa	19%

Approximately half of them were sponsored by an organization, either public or private, in the United States. The private organizations were educational institutions or church-related agencies. Another 30% were sponsored by the host country. The majority of the consultations were related to practice, education, research, and administration. Andrews concludes that because there are many opportunities for American nurses to participate in nursing around the world, nursing curricula should include a component on international health. According to Andrews, "traditionally educational programmes do not prepare nursing students for international health."

Henkle, from a survey of 78 nurses working internationally and administrators of four nonprofit agencies with nurses abroad, suggests content for preparing nurses to practice abroad. Those already working outside of the United States said that an international nurse should have the following:

1. Knowledge of the specific culture where she/he will work
2. Knowledge of international health issues
3. Understanding of the health needs and priorities in developing countries
4. Understanding of the influence of politics on health services
5. Familiarity with the differences in nursing roles and systems in other countries
6. Skills in cross-cultural communication
7. Problem solving skills
8. Skill in the decision making process
9. Adaptability and flexibility in nursing care

Like Andrews, Henkle concludes that nurses working internationally need special preparation that should at least be introduced during their basic education. Mooneyhan et al.[32] report from a survey of 330 National League for Nursing (NLN) accredited baccalaureate and higher degree nursing programs that students often graduate with little awareness of or sensitization to health concerns in other countries. Lindquist[27] conducted a survey to identify ways in which baccalaureate schools of nursing were internationalizing curricula. She concludes that although the number of schools is small, creative approaches are being used. Lindquist suggests that schools with an international component in their curriculum share their experiences and ideas with other educators.

Masson[29] outlines practical suggestions for the nurse preparing for work in another country. She emphasizes the importance of gaining a conscious awareness of one's own cultural beliefs and professional values. In addition, Masson stresses the need to be knowledgeable about the health system and, specifically, the nursing system of the country in which a nurse will work. She also includes a helpful framework for studying each of her suggestions mentioned previously.

• • •

Many nurses work abroad. In fact, several nursing leaders suggest that international nursing is a new specialty.[3,19] The opportunities are exciting but require specialized preparation. To be an effective international nurse demands study in several areas, including cross-cultural communication and possibly a foreign language, issues of international health, and health and nursing systems in other countries. The nurse aspiring to international practice must evaluate potentials for enjoying creativity and flexibility while learning from and working with people of unfamiliar cultures and health care systems.

The specialty of international nursing can be summarized by three words that characterize this expanding career option—Diversity, Challenge, and Opportunity.

STUDY ACTIVITIES

1. What forces currently affect nursing internationally?
2. What is meant by primary health care (PHC) and how can nurses function in PHC?
3. Name at least four international nursing organizations.
4. What is the WHO and how do nurses help that organization fulfill its mission?
5. Research several current nursing journals for job opportunities abroad.

REFERENCES

1. Abu-Saad H: Nursing a world view, St. Louis, 1979, the CV Mosby Co.
2. Almeida MC and Rocha JS: O saber de enfermagem e saber de enfermagem e sua dimensao practica (Nursing knowledge and its practical dimension), Sao Paulo, 1986, Cortez.
3. Amin AE: Cross-cultural awareness: a nursing imperative, Internat Nurs Rev 31(1):9-10, 1984.
4. Anderson S: Response of nursing education to primary health care: the training and practice of post basic community health nurses in Botswana, Internat Nurs Rev 34(1):17-26, 1987.
5. Andresen B: The negotiating machinery of the Danish Nurses' Organization, Internat Nurs Rev 33(6):174-177, 1986.
6. Andrews MA: US nurse consultants in the international marketplace, Internat Nurs Rev 33(2):50-55, 60, 1986.
7. Chamberlain MC and Beckingham AC: Primary health care in Canada: in praise of the nurse? Internat Nurs Rev 34(6):158-160, 1988.
8. Chokrieh AC and Adebo EO: Evaluation of nursing knowledge and skills in Nigeria, Internat Nurs Rev 24(2):55-60, 1977.
9. Collins S: Nursing—the European dimension, Internat Nurs Rev 30(6):178-180, 1983.
10. Conselho Federal de Enfermagem (COFEN): O exercicio de enfermagem nas instituicoes de saude do Brasil; 1982-1983: forca de trabalho em enfermagem (Nursing practice in health institutions in Brazil; 1982-1983: the nursing work force), Rio de Janeiro, 1985, COFEN.
11. Das U: Basic steps in the review of Nepal's nursing curriculum, Internat Nurs Rev 33(3):87-89, 1986.
12. Davis A: Health problems and nursing practice in sub-Saharan Africa, Internat J Nurs Studies 12:61-64, 1975.
13. Davis JH and Dietrick EP: Unifying the strategies of primary health care in nursing education. Internat Nurs Rev 34(4)102-106, 1987.
14. Easson GA: Professional nursing in the Soviet Union, J Nurs Ed 16(7):23-26, 1977.
15. Fadayomi TO and Oyeneye OY: The demographic factor in the provision of health facilities in developing countries: the case of Nigeria, Soc Sci Med 19(8):793-797, 1984.

16. Fukuda H, Ebina M, and Shikamura M: The roles of nurses in various settings in Japan. In the report of the First International Seminar on Nursing and Nursing Education at Kasatsu, August 15-18, 1986, Kusatsu, Gunma.
17. Germano RM: Educacao e ideologia da enfermagem no Brasil (Education and ideology of nursing in Brazil), Sao Paulo, 1985, Cortez.
18. Harnar R: Nurses: a resource to the community, Contact, No. 87, 1-15, 1985.
19. Henkle JO: International nursing: a specialty? Internat Nurs Rev 26(6):170-173, 1979.
20. Inoue I: Attendance care at hospitals in Japan, Internat Nurs Rev 30(6):172-174, 1983.
21. Jamison S: Forces perceived to influence implementation of curricular changes for primary health care in basic nursing education in Thailand, Unpublished doctoral dissertation, 1988.
22. Jinadu MK and Adediran S: Effects of nursing education on attitudes of nursing students toward dying patients in the Nigerian sociocultural environment, Internat J Nurs Studies, 19(1):21-17, 1982.
23. Kamigori H, Seto M, and Tokuzawa: Conceptual overview of Japanese Nursing. In the report of the First International Seminar on Nursing and Nursing Education at Kasatsu, August 15-18, 1986, Kusatsu, Gunma.
24. Kojima M: Nursing education in Japan and its future trends, Internat Nurs Rev 34(4):94-101, 1987.
25. Kurtzman H et al.: Nursing process at the aggregate level, Nurs Outlook, 737-739, 1980.
26. Lindquist G: Primary health care in four countries, J Prof Nurs 2:4:203, 1986.
27. Lindquist G: Programs that internationalize nursing curricula in baccalaureate schools of nursing in the United States, J Prof Nurs 2(3):143-150, 1986.
28. Mahler H: Action for change in nursing, World Health 12:1-2, 1978.
29. Masson V: International nursing, New York, 1981, Springer Publishing.
30. May K and Meleis A: International nursing: guidelines for core content, Nurse Educator 12(5):36-40, 1987.
31. Messias D: Nursing in Brazil, Unpublished manuscript, 1988.
32. Mooneyhan EL et al.: International dimensions of nursing and health care in baccalaureate and higher degree nursing programs in the United States, J Prof Nurs 2(2):82-90, 1986.
33. Morakinyo O and Johnson MN: Role perception and role enactment of the nurse and their determinants in a teaching hospital in Nigeria, Int J Nurs Studies 20(4):201-214, 1983.
34. Mule G: Nursing education in Kenya: trends and innovations, Internat Nurs Rev 33(3):83-86 1986.
35. Ngcongo N and Stark R: The development of a family nurse practitioner programme in Botswana, Internat Nurs Rev 33(1):9-14, 1986.
36. Nousianen T: Story of a strike, Internat Nurs Rev 31(6):184-186, 1984.
37. Quesada M: The PNA's primary health care project—two years after, Philippine J Nurs 49(3):115-123, 1979.
38. Quinn S: Nursing: the European Economic Community Dimension, J Adv Nurs 4:439-452, 1979.
39. Quinn S: The other side of the pond: news of nursing in the United Kingdom, J Prof Nurs 1(5):260-261, 1985.
40. Rodrigues MA: Enfermeira na saude escolar (The nurse in school health), Rev Paulista Enfermagem, 3(2):50-53, 1983.
41. Roemer, MI: National strategies for health care organization: a world overview, Ann Arbor, MI, 1983, Health Administration Press.
42. Roettger S: Nursing in India and Bangladesh: an overview, Unpublished manuscript, 1988.
43. Rowe EL: The knowledge of American nurses serving in Ethiopia, Nigeria, and Liberia concerning the etiology and treatment of typhoid, typhus, and malaria, Doctoral dissertation, 1975.
44. Schmidt MJ: Natureza das condicoes de trabalho da enfermagem (Nature of nursing working conditions), Rev Paulista Enfermagem 4:(3):89-94, 1984.
45. Settachen P: Nursing education, nursing services, and primary health care in Thailand, Unpublished manuscript, 1986.
46. Silva GB: Enfermagem professional: Analise critica (Professional nursing: a critical analysis), Sao Paulo, 1986, Cortez.

47. Stockler A: Nursing in Israel: a review of the past, pre-state and early post-state period, Internat Nurs Rev 33(3):76-78, 1986.
48. Stovring T: Changing scene in Norway, J Prof Nurs 2(5):173, 1986.
49. Tornbjerg A and Jacobsen L: Violation of human rights and the nursing profession, Internat Nurs Rev 33(1):6-8, 1986.
50. Ukatu BO: Nursing as a profession in Nigeria, New Era Nurs Image Int, 2(2):12-18, 1986.
51. UNICEF: The state of the world's children, New York: 1987, 1988, UNICEF.
52. World Bank: Health sector Policy paper, Washington, D.C., 1980, World Bank.
53. World Health Organization: Alma-Ata 1978: primary health care ("Health For All" Series, No. 1), Geneva, 1978, World Health Organization.
54. World Health Organization: Leadership in nursing for health for all: a challenge and strategy for action, Geneva, Switzerland, 1986, World Health Organization.
55. World Health Organization: Nursing Services: report on a WHO symposium, EURO Reports and Studies 22, Copenhagen, 1980, WHO Regional Office for Europe.
56. World Health Organization: Regulatory mechanisms for nursing training and practice: meeting primary health care needs (Technical Report Series No. 738), Geneva, 1986, World Health Organization.
57. World Health Organization: Report on consultation on women as providers of health care, Geneva December 17-19 1980 (unpublished WHO document HMD/81.2.).
58. World Health Organization: Report on the education and training of nurse teachers and managers with special regard to primary health care (Technical Report Series No. 708), Geneva, 1984, World Health Organization.
59. World Health Organization: Report on the second WHO consultation on women as providers of health care, Geneva, August 16-20, 1982 (unpublished WHO document HMD/82.10.).

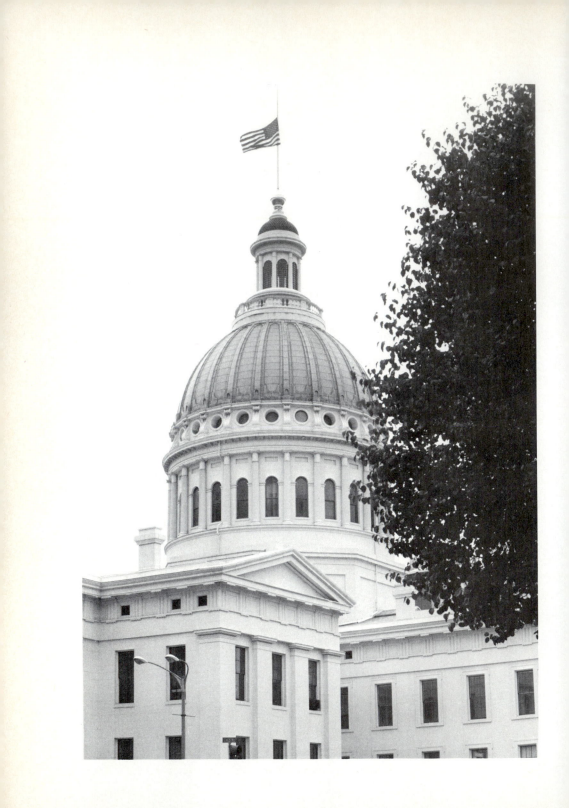

CHAPTER 14

IMAGE OF NURSING

Vicki L. Black
Carmen Germaine-Warner

OBJECTIVES

After completing this chapter the reader should be able to:

- List at least four societal expectations of women that give impetus to the traditional image of nursing

- List and describe five time periods in nursing history and their individual societal image of nurses

- Discuss the image of nursing perceived by physicians, other health professionals, and nurses, and the group that perceives the lowest image of nurses

- Name and discuss positive moves made by nurses that improve autonomy and status

- Describe how the title *nurse* originated and what it means

- Discuss the role of men in nursing and their history and potential contributions to the image of nursing

- Discuss how nursing behaviors and attitudes can be changed to enhance the nursing image

Professional nursings' image continues to be a major challenge for all nurses, individually and collectively. The chapter briefly reviews the historical development of nursings' image and discusses and evaluates Kalisch and Kalischs' five periods of nursings' image, incorporating the effect of mass media on the image. Nursings' image is analyzed—what nurses think of themselves and the effect that this image has on the image of the profession. The title *nurse* is scrutinized also.

Solutions and strategies for improving the profession's image are included and subsequently discussed in the chapter that follows. Collective bargaining, computerization, elimination of internal sexism, media committees, education, and marketing strategies are discussed as areas that affect the image of nursing. Comments made by nurses during a research survey regarding the image of nursing are also incorporated.

Historical Development of Nursing's Image

Credit is given to Florence Nightingale for the written history and development of modern nursing; O'Brien[27] suggests that the image of nursing also has its roots in the Nightingale era. At that time, men were the laborers and the bread-winners, and almost all women were socialized into becoming wives, mothers, and housekeepers. Nursing was perceived as "women's work"—a natural extension of all of the altruistic qualities valued in women.[31]

Women were expected to lovingly devote themselves to the health and well being of other people, and they were also expected to do this without any thoughts of autonomy at the bedside or in their identified professional activities. In the hospital setting, nurses were recognized as physician extenders. Unlike today, physicians in the past were exclusively male and nurses were female. The expectations of nurses were altruism, sacrifice, and submission. These expectations were not only encouraged but demanded. Obligation and love, not a need to work, were required to bind the nurse to her patient. In a society thus oriented, it was natural that women viewed nursing as a means of manifesting their love to others; such a noble characteristic was attractive to many women and drew them into nursing. An extension of this thought process became a part of a girl's upbringing, and nursing skills were integrated into the teachings passed from mother to daughter.

The usual image of Florence Nightingale is a self-sacrificing young woman with no desire or need of money, rest, or recognition. Actually, she was a courageous, liberated, independent woman who may be credited with leading nursing out of the Dark Ages.[25] Ms Nightingale had strong convictions about what nursing should be and fought hard to see that certain clinical and educational standards were maintained.[28] Even today the image of Florence Nightingale as the "lady with the lamp" remains perhaps the most popular public image of the founder of modern nursing.

Linkage Between Mass Media and Nursing Image

Extensive research on the image of the nursing profession has been done by Kalisch and Kalisch.[14,16,17,18] Although somewhat harsh at times, these authors make some worthwhile statements that can help the nursing profession view itself more objectively. They identify five periods of time during which distinct corresponding images of the nursing profession can be seen. These periods are reviewed here with emphasis on the effect that mass media had on the image of nursing during these periods. The following material is condensed and simplified to conserve space and time for the reader.

Period 1: Angel of Mercy (1854-1919)

In the pioneer days of nursing, there were two eminent images of nurses. One image, in a Charles Dicken's novel, was Sairy Gamp, the poorly educated alcoholic nurse who worked in primeval conditions primarily performing domestic chores. The second prevailing image was Florence Nightingale, the original "Angel of Mercy."

In the early 1900s, nurses were viewed as honorable, moral, spiritual, self-sacrificing, and ritualistic. World War I media representations continued the "Angel of Mercy" image, idealizing nurses and making them a token of exemplary moral purity.

This time period corresponded with the silent era of the film industry. The nurse served a symbolic function more than any other useful function. Neither the role of the nurse nor the educational preparation were well presented. The nurses' role in films was influenced by a moral code from the Victorian era. Just as in society in general, the image of women in films was primarily defined by their economic and marital status. A female nurse was almost always depicted in relationship to a male. A familiar theme in the motion pictures was that of the male patient falling in love with his nurse. Amusement was frequently derived through the antics resulting from a nurse being pursued by an ardent admirer.

During the "Angel of Mercy" era, nurses appeared in a substantial number of literary endeavors. Nurse heroines were characterized as being involved in a dual search: (1) success and meaning in nursing and (2) happiness and fulfillment through love and marriage. This dichotomous representation often resulted in a mixed image. Conflict within the nurse herself often ensued because success as a nurse meant intelligence, expertise, and preserverance, whereas success at love and marriage demanded the conventional feminine qualities of faithfulness, compliance, and obedience. Perhaps the resulting paradox was as confusing for the nurse as it was for the public.

From 1916 to 1918, the nursing profession received its greatest attention in the propaganda films of World War I. Nurses were consistently cast as Red Cross nurses and represented an idealized and almost mythical womanhood. The extent to which nursing activities were illustrated was largely limited to gentle, maternal concern for the patient's comfort. Films generated from Hollywood emphasized nursing as it was during the war. The war provided an improvement of the professions' image in novels. Although skilled nursing activities and knowledge were seemingly deemphasized, the image of the nurse was projected as an autonomous and intelligent health care provider.

Period 2: Girl Friday (1920-1929)

With the passage of the Womens' Suffrage Reform in 1919, women entered a new domain of professional endeavors and activities. Unfortunately, at the same time, nursing education regulations were lowered and students were exploited as cheap labor, literally staffing entire hospitals. Nurses were described as "faithful, dependent, cooperative, long suffering, and subservient." Their careers culminated in marriage, which represented a woman's only legitimate destiny. This attitude was conveyed in the enterprises of Hollywood in which nursing was depicted as a conscientious and admirable choice but acceptable only until time for marriage. In films of this era, nurse heroines were not cast as career nurses. Nursing was simply a means to an end.

In novels written after World War I, nurses diminished in importance. They were depicted as remedies for the emotional turmoil that active soldiers suffered and endured, and the nurse's duty was that of instilling hope into the lives of wounded soldiers.

Period 3: Heroine (1930-1945)

For the next 1 1/2 decades, nursing was acknowledged as a worthy and important profession that enabled women to earn an honorable living. Nurses were identified as educated and owning certain abilities. Adjectives such as courageous, chivalrous, fearless, reasonable, clear-headed, humanitarian, and magnanimous were used to illustrate and portray nurses.

The only feature length films ever produced, seven in number, that focused entirely on the nursing profession were released in the 1930s. These films stressed the education and work of professional nurses. Attractive young women were portrayed as putting the demands of their profession before personal ambitions. One of the most popular films, nominated for the 1934 Academy Award for Best Picture, was *The White Parade*. Loretta Young provided audiences with a realistic portrayal of the challenges and problems encountered in becoming a nurse in a large hospital school. The plot stressed that not every woman was destined to become a nurse, but those that were could expect a life of hard work, minimal monetary reimbursement, and immense personal satisfaction. The heroine of the film rejected the offer of marriage by a millionaire to continue her career as a nurse.

In the Depression years of the 1930s, such devotion and selflessness meant a great deal. The viewing public understood that the nursing profession maintained high standards and insisted on rigorous self-restraint from its practitioners and students. Hollywood ceased to present nursing as a short-lived humanitarian hobby for rich girls before their more permanent status as wife and mother.

During World War II, the perceived worth of professional nurses by American society intensified tremendously. This was magnified on the screen as nursing assumed a loyalist and activist character never before or since matched in feature films. In 1943, at the zenith of the war, the studios produced their greatest accolade to the profession. *So Proudly We Hail* (1943), a Paramount release based on the experiences of nurses on Bataan and Corregidor when the war began in the Philippines, was one of the biggest successes of the year. The image of nursing was very positive.

Period 4: Mother (1946-1965)

It may have been a natural development after World War II that a major goal for many American women was to stay home and care for children. Nurses during this period were chronicled as maternal, compassionate, unassertive, submissive, and domestic. Postwar society would not support independent and autonomous women. Their place was typically perceived as being in the home raising children.

During the 1950s, television programs usually portrayed nurses as worthy of respect and appreciated for their skills. They were depicted in roles subordinate to physicians and employed in positions that they would easily surrender for marriage or children. Work as a nurse was often seen as a means to obtain amenities such as vacations or luxuries for the home and family.

The American public was captivated by the medical world in the figures of Ben Casey and Dr. Kildare in the 1960s. Although the nurse was positively portrayed in these films as intelligent, altruistic, perceptive, and energetic, there was a subtle erosion of the nurse's image.

Period 5: Sex Object Image (After 1966)

After 1966, the mother image of the nurse, which was popular in the mid-1940s, changed to the sex object image. Nurses were increasingly depicted as being sexually promiscuous, self-indulgent, superficial, and unreliable. Nurses became "sexual mascots" for health care teams and seen in X-rated movies. They were often depicted as more interested in linen closet trips than in professional growth and development. Eventually, nurses were portrayed as cold, uncaring, power hungry, and unmotivated persons, and the once honored and virtuous film image of the nurse was a thing of the past.

Television censorship standards were lax in the early 1970s. Nurses who were portrayed inappropriately or provocatively dressed were no longer censored. During this decade, nurse figures were primarily cast in series that accentuated the medical model and physicians as almost superhuman. In films of these years, nurses were undervalued and poorly represented. Their contributions to health care were not addressed.

EXAMPLE: Major Margaret Houlihan on *MASH* was technically competent but had little effect on patient welfare. As a surgical nurse, she was supportive to the surgeons, but they were clearly the "heroes." The scene was further skewed by the fact that the patient received little emotional support or physical comfort by the nurse and was rarely seen by Major Houlihan.

The television show closely associated with scientific endeavors was the portrayal of the nurse in *Doctors' Private Lives*. In her off duty hours, the nurse served as an assistant to a physician-researcher. The nurse was often chastised, insulted, and sexually manipulated by the physician.

The 1970s represent the lowest point in film history for the nursing profession. Certainly, nurses were not portrayed as altruistic, intelligent, and virtuous. Instead, a new nurse characterization appeared—that of the malevolent and sadistic personality.

EXAMPLE: The highly acclaimed *One Flew Over the Cuckoos' Nest* (1975) depicted Nurse Ratched as a soul-destroying, castrating mother figure. She abused her position as a psychiatric nurse to arrange cruel punishments. In one scene, she has a patient loboto-mized, McMurphy, to demonstrate her ultimate power over the patients. In another box-office hit, *Coma* (1978), a nurse plays a key role in the murderous conspiracy to sell needed transplantable organs to unethical and ruthless surgeons.

The mass media of the 1980s has not improved the image of the profession. Movies such as *Terms of Endearment* endorse the image of the cold-hearted, punitive sadistic nurse who derives perverse pleasure from patient suffering.[5,6]

Bumper stickers and T-shirts claiming "Nurses Call the Shots" and greeting cards that depict nurses who derive pleasure from the discomfort of patients may, on the sur-face, appear fairly innocent and cute, but they relay a subtle message to those who inter-pret them in various ways. Television shows during the 1980s decline to promote a posi-tive professional image of nursing. Shows such as *St. Elsewhere, Trapper John, MD,* and the daytime dramas depict nursing in an unfavorable and unprofessional light. Perhaps the television show that blatantly demoralizes and insults nurses is *Nightingales* (1989). In this film, student nurses, five single females, are cast as brainless male-chasing dum-mies who wear skimpy underclothing or bathtowels. They demonstrate no clinical com-petence or expertise but exhibit playful sexual escapades in the linen closet.

NURSING'S IMAGE OF ITSELF

Nurses may sometimes feel that it is not important how they perceive nursing—their 8, 10, or 12 hour days should speak for them. However, individual attitudes, feelings, and perceptions are reflected in one's appearance, behavior, and outcome from interac-tions with others, including patients, peers, and the public. Collectively, these individual nurses' attitudes, behavior, and interaction constitute nursing's self-image. The image of nursing by nurses is cited as perhaps the most damaging influence affecting the profes-sion's image.[3,37,41] Until the profession changes its self-image, it is unlikely to persuade the public to do so. Nurses who verbalize comments such as "I'm only a staff nurse" or "I was just following the physician's order" are not improving the image of nursing.

To examine issues surrounding the image of nursing, Strasen[38] suggests the incorpo-ration of Rogers' principles of self-image psychology that focus on the self-concept of the individual nurse. Tracy[39] explored specific principles of the self-concept model and studied how these principles actually determine individual achievement. Tracy[39] describes two basic principles that Strasen[38] believes have significant implications for improving the image of the nursing profession.

A major principle of the model, the law of belief, declares that whatever an individu-al strongly believes is actualized. This principle may be commonly known as the *self-fulfilling prophecy*.[38] Everything an individual subconsciously believes becomes reality.[34] Only information consistent with internal beliefs is allowed to pass through to the con-scious mind. Therefore the self-concept affects one's image of self and thus one's profes-sional image. Actualized feelings are reflected. The key, Strasen emphasizes, is to focus one's energy on oneself and not on external factors over which one has no control.

Another construct that applies to the model is explained by Strasen as the *responsibility/achievement relationship*. This model states that an individual experiences a confident self-concept, the attitude of being in control, and achievement in equal proportions to the willingness and ability of that individual to take responsibility for his or her own life without blaming external factors. Applied to the nursing profession, the concept implies that until nurses internalize feelings of control and professionalism, the group will continue to act as if they are powerless and not in control of their own destiny. Nurses must believe that they are meritorious professionals willing to accept accountability for their lives and practices no matter what external factors are present. Strasen suggests that full professional potential for nursing will not be attained until these beliefs are internalized and incorporated into each nurse's daily professional practice.

Nurses frequently become trapped in one particular image. They may believe that to be a "real" nurse one must work in a hospital providing direct patient care and that when one moves away from the bedside or the hospital setting, status as a "real" nurse is lost. Nurses must begin to educate members of the profession, the public, and nursing students that "real" nurses are involved in a variety of interesting and valuable professional activities in many diverse settings. The belief that it is acceptable not to be at the bedside must be generated, discussed, encouraged, and disseminated. Real nurses engage in research, deliver babies, consult, participate in ministry, administer anesthesia, provide psychotherapy, collaborate with administration, and teach. Real nurses also work in jails, homes, clinics, hospice settings, colleges, industries, private businesses, reservations, and in rural and urban areas. Nurses participate in all arenas of life.

There is a dearth of research in the United States on the perception of nurses as a group and virtually no research on nurses' perception of their self-image as compared to their individual "ideal self-image." Zalar and Suter[41] developed the Nursing Image Survey and completed a study that includes 486 working nurses and nursing students in Northern California. The survey indicates a difference between nurses' self-image and ideal self-image, specifically in the areas of professionalism and stress.

Porter, Porter, and Lower[30] designed a study to evaluate the public's perception of the nursing profession. The study includes three groups (registered nurses, physicians, and the general public) who were asked to describe their image of nursing in one word. Analysis of the data indicates that the nurse group demonstrated the lowest percentage of positive responses (72%) in comparison with physicians (100% positive) and the general public (84% positive). Predominantly all subjects used the following adjectives to illustrate their image of nursing:

Caring	Warm
Empathetic	Concerned
Nurturing	Sensitive
Compassionate	Patient

Twenty-three percent of physicians labeled nurses as "efficient, competent, professional, responsible, and organized." In sharp contrast only 11% of the nurses used similar terms to describe themselves. In addition, 23% of the physicians characterized nurses as "superlative, indispensable, essential, valuable, and admirable," whereas only one nurse employed analogous terms. The registered nurse respondents used words such as "overworked, chaotic, harried, overstressed, moody, underestimated, ignored, under-rated, underpaid, disillusioned, indifferent, and oppressed."

A study by Martin[22] examines job characteristics responsible for nursing prestige as perceived by practicing health care professionals; registered nurses (n = 30), hospital administrators (n = 154), and physicians (n = 300). The respondents' perceptions of nursing were compared to their perceptions of other health care professionals. The results reveal the following:

1. Physicians ranked nursing education significantly higher than did nurses and administrators.
2. Administrators rated nursing income higher than did nurses or physicians.
3. Administrators and physicians ranked nursing authority and prestige significantly higher than did nurses.
4. Administrators rated nursing importance significantly lower than did nurses and physicians.
5. Nurses viewed their occupation as one with great social expectations and requirements (importance, complexity, difficulty) but with few social compensations (income, authority, general prestige). This view was consistent among the nurse respondents.

Participants throughout the nursing community were asked to share their image of nursing 10 years ago and their current image of the profession.

Ten years ago I felt that nursing was being victimized much like women in society. Today, I feel positive changes are happening and will continue to develop.

Kathy Anderson, RN
Clinical Staff, Critical Care
Torrington, Connecticut

In the 1970s, I perceived nursing mainly as a hospital-based provider with little influence on health care delivery and I saw nurses as unwilling to change or "rock the boat." Today, I see nurses as *the* providers of care throughout the system and as change agents capable of capsizing the boat!

Tracy Carlisle, RN, MSN
Neuroscience Clinical Nurse Specialist
Gainesville, Georgia

My image of nursing 10 years ago was that of a direct caregiver and physician-order executor. Nursing provided care and comfort to the patient. Now I believe that nurses are autonomous, problem solvers, and leaders, besides providing direct patient care.

Peter Koch, RN, MS
Instructor of Nursing
Houston, Texas

My personal image of nursing was that we were a group of professionals who had much to contribute to the care, safety, and health of the world and I liked being part of that. Now I am somewhat disillusioned when I see most of the goals I thought we had as an organization have not been accomplished and I am worried.

> Elaine Slocum, RN, BS
> Director of Nursing
> Starke, Florida

These nurses were also asked to describe their perceptions of the nursing image for the late 1990s:

Because of all the poor publicity that we seem to be getting from shows such as "Nightingales" and coverage from the nursing shortage, I fear our image will be more tainted than in the past 2 decades.

> Elaine Slocum, RN, BS
> Director of Nursing
> Starke, Florida

I see many free-standing clinics and practices owned and operated exclusively by nurses. I see improvement in the health of the nation as nurses will stress these basic health imperatives: health prevention, education, alternative treatment, taking charge of one's own body.

> LaFelle Blust, RNC, MA, NP
> Ethics Consultant

In the 1990s, nursing will have developed solutions to the problems of nursing shortages, entry into practice, and nursing autonomy. More importantly, there will be a concise definition as to the meaning of nursing. This will improve our image to other health care providers and to the public. A new term may be developed to describe clinical nursing activities theory. As a profession, we will be closer to the acceptance of...a single paradigm within the profession of nursing. This will occur as a result of increased research and a meta-analysis of the completed research.

> Peter Koch, RN, MS
> Instructor of Nursing
> Houston, Texas

Unless we work to improve our image and define our practice, the image will remain the same or deteriorate.

> Coleen Cahill, RN, BS
> Staff Nurse
> San Diego, California

Will probably be diluted maybe to oblivion by internal disputes, no role clarity, unacceptable conditions, and lower paid technicians to replace them.

> Gail Walraven, RN, MS, CEN
> Consultant, Health Systems Management
> Past Corporate Vice-President Intelligent Images
> San Diego, California

NURSE—BEST TITLE FOR THE PROFESSION?

In past years, the various nursing organizations have discussed appropriateness and validity of the title *nurse*. Questions from these discussions include:

1. Does the title do justice to the profession?
2. Is the title sexist, a barrier keeping men out of the profession?
3. Would changing the title help the profession's image?

Before these questions can be adequately considered, the word "nurse" and its effect on the profession's image must be examined. *Nurse* is derived from the Latin word *nutricus,* meaning that which nourishes, fosters, and protects.[10] The *American Heritage Dictionary* defines nurse as (1) a person trained to care for the sick or disabled under the supervision of a physician; (2) a person employed to take care of a child, nursemaid; and (3) a worker ant or bee that cares for the young.

Fagin and Diers[10] suggest that nursing is a metaphor and metaphors influence language, thought, and action. They consider nursing to be a simile for mothering; therefore one associates nursing with nurturing, solacing, caring, the laying on of hands, and other maternal behaviors.

These behaviors are sometimes viewed in the context of current society's values and mores as humdrum and ordinary. The authors suggest that too little of these nurturing characteristics are experienced in society and that, as a result, many children and adults feel alone and unloved. Fagin and Diers suggest that adults in contemporary society may not like to be reminded of the child within by being told that someone's profession is nursing.

Fagin and Diers[10] also note that nursing is a metaphor for equality. They believe that nursing not only symbolizes women's struggles for equality but that the profession itself represents the typical figure of the "underdog" in its struggle to be heard, approved, recognized, and appreciated. One can only wonder how that can be so, when nursing composes the largest occupational group in the health care system.

Nursing is also closely associated with intimacy. By virtue of their work, nurses are involved in private, personal aspects of people's lives. Nurses do for others publicly what healthy persons do for themselves behind closed doors. Many patients are vulnerable and frequently depend on the nurse and the nurse's physical, emotional, and spiritual strength. After recovery, the patient may feel as if the nurse knows all of his or her secrets. It can be disconcerting for an individual to have been so intense and intimate with a virtual stranger.

Nurses see and touch the bodies of strangers during the course of their work. Unfortunately, somehow nursing as a role and an occupation became affiliated with the broad term of *sex.* Undoubtedly, advantageous circumstances were involved and, from a seemingly virtuous caring for human beings, there were those who began to expand and fantasize, resulting in an image of nurses as knowledgable, willing, capable, and experienced sexual partners. Although every occupation has individuals who fit the misinformed stereotype, most nurses are embarrassed by this development. Unfortunately, this image is one perpetuated by the mass media and encouraged by the sexist faction of our society.

The title of nurse is all inclusive. It incorporates many positions—registered nurse, licensed practical or vocational nurse, nurse assistant, nurse practitioner, and others. It does not discriminate between educational levels of preparation. Educational background usually creates differences in language, behavior, tastes, and thought processes. The lack of differentiation often contributes to the impression that "a nurse is a nurse is a nurse." One recommendation by Vann[40] is to revamp the current system so that newly graduated nursing students can take an initial state-sponsored examination focused on nursing theory. If successfully completed, this examination would entitle the graduate nurse to use the title *Nurse-in-training*. The individual would work under the direct supervision of professional nurses. After 4 or more years of clinical experience, they would be eligible to take a state-sponsored examination focusing on nursing practice. Successful completion of this final examination would result in the right to be called *Professional Nurse*. This model is based on a concept employed by the engineering profession.

The authors conducted a study in California to determine the opinion of nurses regarding the proposal of changing the title of nurse. Reactions were varied. Individuals opposing the name change believe that changing the name would do nothing to enhance the professional image of nursing. Suggestions from this group include (1) working to standardize the profession by elevating the entry level to the baccalaureate level and (2) increasing salaries. This group did not perceive that the title nurse excluded men from nursing, but one participant suggested that men could assume the title *male registered nurse* (MRN). Others felt that there are too many new titles in hospitals and that patients still have the most confidence in nurses.

Nurses approving a name change believe that the title nurse is sexist and connotates subservience and passivity. One participant notes that the term *nurse* is "one of the most overworked, ill-defined terms in the English language"[4] and that it implies reference to the mammary glands. Also noted was "nurse implies that a client is going to be taken care of in an all-encompassing, infantile way. There is no recognition that he must do his part in getting well".[4] Others felt that the title nurse is sexist, stereotypical, and archaic. The 48 suggestions for a title change include the following:

1. Clinical coordinator
2. Health care professional
3. Medical care worker
4. Licensed health advocate
5. Patient care coordinator
6. Person caregiver
7. Primary health care specialist
8. Registered health care facilitator
9. Trained observer patient advocate

The following comments were elicited from the participants....

No, I don't think the title nurse should be changed. It would create more confusion in the public's mind and would not be in the public's interest. More energy should be directed toward educating the public about the nurse's role in health care. Also, as a profession, we should once and for all finalize decisions concerning entry level into practice.

> Peter Koch, RN, MS
> Instructor of Nursing
> Houston, Texas

I really do not believe our title needs to be changed as much as our image. The only way to change our image is to define our practice. I believe that the public in general still perceives nurses as the handmaidens of the doctor. In fact, some nurses see themselves as handmaidens; so I suppose we also need to define our practice to our own profession. Nursing is a female-dominated profession and as a female-dominated profession we will probably be wrestling with our image for a long time.

> Colleen Cahill, RN, BS
> Staff Nurse
> San Diego, California

Yes, I think the title nurse should be changed because the public gets confused. They perceive that all nurses are the same. We all get lumped together because there is no clear definition of nursing.

> Mary Burch-Lein, RN, BSN
> Staff Nurse
> San Diego, California

MEN AND THE IMAGE OF NURSING

The literature indicates that the nursing profession would benefit from a large influx of men into the profession.[1, 21] But, if a man decides to enter the profession, he is plagued by social stereotypes; male nurses are often considered social misfits unable to fit into a "real man's" job. Again, the media is detrimental in its portrayal of men in nursing.

EXAMPLE: An episode of the prime time sit-com, *Mr. Belvedere,* caricatured a family confronting its preadolescent boy for indicating his aspiration to become a nurse. The audience was left with an acute sense that nursing was an inappropriate choice for young men.

A fallacy about men in nursing is that men are new to the profession. When reviewing nursing history, one finds repeated documentation that men were the first nurses to experience large-scale conventional education in Western civilization. Men supplied one half of the nursing care provided in the eleventh, twelfth, and thirteenth centuries. Until the late nineteenth century, nursing was considered as much a male profession as a female one. The profession was genderless. There were several circumstances that led to the decline and near extinction of men in nursing. Ironically, Florence Nightingale was responsible in part because she consciously defined nursing as female. She worked tire-lessly to establish nursing as a worthy career choice (outside the home) for respectable women.[11, 24]

The Industrial Revolution is responsible also for the lingering gender-specific stereo-types that exist within nursing today. Science, technology, and business became the accepted standards for aspiring men in the nineteenth century. Medicine was also a valu-able vocation, causing further division of the health occupations into sex-specific roles. Men chose medicine; women chose nursing. It is proposed that this, and the restriction of men from the nursing profession, ultimately influenced the subordinate role that nurs-ing assumed in relation to medicine.

In 1901, a single event resulted in making nursing gender-specific. The US Congress created the Army Nurse Corps and designated it female. Seven years later the Navy Nurse Corps followed suit. Therefore after 1901, a young man entering nursing became an oddity. The percentage of male nurses in the United States diminished from 7.6% in 1910 to 3.8% in 1920. In 1989, male nurses composed only 3.1% of the nursing force in America.[24]

As previously mentioned, a reason often cited for the continued voluntary exclusion of men in nursing is the image of the profession that is a definite feminine nurturent one. This image creates difficulty for some men who might otherwise be attracted to the field. Holleran (1988) suggests that internal sexism keeps men out of nursing, whereas others suggest that changing the title of nurse to a less female-oriented name might eliminate barriers to the successful recruitment of men into nursing.[33]

Comments from our participants include the following:

I feel men in nursing, just as male elementary school teachers, will have a positive effect on the profession. It will reduce the stereotyping of female and male professions and will develop a collegiality that should benefit everyone.

LaDelle Blust, RN, MA, NP
Ethics Consultant

Miniscule minority in the ranks but inordinately represented in management.

Gail Walraven, RN, MS, CEN
Consultant, Health Systems Management
San Diego, California

The visibility of men has increased over the past 10 years within the nursing profession. More men are pursuing a career in nursing. However, as there were few men in staff nurse positions 10 years ago, there are few men in leadership positions presently. I believe that as men enter nursing, leadership positions will be occupied by men in equal proportions. The stigma attached to men in nursing will decrease with time and as increasing numbers of men enter the profession. Visibility is a key factor in their acceptance.

Peter Koch, RN, MS
Instructor of Nursing
Houston, Texas

STRATEGIES FOR IMPROVING THE IMAGE OF NURSING IN THE 1990S

The nursing profession faces some difficult issues and challenges as it relates to image building. Many of these controversies must first be addressed and settled within the nursing community. Nurses need to assume responsibility and accountability for their profession and their professional image (see box).

Collective Bargaining

Collective bargaining is defined as the process by which unions participate in administrative decisions involving the terms of employment and the price of labor. Most nurses seek improvements in salaries, hours, and overall working conditions. Thus collective bargaining for a time became an attractive possibility as a positive and powerful organizational tool. Currently, approximately 120,000 RNs are represented and work under contracts arbitrated by state constituents of the American Nurses' Association. These nurses, in conjunction with others represented by different labor unions, encompass a considerable percentage of the nations 800,000 RNs employed in hospitals.[43]

Labor groups who seek to represent RNs attempt to counteract the hackneyed image of the nurse as an acquiescent, powerless, and passive "handmaiden" in the work environment. Certainly labor unions that are vying to expand and strengthen their position see nurses as a large, potentially strong, and powerful group of professional people. However, nurses are also vulnerable when they attempt to find fast solutions through this channel. Nursing must continue to foster a positive powerful image and continue to organize. However, the question remains whether it is best done through other means than unions. Many promises by unions to potential members become idle after the contract is signed. Sometimes nurses find themselves in worse conditions than before they signed with a union.

Computer Technology

Experts are convinced that the development and implementation of computer technology enhances the management and delivery of health care and will continue to do so in the future. Nurses must become computer-literate and more knowledgable regarding computer use so that the profession will be in a proactive position to influence rather than be influenced by (reactive position) computer implementation.[13,42] An institution that does not invest in the costs of technology may become antiquated in a relatively short period of time. Nursing must be aware of this. Nursing simply cannot afford to lose this important opportunity to mainstream the profession.

The image of nursing can be influenced by the increase in computer technology. Documentation, care planning, "trending" of patients' laboratory values, quality management, committee work, and administrative records can be computerized. Nurses save time by accessing a computerized system.

To acquire the necessary skills, nurses must become educated and proficient in com-

NURSINGS' RESPONSIBILITIES FOR IMPROVING ITS OWN IMAGE

Recognize that an image problem does exist and that each individual nurse has a responsibility to improve the profession's image.[37]

Strengthen involvement in professional organizations; collectively, nursing is extremely powerful.

All nurses, including staff nurses, should be provided the opportunity to become salaried staff members rather than hourly wage earners.

Nurses must become politically active and politically knowledgeable; nurses should run for office.[19]

Documentation is crucial, shifts the balance of power, and allows nurses to state their case on a rational basis; documentation is also essential for third party payment.[23, 29]

Write and submit feature stories on nurses for local media.[15, 30]

Demand that nurse authors be considered for editing health columns.[16, 30]

Provide technical assistance to media.

Provide ongoing public service announcements; focus attention on well-defined services created and controlled by nurses: case management, nurse-managed homeless centers, wellness centers, birthing centers.[9, 26]

Create public forums—"spend a day with a nurse."[9, 32]

Have nurses present educational talks at local shopping malls, public education series.

Establish a speakers bureau for local elementary, junior, and high schools.

Improve the community image; volunteer for community sponsored activities (Big Sister League, American Heart Association, AIDS Project).[8]

Nursing career literature, especially books in schools and public libraries that introduce the profession to prospective nurses, need to be revised and updated by nurse authors.[16, 35]

Health care texts must be improved and updated to reflect the 1990s image of nursing.[35]

Nurses must become more active as authors and as collaborators with established authors to receive accurate and quality literary portrayals.[18]

Monitor the "get well" cards found in hospital gift shops and in local card shops; any adverse portrayal of nurses should be protested verbally and in writing.

Establish schools of nursing as research and information centers for people experiencing critical health care issues, i.e., AIDS, homelessness.[26]

Increase staff nurse involvement in scholarly activities such as research.[16]

Never allow the nursing profession to be portrayed as physicians' handmaidens; insist, instead, that nurses be portrayed as physician's peers.

---

puter technology. Hospital and nursing school libraries should maintain subscriptions to computer journals, especially those designed for nursing, so that nursing can keep abreast of current trends and knowledge. Nurses should develop their expertise in computers and participate in their institution's system. Nurses must be included in every aspect of the system, including the decision of which system to purchase, which packages to acquire, and how programs should be used and implemented. Nurses can also enhance the image of nursing in the business community by marketing their expertise to leading computer-oriented companies, e.g., IBM. These companies need nursing input in the development, implementation, and marketing of health care packages. Nursing also needs input and should seize this opportunity before someone unqualified speaks for the profession. The participants in our research survey were asked to reflect on how the explosion of technology affects the image of nursing. The following are samples of the responses that were most representative:

Will continue to increase and create more demands on knowledge and performance.

> Mildred K. Fincke, RN, BSN
> Vice President
> Allegheny General Hospital

Both an opportunity and a challenge. For the average nurse, it represents only added stress and pressure.

> Gail Walraven, RN, MS, CEN
> Consultant, Health Systems Management
> San Diego, California

Individuals who are interested in nursing are often people oriented versus machine or object oriented. Consequently the demand by technology to become involved can be unattractive and cause some not to enter the profession and others to leave it. The challenge is how to use the technology to enhance what nurses enjoy most.

Elimination of Internal Sexism

One author states, "It is ludicrous to think that the wholesale addition of men into nursing will make the nursing profession a better one."[11] It is suggested, however, that increasing the number of male nurses will make the profession a different one. Patients may experience a fuller range of professional interventions for their human responses.[20] The nursing profession and practice will become balanced. In some occupations, the balance is improved with the admission of more women. Nursing will become balanced with the admission of more men.

Sexism, antifemale and antimale, must be eliminated from society and from the nursing profession. Sexism continues to harm and disrupt the professional image of nursing. It is time for each individual nurse, each nursing organization, and each nursing school to examine internal beliefs about each patient, each member of the health care delivery system, and the general public. Nursing is not limited to one gender; it is a profession with room for all contributors of knowledge and patient care delivery. Nursing is genderless and its potential is equally as limitless.

Development of Internal Media Committees

Almost every health care institution and organization generates internal media. Internal media, in the form of catalogs, brochures, newsletters, annual reports, program publicity, advertisements, films, and educational material are important to the institution's public relations but should be viewed as having equal importance to the image of nursing. Nursing, usually the largest group of employees in a health care facility or organization, often is not included in essential documents such as annual reports. This must not continue. Nurses are more cognizant of their role, their contributions, and what their services cost their patients; to be silent is unfair to consumers, as well as to nursing.

It is suggested that health care facilities have an internal media committee, and many have had such a group for years. They have not always had the strong nursing representation that they should have. Nurses must become active in such committees and actively review all materials, paying special attention to the effect these materials will have on the image of nursing. For example, the visual and verbal message of recruitment materials reflects the institution's beliefs and attitudes about nursing. Furthermore, means of communicating information that is generated should be examined and the following questions asked:

1. Is nursing included in all significant materials, including the annual report? If not, deficiencies should be noted and relevant recommendations forwarded to the appropriate people.
2. If nursing is referred to, are the references accurate and appropriate?
3. What pictures of nursing are included? Are nurses shown interacting with patients or are they shown following physicians?
4. What image of nursing is portrayed by the advertisements and recruitment of the institution? Do they illustrate nurses as cartoon characters or as professional autonomous care providers?
5. Do the advertisements use professional language? Are there references to professional nursing practice?

Nursing must work with public relations (PR) committees to ensure that nursing is represented in a positive professional manner to people and groups using the services of that facility or organization. Nursing can establish a PR liaison role to accomplish this. The PR liaison consultant can provide the PR department with accurate written materials and photographs when needed. Nursing must become proactive within the institution's marketing departments. To enhance the image of nursing, it is imperative that the profession receive acknowledgement for its many contributions to the health care delivery system.

External Media Committees

The mass media, print and broadcast, are the most pervasive influences on attitudes and opinions in contemporary life. As previously discussed, this has not always been in the nursing profession's favor. Nursing has been and unfortunately still is misrepresented and often cast in an unfavorable light. Unfair portrayal of the nursing profession makes recruitment of potential candidates difficult but also adversely affects the decision-making process of policy makers who decide what scarce resources the nursing profession will or will not have. One cannot expect the best individuals to aspire to a profession unless they are consistently shown to be intelligent, competent, autonomous, and professional.

What can nursing do to counteract and stop a seemingly pervasive negative image? Numerous nurses and groups of nurses suggest that external nursing media committees be organized within every hospital, every school of nursing, and at each level of every nursing organization. These media watch groups must take responsibility for monitoring the media for all references to nursing. The groups must respond to the media for positive and negative referrals to nursing. It is their responsibility to write letters to producers, television networks, and advertisers. Several groups develop awards to give to journalists for accurate portrayals of nursing.

These media watch groups can also offer technical assistance to the media. They can volunteer to review materials for relevancy and accuracy. This type of review provides nursing with the opportunity to alter stereotypical and inappropriate images and replace them with positive accurate portrayals.

Education

One area that has done little to unify the profession relates to educational levels. Entry into practice is remarkably controversial and divisive within and outside the profession. Internally, the entry-into-practice question has divided the professional group. There are many educational differences between nurses; it is confusing for the public and often for future nurses themselves.[22] It may be inappropriate to lump all levels of education—nursing assistant (NA), licensed practical nurses (LPNs), diploma, associate degree (AD), and baccalaureate (BSN) prepared nurses—under one title "nurse."

It is becoming more and more common that a BSN degree is the beginning educational level for entry into professional nursing practice. Donley[7] suggested that nurses have let the lowest common-denominator–theory shape their present and forecast their future. Persons trained for 3 months to 3 years, included under the same title of "nurse", are a detriment of the profession. Upward mobility programs for students and practitioners of technical and associate degree programs are at last making it possible for many nurses to earn the baccalaureate degree expeditiously.

There are many well-educated, politically knowledgeable nurses who practice in America in a variety of arenas. These nurses need to demand more attention within health care institutions. The public needs to be more aware that endeavors such as nursing research exist and are important to patient health. Nursing is becoming more scholarly. It should be publicized as such.[4]

In the California research study referred to earlier (p. 383), nursing colleagues reflected on how increasing educational demands have influenced the image of the profession:

The expectations of nursing today calls for educated and motivated individuals. The image of nursing is changing due to the elevated efforts of our nursing leaders to attain the highest level of competency possible for our profession.

Kathy Anderson, RN
Clinical Staff, Critical Care
Torrington, Connecticut

It has divided nursing along several lines. However, with time, the idea of a baccalaureate degree to practice nursing will be accepted. This is an evolutionary process much like the phasing out of diploma schools. Nursing will begin to see the necessity for a baccalaureate degree to practice nursing.

> Pete Koch, RN, MS
> Instructor of
> Nursing
> Houston, Texas

I think it has helped and will continue to help nursing—I can't believe how much more respect I get from my colleagues in medicine now that I have MSN behind my name.

> Jane Schiavo, RN, MSN
> Cardiothoracic Clinical Nurse
> Specialist
> Camden, New Jersey

The profession increases its demands/standards in an effort to make itself more "legitimate," but it is treating the symptom, not the disease. The disease is a lack of role clarity–lack of a valued role. Unfortunately, nursing, like teaching, is essential to this society, but not valued as much as the most menial male-dominated field.

> Gail Walraven, RN, MS, CEN
> Consultant, Health Systems Management
> San Diego, California

The only way to change the image of nursing is to require a BSN as minimum entry level into the profession.

> Colleen Cahill, RN, BS
> Staff Nurse
> San Diego, California

MARKETING

Historically, nursing has not perceived a need to market itself as a predominantly female vocation. This need has only recently become evident.[2] As the profession works to upgrade its image, marketing strategies are important. For an occupation to attain the status and power of a profession, the public must perceive it as such. The public can be informed by successful marketing. To change perceptions, a desirable image of nursing must be effectively and efficiently communicated. It is crucial that nursing services, nursing programs, and the nursing profession is strategically marketed to a wide range of audiences to promote nursing excellence and to project an achievement-oriented professional image of nursing.

Stanton and Stanton[36] suggest that the following important areas are critical to market nursing as a positive powerful profession:

1. Marketing of a more positive image
2. Marketing of the profession as a collective group
3. Marketing of nursings' unique role in health care delivery
4. Marketing of the profession in general to attract qualified candidates and to retain existing professionals
5. Internal marketing of the profession to ensure that all health care professionals and administrators realize how essential nursing is to the advancement and survival of health care institutions
6. Educating entry level professionals to marketing strategies
7. Successful marketing of nursing products and services that have been used, tested, and evaluated
8. Conducting nurse-driven marketing research with networking and dissemination of results
9. Through research and education, marketing trends must be evaluated in relationship to their effect on nursing

Before nursing can be marketed adequately, the profession must begin to "cost its services" out. It is impossible to market what one cannot measure in terms of dollars. Historically, nursing is considered a cost center instead of a generator of revenue. The largest group of health care personnel are classified as "nursing." This may and usually does include all levels. To project a healthy internal, as well as public, image, it must be obvious that consumers are getting what they are paying for. The health care organization must show that this group is not a liability but that it generates revenue/business. Nursing can not afford to be a charitable magnanimous profession. Health care is big business, with astronomical revenue turnover. To survive in such a highly competitive environment, nursing must also become profit oriented.

Dress for success

In the business world there are dress-for-success rules. To be successful in business, one plays by the rules. Many nurses seem affronted by the dress-for-success rules, but personal appearances certainly set the tone for the image portrayed. One's appearance must inspire confidence in one's ability or the odds are automatically stacked against success. Dress is a powerful form of self-expression. Imagine being in a place where gum-chewing nurses wearing stained drab uniforms are in charge of care. Regardless of how talented or how technically knowledgable, one's professional image and credibility can be sabotaged by the way one projects to others. It is a simple rule but easily ignored or minimized by some members of all professional groups.

People derive images of nursing from a variety of sources, including personal acquaintances and contact during their own or someone else's illness or experience of nurses. Nurses need to present themselves as professionals to all with whom they come in contact. This is not limited to the patient's room or nurses station but includes the

hallways, elevators, and cafeteria. It extends to the supermarket and social activities—
any of the places that a nurse may come in contact with those who will influence the
public or the media.

•   •   •

The authors gratefully acknowledge the following people for their participation in this chapter on the image of
nursing:

Kathy Anderson, RN
Clinical Staff, Critical Care
Torrington, Connecticut

LaDelle Blust, RNC, MA, NP
Ethics Consultant
Producer: Biweekly Consumer Health Program

Mary Burett-Lien, RN, BSN
Staff Nurse
San Diego, California

Colleen Cahill, RN, BS
Staff nurse
San Diego, California

Tracy Carlisle, RN, MSN
Neuroscience Clinical Nurse Specialist
Gainesville, Georgia

Mildred K. Fincke, RN, BSN
Vice President
Allegheny General Hospital
Pittsburgh, Pennsylvania

Peter Koch, RN, MS
Instructor of Nursing
Houston, Texas

Jane Schiavo, RN, MSN
Cardiothoracic Clinical Nurse Specialist
Camden, New Jersey

Elaine Slocum, RN, BS
Director of Nursing
Whispering Pines Care Center
Starke, Florida

Gail Walraven, RN, MS, CEN
Consultant, Health Systems Management
Past Corporate Vice President, Intelligent Images
San Diego, California

STUDY ACTIVITIES

1. Provide specific examples of ways in which the image of nursing is positively or negatively influenced,
   e.g., T-shirts with captions.
2. Discuss examples and then provide approaches and actions that the nurse can take when negative images
   are portrayed in written media, television, and elsewhere.
3. List factors about "appearance" that nurses should consider when "on the job" and "off the job" to enhance
   public perception of nursing's status/image.
4. Describe a well-dressed/educated nurse who portrays the optimal image to others.
5. Describe how (you) would like the profession of nursing to be perceived by society, and what will be necessary to achieve that level. Compare your description with that of several of your friends or classmates.

REFERENCES

1. Alvarez AR: Selected characteristics of male registered nurses in New Jersey, Nurs Forum 21(4):166-73,
   1984.
2. Auttonberry DS: The role of the master's-prepared nurse in marketing, Nurs Manage 19(9):40-42, 1988.
3. Bille DA: The nurse's image—a mirror of the self, Today's OR Nurse 9(8):7-8, 1987.
4. Bower FL: Image making for nursing, Calif Nurs Rev 11(3):10, 29-30, 1989.
5. Curran CR: Effective utilization of the media. In McCloskey JC and Grace HK, eds.: Current issues in
   nursing, ed 2, Palo Alto, 1985, Blackwell Scientific.
6. Curran CR: Shaping an image of competence and caring, Nurs Health Care 6(7):370-373, 1985.

7. Donley SR: Strategies for changing nursing's image. In McCloskey JC and Grace NK, eds.: Current issues in nursing, ed 2, Palo Alto, 1985, Backwell Scientific.

8. Eichenberger J and Parker JE: The making of an image, AAOHN Journal 35(3):113-115, 1987.

9. Evans D, Fitzpatrick T, and Howard-Ruben J: A district takes action, Am J Nurs 83(1):52-54, 1983.

10. Fagin C and Diers D: Nursing as a metaphor, N Engl J Med 309(2):116-117, 1983.

11. Halloran EJ: Men in nursing. In McCloskey JC and Grace HK, eds.: Current issues in nursing, ed 2, Palo Alto, 1985, Blackwell Scientific.

12. Holleran C: Nursing beyond national boundaries: the 21st century, Nurs Outlook 36(2):72-75, 1988.

13. Johnson-Hofer P and Karasik S: Learning about computers, Nurs Outlook 36(6):293-294, 1988.

14. Kalisch BJ and Kalisch PA: Anatomy of the image of the nurse: dissonant and ideal models. In Williams C, ed.: Image making in nursing, Kansas City, 1983, American Nurses' Association.

15. Kalisch BJ and Kalisch PA: Communicating clinical nursing issues throughout the newspaper, Nurs Research, 30(3):132-138, 1981.

16. Kalisch BJ and Kalisch PA: Improving the image of nursing, Am J Nurs 83(1):48-52, 1983.

17. Kalisch PA and Kalisch BJ: Nurses on prime time television, Am J Nurs 82(2):264-270, 1982.

18. Kalisch PA and Kalisch BJ: The image of nurses in novels, Am J Nurs 82(8):1220-1224, 1982.

19. Kelly LS: Agenda for tomorrow, Nursing Outlook 35(5):215, 1987.

20. Kus RJ: A challenge to nursing: eliminating anti-male sexism in American society. In McCloskey JC and Grace HK, eds.: Current issues in nursing, ed 2, Palo Alto, 1985, Blackwell Scientific.

21. London F: Should men be actively recruited into nursing? Nurs Admin Quarterly 12(1):75-81, 1987.

22. Martin E: The prestige of today's nurse, Nurs Management 20(3):80B-80P, 1989.

23. Maxson-Ladage W: What image do you display? AD Nurse 3(2):26-28, 1988.

24. Miller T: Men in nursing, Calif Nurs Rev 11(2):10-12, 14-16, 33-36, 1989.

25. Nauright L: Politics and power: a new look at Florence Nightingale, Nurs Forum 21(1):5-8, 1984.

26. Naylor MD and Sherman MB: Nurses for the future: wanted—the best and the brightest, Am J Nurs 87(12):1601-1605, 1987.

27. O'Brien P: All a woman's life can bring: the domestic roots of nursing in Philadelphia 1830-1885, Nurs Research 36(1):12-17, 1987.

28. Palmer IS: Origin of education for nurses, Nurs Forum 22(3):102-110, 1985.

29. Perry J: Creating our own image, New Zealand Nurs J 80(2):10-13, 1987.

30. Porter BJ, Porter MJ, and Lower MS: Enhancing the image of nursing, J Nurs Adm 19(2):36-40, 1989.

31. Reberby S: A caring dilemma: womanhood and nursing in historical perspective, Nurs Research 36(1):5-11, 1987.

32. Scherer P: When every day is Saturday: the shortage, Am J Nurs 87(10):1284-1290, 1987.

33. Shiffer SW: California men in nursing, Calif Nurs Rev 11(2):6, 1989.

34. Sinetar M: Do what you love, the money will follow. Discovering your right livelihood, New York, 1987, Dell Trade.

35. Smith MK and Smith MC: What high school texts say about nursing, Nurs Outlook 37(1):28-30, 1989.

36. Stanton M and Stanton GW: Marketing nursing: a model for success, Nurs Management 19(9):36-38, 1988.

37. Stewart-Amidei C: From bedpan to…? J Neurosci Nurs 20(3):139-140, 1988.

38. Strasen L: Self-concept: improving the image of nursing, J Nurs Adm 19(1):4-5, 1989.

39. Tracy B: The psychology of achievement, Chicago, 1984, Nightingale-Conant.

40. Vann DS: Essay on the title "professional nurses," Nurs Forum 23(2):69, 1987-88.

41. Zalar MK and Suter WN: Studying the image of nursing, Calif Nurs Rev 83(7):2-4, 1987.

42. Zeilstroff RD: Cost effectiveness of computerization in nursing practice and administration. In McCloskey JC and Grace HK, eds.: Current issues in nursing, ed 2, Palo Alto, 1985, Blackwell Scientific.

43. Zimmerman A: Collective bargaining in the hospital. The nurse's right, the professional association's responsibility. In McCloskey JC and Grace HK, eds.: Current issues in nursing, ed 2, Palo Alto, 1985, Blackwell Scientific.

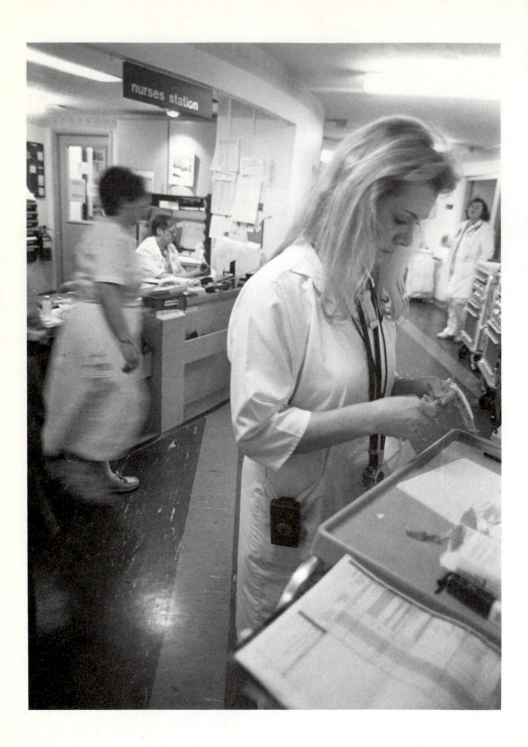

15

THE FUTURE: A CHALLENGE FOR NURSES AND NURSING

Luther Christman

OBJECTIVES

After completing this chapter the reader should be able to:

- Describe ways in which patient care will be changed by technological advances

- Identify new societal dynamics/problems that may create challenges to nurses and other health care professionals in the next couple of decades

- Propose changes in educational preparation for nurses that will provide greater congruency with educational levels of other highly respected professions

- Discuss how nurses are socialized into the profession through exposure in clinical settings and into nursing practice through interdisciplinary approaches

- Describe approaches to doctoral education that may be taken by nurses and the emphasis of these programs of study

The future promises exciting and stimulating changes in the health care delivery system. The nursing profession is faced with the challenge of taking an active part. The future image of nurses depends on how quickly and effectively nurses can lose the lethargy that is a major restraining force in their professional growth and development.

EXPANDING TECHNOLOGY

Every person involved in health care delivery is well aware of the economic, political, professional, scientific, and technological forces that exert pressures on the system. For example, many nursing activities are already being done by technology. Vital signs will be monitored more accurately by machine than by clinicians. Alerting mechanisms will be built into monitoring devices to warn health care team members about deteriorating changes so that lead time for action will be available. Anxiety levels of patients will be assessed in a similar fashion. Software will be devised so that patients can perform much of their own psychotherapy without clinical assistance. Teaching machines will be available for patients to learn about their disease process and how to manage it. Sensors will monitor therapeutic drug levels and automatically replenish them without clinician interface. All clinical records will be automated. Eventually all the scientific and clinical information generated by worldwide research will be on line and available to clinicians of all types.[3,4] The key to using this immense bank of knowledge will be the ability to ask the correct questions. Many persons will manage their personal health through home computers and access to this knowledge bank. As software becomes more sophisticated, each person will be able to have a highly individualized program for maintaining good health. Similarly, every clinician will have a personalized continuing education program tailored to knowledge deficits and to new and emerging knowledge needed to maintain competence.

COMPUTER ASSISTANCE

Computer–assisted patient care can reduce error and give certitude to the clinical planning process. It can be used also to evaluate patient care. It will be possible to develop methods to assess the quality of performance of each practitioner and the cumulative performance of the staff. A complete audit trail may be kept on each clinician. At the end of the year a performance score for each clinician of every type will be available. Licensure renewal will depend on performance based on national norms rather than some perfunctory protocol.[1,2] All these developments will lead to the reorganization of hospitals into clinical and nonclinical entities. This approach will conserve considerable nurse time, increase productivity, require more competence, lower the costs charged against the nursing budget, and reduce the total numbers of employees.

NEW THREATS TO HEALTH

Some future forms of illness will require a multiprofessional approach. Many health problems will result from the environment. For example, the depletion of the ozone layer may precipitate new forms of pathology. Problems secondary to waste disposal inevitably will arise. The disturbance created by disruption of natural ecological balances may become significant avenues of future disease processes. An increasing density of the world's population may provide built-in incubation media for fostering new diseases. The movement of humans and animals by air travel around the world may circulate and transport vectors that may soon be evident. There is a reasonable possibility of more retroviruses emerging that are not dependent on sexual transmission. Longer life spans may result in the manifestation of more genetically influenced diseases. The list of new impingements on good health is growing.

The contradictory states of loneliness and population density may cause new varieties of psychosocial/biological stresses. Persons may work in a more socially isolated environment resulting from sophisticated technology. The automated office is an example of a place in which a person may have no other human contact. As the social densities of the world's population nearly doubles, there may be many forms of sociological pressures with concomittant disruption in human functioning. All of these suppositions are based on trends in evidence.

Patients who experience disturbances of loneliness and population density have sociological, anthropological, and psychological problems. Managing the patient in her or his setting presents an opportunity to treat the holistic pattern of disarray instead of just psychological reductionism. This form of care, properly managed, will require clinical training at the doctoral level to produce the best outcomes. Nurses who perform well in this role build confidence in patients.

NURSES ENTER PRIVATE PRACTICE

Nurse–owned health care organizations also can satisfactorily and effectively deliver health care services to the public. A probable national health insurance, with all the bureaucratic controls inherent in such a system, may result in the elimination of fee for service for all forms of clinicians. Contractural arrangements will be one of the chief means of reimbursement. Nurse-owned businesses could flourish and be a strong component of care.

The care of patients in hospitals of the future will be different. Only the acutely ill who require all of the advantages of the automated hospital will be hospitalized. To keep pace with technology, nurses will have to perform far beyond the level of technology. In all likelihood, nurses will be able to manage only one patient or very few patients under these conditions. The closeness and constancy of interaction will change perceptions of the capability of nurses because nursing care may be the prime need for hospitalization.

COLLEGIALITY AMONG HEALTH PROFESSIONS

Acceleration of technology and economic crises in the health care field require the ability to shape and modify various pressures positively and depends on how much cohesion exists within each respective group of workers and/or clients within the system. Those with a strong public image can use their strength to influence the format of health care delivery, are better able to attract intelligent and career-oriented students, be appointed to key commissions, and foster collegial relationships with important power groups.

All clinical professions will find it increasingly necessary to function as multidisciplinary units. The movement toward doctoral preparation for all will result in large overlap of knowledge content between them. It may be that ultimately there will be mergers of professions and a reduction in number.[2] It is not possible to predict in which direction these mergers will go. The chief influence will be the state of scientific and clinical knowledge at the time these may occur.

EDUCATIONAL PREPARATION: BUILDING TOWARD UNITY

Many studies about nursing are done by researchers outside the profession, and each study strongly recommends that preparation for nursing be in institutions of high learning. Although some progress has been made, educational preparation continues as the major point of division. Nurses appear to insist on the weakest preparation of any of the members of the health professions; 70% had less than baccalaureate education in 1988. The educational process is crucial because it establishes the base around which a profession can rally its strengths and plan for advancement. To understand why it is currently a problem, it may be helpful to consider several significant factors.

The concept of nursing education was imported from abroad and lacked the predisposition to migrate to universities, a mark of the professions that developed out of higher education in this country. Customarily, nurses were trained in small neighborhood schools, where nursing students were kept in isolation from students of the other various health professions. This contributed to a lack of understanding. Nursing students gained only a rudimentary notion of the competencies of the members of the other professions. More serious, however, was that the members of other professions poorly understood nurses—a fact still evident in many situations. Thus the educational isolation of nurses is disadvantageous for all.

The pattern of an abundance of small schools tied to local communities continued with the advent of community college programs. Although the form of preparation changed, the substance remained essentially the same. Community control and local employment opportunities continued to dominate. Career orientations were thwarted without further education. Employment histories of nurses display a series of jobs rather than a professional career. Hospitals and other local employers, in turn, were subject to local supplies of nurses. This relationship became a strong barrier to innovation and change and the effect on nurses' incomes was profound. A few employers could quietly agree on nurses salaries and mute the effect of supply and demand over a long period of time. These same employers paid salaries that were nationally competitive to persons in the other professional groups. All had to recruit from the same university campuses.

Thus the ground rules for professional income took different directions. This set of circumstances probably is a major reason for the nurse shortage.

This author believes that only on university campuses can students learn the political and organizational skills needed to effectively deal with the complexities of the world of health care. The comparative strengths of nurses compared to others grew in an unfavorable ratio as a result of the relative deprivation in education. Without a uniform educational base, it may be impossible to (1) inform the public about what nurses do, (2) stabilize colleagueships with other professions, and (3) set clear standards of care.

As the various clinical professions increase their respective knowledge bases sufficiently to manage the rapidly enlarging scientific core, the differences between them may become less. Merger of some, most, or all is one of the possible outcomes. The enlarging scientific core for all the clinical professions takes different directions and results in the total knowledge content that prepares individuals in a unique clinical profession. Nursing is perceived as developing from a scientific core shared with other clinical professions into a profession in its own right with goals and skills that make it "nursing."

In all likelihood, the Doctor of Nursing degree as pioneered at Case Western University will be the minimum entry. It is the analog of the Doctor of Dentistry or Doctor of Medicine degree. The clinical doctorate, as advanced preparation, is the analog of clinical boards. Adopting this format will enable nurses to keep pace with the expanding theory and content of science.

CHANGE IN ROLE IMAGE

Professional practice laws and licensure restrictions are based mainly on the level of professional preparation. This mode of recognition is deeply embedded in the American culture. Significant changes in the level of recognition, notably a positive change in image, will come if the vast majority of nurses are rigorously educated.

Nursing has the stigma of inertia; part of this inertia results from the role-socialization process. Many nurses have not undergone the role-professionalizing process of the university-based professions. Nurses' role socialization occurs, for the most part, in isolation from others in relatively restricted educational and clinical settings. Because of the paucity of fundamental sciences, their preparation is more task-oriented, with emphasis on motor skills rather than thoughtful analysis of the clinical scene. Heavily entrenched "ward routines" and procedure-book ideology helps to condition them to almost automatic behavior with little variation at any time.

The heterogeneity of preparation by different routes lessens role empathy between them and saps the ability to mobilize for improvement. Thus several images of what is nursing practice and what is a nurse is indigenous to the profession. Clarification of male image cannot result until homogeneity of preparation is achieved.

Role empathy, or taking the role of the other with all the insight that is required, is a means of assisting easy communication within the profession. It is, essentially, a form of social fit in which all the role dimensions are clear and each nurse can adjust with some degree of freedom instead of stereotyped preconceptions. Clarification of role image cannot result until homogeneity of preparation is achieved. Nurses also need to use professional organizations to influence society, instead of as a platform for divisive debate.

One way to explore improvement of the nursing image is to examine professional preparation from an ethical perspective. From that perspective, nurses must fulfill professional responsibility to the public. They cannot maintain their ethical commitment to patients if they do not keep pace with the burgeoning output of science and technology. Condensing it to its final outcome, faculty members of schools with less than university standing are withholding the rich benefits of the growth of science from patients. By a mere matter of logistics, less than half the scientific content can be taught in 2-year programs as in university programs. The advanced levels of science in the upper division are planned to be richer in content than introductory courses. Because no one can use knowledge one does not have, no matter how highly motivated, graduates of nonbaccalaureate programs can give patients care only from this restricted base. Education that narrowly restricts the ability to serve patients must be questioned in the growing ethical climate of the nation. The insidious comparison of a reduced scientific base for nursing education, compared to all other clinical providers, surely poses an ethical and moral dilemma. Withholding scientific content through curriculum offerings almost invites an ethical probe to examine the ultimate outcomes for patients. A rigorous assessment may reveal these ethical flaws. Intertwined with these are economic implications with the increased overhead involved in maintaining large numbers of small schools. It appears that no one has assessed this economic cost because the pattern continues. However, if assessed and planned in large scale, there may be enough in overhead costs used to maintain this large number of small schools to pay for most nurses to complete much of their graduate education. To project overall, only 150 large university schools are needed to turn out more numbers of well-prepared nurses than can be done by the existing splintered, nonarticulated system. The whole system also raises ethical questions of all sorts regarding use of resources and suggests solutions.

The nursing profession has a monopoly on its practice granted by means of licensure or registration. It also has a concomitant obligation to supply high standards of service to the public. One cannot avoid the ethics of this position. Only professions that maintain high public trust can expect to wield strong social influence in the affairs of health. This influence is not a condition granted in perpetuity by society but must be earned continually and achieved by unstinting effort by those who make the profession a career. One of the easiest ways to spark this growth is to urge every new baccalaureate graduate to immediately enroll in graduate study. Within 5 years, an entirely new crop of nurse careerists could be in place. A new plateau would be a reality and act as catalyst to keep the flow of energy focused on high goals. The image of nurses as a superb public resource would be potentiated and recognized as a professional knowledge system able to keep current with the burgeoning of scientific knowledge and human needs.

UNIFICATION OF PRACTICE AND EDUCATION

As discussed previously, nurses wishing to move to full professional status must strengthen their role. The full professional role for any of the clinical professions encompasses the activities generally listed under the concepts of practice, education, research, management, and consultation. When nurses adopt only one of these sub-roles and try to force that sub-role into a full role activity, a diminution in quality occurs. Additionally, when large numbers of nurses make this decision, the profession is atomized. The growing edge of each part is narrowed and lacks stimulation. The growing edge has a far different quality when the full professional role is achieved. It compares favorably with the progress identifiable in the other major clinical professions such as medicine and psychology.

The role induction of student into the profession is in many respects as critical to their development as is the academic program. Reality shock is a recurrent theme. A useful hypothesis for investigation is whether students experience less reality shock in settings conditioned by the unification of service and education. The induction process produces qualitative differences for students in settings in which studied aloofness, scapegoating, or any other forms of less than peaceful coexistence is present among nurses in contrast to where service and education activities are mutually facilitative. In one setting, students perform under wraps and must choose sides; in the other, the milieu encourages students to be expressive users of knowledge. Furthermore, the sensitive issues of ethical practice can be more thoughtfully examined when service and education are integrated components. The establishment of healthy learning environments for student nurses is a current challenge within schools of nursing, and the status quo is varying degrees from desirable.

If nursing education and practice become unified, an excellent means of socializing students is possible because behavioral models of excellence are in place; it fosters commitment as a lifestyle dominated by a set of values that stimulates the growth and formation of a professional conscience, an inner voice that guides and monitors behavior. In addition, it provides mentors capable of stimulating students to think big about career choices and, finally, the way is paved for better interprofessional efforts to improve patient care.

The amount of scientific knowledge a practitioner possesses is set by the individual's level of professional preparation. Clinical behavior is a direct outcome of attained preparation because the predispositions to act in the clinical situation are formed, limited, and defined by the quantity of knowledge possessed by each practitioner. The total role expression of knowledge and the quality of individual practice correlate one to one with individual knowledge systems. The variation in practice at each level of preparation is likely a result of the variation in one's ability to apply possessed knowledge in the practice arena. There can be no guarantee that individuals will use the knowledge they possess. However, the structural variables for organizing care are highly influential on the types of expressive behavior. An entirely different outcome is possible when the structure enables synchronized effort in contrast to settings where there are built-in constraints. Therefore when service and education are not artificially limited and isolated entities, the full use of knowledge can be mobilized. This is in contradiction to settings in which polarization of these entities hampers the innovative use of knowledge.

The full use of knowledge is an obligation the nursing profession owes to the public it serves. Artificial constraints on full professional competence result in disservice to the public. The academic enterprise cannot remain encapsulated from the empirical use of knowledge, and the service system cannot remain insulated from the source of most knowledge and still produce professional nursing services that will be highly valued by society. When the two elements of practice are welded together in a unified whole, a linkage system results in the rapid dissemination of new knowledge, for the examination of novel and more sophisticated practice issues, and for the growth of a rich media to support more strength and vigor in clinical efforts. This unification is the absolute basic requisite for the creation of centers of excellence in nursing. Clinical research cannot thrive without easy entry to the care arena, for that is where the exciting research problems are.

Nurses in service roles and educators must work together to improve the educational nursing environment. Improvement may result in a higher percentage of nurses extending their education. Besides a low number of candidates for higher degrees as compared to all other clinical and scientific disciplines, nurses tend to further their education at a later period in life. The bulk of persons earning doctoral degrees in most other professions and disciplines generally do so by their late twenties. They launch their careers when they are young and energetic. The small percentage of nurses at the doctoral level is combined with an older age of attainment, a situation that is not conducive to building leadership strength. Clinical research as a means of enriching practice remains at low ebb, important positions in the profession are filled with less strongly prepared nurses, and collaboration with other major providers is hampered by inequalities in sophisticated knowledge. The reuniting of education and practice is a powerful means of enhancing the strength of the profession.

SELF-GOVERNANCE

Self-governance is another means of consolidating professional pride, self-imagery, and clinical visibility. Nurse faculty members generally function under self-governance structures. Nurses who are in service agencies can use self-governance staff organizations as an organizational device to consolidate the strength of nursing management with that of the clinical vigor of the nursing staff. The rights, responsibilities, and obligations of this pathway should enable nurses to serve their patients through the standards emanating from a unified effort. Participation in this endeavor can result in new vistas of self-direction and augment the professional growth of each nurse.

RECRUITMENT OF THE BEST CANDIDATES INTO NURSING

A structural factor that affects nursing is the strong adherence to a single gender profession. The recruitment of other than white women into schools of nursing is very noticeable. There is a slight increase of nonwhite women since President Johnson's administration and the advent of affirmative action legislation. An even distribution of sexes in the nursing profession lacks affirmative action. The small percentage increment in men seems to be more by chance than by concentrated effort and selective by schools rather than a measured and united effort. Continued democratization of health personnel and persistent efforts by nurses to become a two-gender profession will result in improved image. It is awkward to insist on affirmative action for women and then not set a good example. A two-gender profession would have all the benefits of balance.

Relatively few studies examine variables related to what attracts and keeps men in nursing. In all probability, the characteristics listed as desirable nursing qualities are not possessed by all the women in the profession, no more than all the needed qualifications to be a competent physician are limited to men. Job opportunity and potential for income growth are probably the two biggest basic attractions that must be present to recruit men. These two features will assuredly also attract more top quality women candidates into nursing.

To ensure that nurses can recruit into the profession as many persons with as many worthwhile attributes as possible, the recruitment net has to be expanded as widely as possible. Men will have to be included or those professions that recruit indiscriminately by gender will have a one-sided advantage. The democratizing of the profession to include minority populations and men would do much to change the image.

The increasing mass of scientific information is leading all of the clinical professions to enrich their respective preparations and to adopt a doctoral degree as the entry level of practice. Clinicians who have rich preparation such as physicians, dentists, and veterinarians are adding fellowships to their residencies. Clinical psychologists are emphasizing postdoctoral training. This movement to enrich basic preparation may be one of the reasons for the drop-off in nurse enrollments. Most parents want their children to attend colleges and universities because higher education is the wave of the future. Because nursing education is not firmly embedded in this movement, students may select those fields that are in step with the future. Just raising the level of preparation to the doctoral level will not be sufficient. Unless the Ph.D. programs offered by schools of nursing facilities become as strong clinically as that of the Ph.D. in clinical psychology, the gain will not be very substantial. Continuing to emphasize research methodology and functional content without a rich clinical base will not enable nurses to gain the strengths of other health teams. The psychologist's model, for example, demonstrates that a strong clinical base and research competence can go hand in hand.

The clinical doctorate in nursing (D.NSc.) comes closer to achieving this end than any other development in the graduate preparation of nurses. The essence of research is asking the right question. Without astute insight into practice there is less possibility of intuitively devising the discriminating question. The rigors of using the methods of science to transform theory and content of scientific knowledge into a social good, called *clinical care,* sensitizes the practitioner to the nuances of correct framing of clinical issues.

Professional degrees are usually regarded by the public as esteemed degrees and are given a higher social rating than academic degrees. Certainly, for the basic biological and behavioral sciences, the academic degree is the major pathway. However, persons with professional degrees can be most useful when people need care, thus generating respect. Although it is not the only reason, it is a chief reason why physicians, lawyers, and theologians occupy the social status they are given. People who have the knowledge to assist the populace are given more recognition than those who are more remote, such as basic scientists, although basic scientists are as vital as applied scientists.

LATERAL MOBILITY FOR NURSES

Another advantage of the clinical doctorate is that it permits the possibility of nurses earning combined doctorates in the manner of the M.D./Ph.D. programs. The combination of a scientific doctorate with the professional one results in use of a wide range of content to develop interesting research problems and to participate with an enlarged contribution to multidisciplinary research. Futurists agree that research endeavors of the future will embrace several disciplines/professions in the research enterprise because no one person will have a broad enough knowledge base to investigate the type of questions that have to be addressed. The first nurse to become a Nobel laureate might emerge from this background. The image of nurses as contributors to the scientific domain would be strongly enhanced by such an event.

•   •   •

Unification of all elements of professional nursing is essential to survival as nurses face the burgeoning entirety of scientific knowledge and instant obsolescence of the world. There is no longer time for division and boundary watching. No one is preventing nurses from obtaining superlative clinical skills except nurses themselves. Clarifying the educational preparation is the most important variable in changing the perceptual scene by which nurses are viewed. All the data collected about nurses show that nurses want respect, desire more input into the patient care structure, and aspire to have more freedom of clinical decision making. All of these concepts can be fulfilled by approximating the scientific and clinical preparation of those persons who have these degrees of freedom.

The current mood of unrest makes the care system vulnerable to change. Developed plans that assist in mobilizing the imaginative qualities of nurses can become built-in catalysts that will surge as an electrifying current throughout the profession. Courage and desire to do what has to be done must be demonstrated. The remarkable increase in the potential for improving the nursing care of patients has such social and moral mandates inherent in the concept that they can flame the desire for change. Nurses have a splendid opportunity to move forward. Massive studies are not necessary. Required is an aspiration to potentiate the competencies of nurses. Although the changes will entail some disruptions in present lifestyles of many nurses, the benefits to patients, the increased social value of the profession, and the self-actualization of each individual has so much promise that the professional gains far outweigh existing rewards. A holistic way of organizing is the most effective means of developing a vanguard profession.

•   •   •

Jesse Scott strove for a goal-directed profession that had a unity of purpose. She had high standards and aspired to fulfill the profession on a grand scale. Nurses compose the largest in number of all the health professions, with a huge potential to be enormously useful to society. If nurses individually dedicate themselves to a unity of purpose, commit themselves to closely adhere to the canons of true professionalism, shake off the doubts and misgivings that are troubling, give leadership to a worldwide strengthening of the profession, and develop scholarship and research at the Nobel laureate level, nursing *will* become a magnificent profession. The urge to serve, the deciding factor that caused each person to select nursing as a life work, can inspire all to unlimited progress. Striving in an organized and cohesive way, nurses can fulfill the desire to serve to a glorious culmination. Now is the time to begin; each one who waits becomes guilty of wasting the greatest opportunity that nursing ever had.

STUDY ACTIVITIES

1. Discuss the pros and cons of having various levels/types of nursing education programs.
2. How does the socialization process for nurses take place? Give examples from experience.
3. What is meant by clarification of role image? How does it occur?
4. Explore the educational level of faculty in your school of nursing. How does it compare with faculty college-wide?
5. What are possible approaches to recruit the brightest and best candidates for nursing into the profession?

REFERENCES

1. Christman L and Counte M: Hospital organization and patient care, Boulder, Colorado, 1981, Westview Press.
2. Misuse of RN's spurs shortage, says new study, Am J Nurs 89:1223, 1989.
3. Lessee S: The future of the health sciences, anticipating tomorrow, New York, 1981, Irvington Publishers.
4. Stevenson J and Woods NF: (1986) Nursing science and contemporary science: emerging paradigms. In Sorenson GE, ed: Setting the agenda for the year 2000: knowledge development in nursing, Kansas City, AAN.

ADDITIONAL READINGS

Bridgman M: Collegiate education for nursing, New York, 1985, Russell Sage Foundation.
Brown EL: Nursing for the future: a report prepared for the National Nursing Council, New York, 1948, Russell Sage Foundation.
Cohen B and Jordet C: Nursing schools: students' beacon to professionalism? Nurs Health Care 9:38-41.
Committee for the Study of Nursing Education: Nursing and nursing education in the United States, New York, 1923, The Macmillan Co.

Committee on the Function of Nursing: A program for the nursing profession, New York, 1949, The Macmillan Co.

Fairchild P: Dictionary of sociology and related sciences, Ames Iowa, 1959, Littlefield, Adams, and Co.

National Commission for the Study of Nursing and Nursing Education: An abstract for action, New York, 1970, McGraw-Hill Book Co.

News: RN's are stars of a multimedia campaign to mend their "Image", AJN 40:128, April 1990.

News Caps: Schools woo new students, AJN 40:130, April 1990.

Royal College of Nursing: In Christman L: In pursuit of excellence: a position statement on nursing, London, 1987.

Sarvimaki A: Knowledge in interactive disciplines (Research Bulletin No. 68), Helsinski, Finland, 1988, University of Helsinki, Department of Education.

INDEX